Artificial Intelligence in Neurosurgery

Artificial Intelligence in Neurosurgery: Bridging Innovation and Practice

The field of neurosurgery stands at the precipice of a transformative era, driven by the rapid evolution of artificial intelligence (AI). From optimizing patient selection and surgical parameters to enhancing intraoperative precision, AI has already begun to reshape the landscape of neurosurgical care. Yet, as these technologies advance from preclinical studies to real-world applications, the challenges of responsible integration, evaluation and safety have become increasingly urgent.

This groundbreaking textbook equips neurosurgeons with the foundational knowledge to navigate the complexities of AI in clinical practice. It explores the remarkable progress of AI systems, from machine learning (ML)–enhanced neuronavigation to agentic systems capable of autonomous, multistep workflows. With a focus on real-world clinical data, fairness and interpretability, the book addresses the critical hurdles of evaluation lag, dataset curation and regulatory oversight.

As AI transitions from passive tools to active participants in medical problem-solving, this text provides a roadmap for neurosurgeons to lead the charge in developing, implementing and critically assessing these transformative technologies. By bridging the gap between innovation and practice, this book ensures that the next generation of neurosurgeons is prepared to harness the full potential of AI while safeguarding patient care.

A must-read for neurosurgeons, researchers and clinicians, this textbook is your guide to the future of AI-driven neurosurgery.

Anand Veeravagu, Associate Professor of Neurosurgery, Department of Neurosurgery, Stanford University School of Medicine. Dr Veeravagu is an expert in the field of minimally invasive spine surgery and serves on national committees. He is the Director of Minimally Invasive Spine Surgery at Stanford University and Director of the Stanford Neurosurgical Artificial Intelligence and Machine Learning Laboratory. He currently serves as the team neurosurgeon for the San Francisco 49ers. He is a leader in the field, having edited and authored a textbook on *Robotic and Navigated Spine Surgery*.

Ethan Schonfeld is a medical student at Stanford University School of Medicine. He is a member of the Stanford Neurosurgical Artificial Intelligence and Machine Learning Laboratory. He has earned a master's degree at Stanford Medicine in Biomedical Informatics where his research focused on the generation of synthetic imaging in neurosurgery. He has authored numerous journal articles and multiple textbook chapters on artificial intelligence in neurosurgery.

AI in Clinical Practice

The Impact of Artificial Intelligence in Radiology
Adam Eltorai, Ian Pan, Henry H. Guo

AI and Precision Medicine in Infectious Disease Management
Jen-Tsung Chen

Digital Healthcare and Artificial Intelligence: A Primer for Clinicians and Students
Clare Rainey, Sonyia McFadden, Jonathan McConnell

Mastering the Art of Facial Soft Tissue Fillers with Artificial Intelligence: The Scientific Way to Avoid a Leap in the Dark with Hyaluronic Acid and AI Predictions
Luigi Cursio, Ciro Cursio, Giuila Cursio

AI and Precision Medicine in Cancer Management
Jen-Tsung Chen

Artificial Intelligence in Neurosurgery: Translatable Technologies and Current Advances
Anand Veeravagu, Ethan Schonfeld

For more information about the series, please visit https://www.routledge.com/AI-inClinical-Practice/book-series/AICLINICAL

Artificial Intelligence in Neurosurgery

Translatable Technologies and Current Advances

Edited by

Anand Veeravagu
Associate Professor of Neurosurgery
Department of Neurosurgery
Stanford University School of Medicine
Stanford, CA, USA

Ethan Schonfeld
Medical Student
Stanford University School of Medicine
Stanford, CA, USA

CRC Press
Taylor & Francis Group
Boca Raton London New York

CRC Press is an imprint of the
Taylor & Francis Group, an **informa** business

Designed cover image: Getty Images

First edition published 2027
by CRC Press
2385 NW Executive Center Drive, Suite 320, Boca Raton, FL 33431

and by CRC Press
4 Park Square, Milton Park, Abingdon, Oxon, OX14 4RN

CRC Press is an imprint of Taylor & Francis Group, LLC

Library of Congress Control Number: 2026939991

ISBN: 978-1-032-74838-2 (hbk)
ISBN: 978-1-032-74837-5 (pbk)
ISBN: 978-1-003-47116-5 (ebk)

DOI: 10.1201/9781003471165

Typeset in Minion
by Apex CoVantage, LLC

Contents

Foreword

"You cannot endow even the best machine with initiative; the jolliest steamroller will not plant flowers."

Walter Lippmann, 1914

I wonder what Mr Lippmann would say if he were to look around a hospital today. In this sacred building, meant to be the paradigm of human connection and emotion, artificial intelligence (AI) has made a bold entrance, and it shows no evidence of slowing down. In the world of medicine and certainly neurosurgery, "machines" are involved in every phase of patient care, including making diagnoses, sifting through treatment options, planning surgeries, providing intraoperative guidance and more recently, predicting postoperative complications. With the addition of large language models (LLMs), technology *has* begun to show its own initiative, in a sense, and it is in fact the human being taking inspiration from the machine he created.

This is an evolution to be embraced. For the modern neurosurgeon, it will be imperative to understand how to best yield AI as both a tool and a partner to provide optimal patient care. This book, written by distinguished leaders in many subspecialties of neurosurgery, highlights the first wave of enhanced possibilities enabled by AI. Neurosurgeons must maintain their role as masters of neural networks, both *in vivo* and *in silico*; in reading this text, we hope you are inspired to incorporate this technology in each aspect of the surgical care pathway.

As a primer, consider the following examples of AI's role in caring for neurosurgical patients.

Diagnostics

There has been a surge in tools devoted to improving both the speed and accuracy of diagnostic tools across neurosurgery. In the fast-paced world of stroke and neurotrauma, with the need for rapid triage, AI-powered tools have shown initial promise; industry partners have created tools to identify thrombectomy candidates and ensure they are brought to institutions with the capability of handling these urgent needs. Additionally, the FDA has already approved machine learning (ML) algorithms to more rapidly diagnose traumatic brain injury (TBI) and prognosticate outcomes. This work has also been extended to low- and middle-income countries, where there exists an even greater need for technology-enabled decision-making owing to the high trauma burden in these regions. In oncology, we now have high-fidelity ML-based brain tumor segmentations, and we are beginning to provide deeper profiling of tumors based on radiomics signatures from imaging. A pediatric patient with a posterior fossa tumor may today benefit from an AI-guided diagnosis of medulloblastoma versus ependymoma to help guide intraoperative decision-making and ultimately influence survival and functional outcomes. Intraoperatively, there are also powerful new technologies using Raman spectroscopy and AI to make real-time tissue diagnoses that previously required several days or weeks to finalize. These examples only scratch the surface. Technology like this will enable more rapid, efficient care and, ultimately, have a greater impact. In this book, look for the commentary of Dr Lissa Baird on the neuro-oncologic diagnostic applications of AI.

Surgical decision-making and outcome prediction

As neurosurgeons' savvy with complex, high-dimensional data continue to grow, we will also make more nuanced and sophisticated surgical decisions. Instead of life-altering decisions, based on fallible measurements of 5 mm of midline shift, 3 cm tumor size, 30 degrees of kyphosis, Pelvic Incidence-Lumbar Lordosis (PI-LL) mismatch of 11 degrees and so many more, consider novel calculators which take in the entirety of the patient's neuroimaging profile combined with their clinical history and neurologic exam to better guide surgical decision-making. Neurosurgeons already do this, though it takes decades of experience and ultimately pointing to a "clinical gestalt" to justify these decisions which are, at best, hard to articulate and, at worst, controversial. There are countless scenarios in neurosurgery, debated annually at conferences, in which even those with such immense experience disagree about whether to do procedures endoscopically, endovascularly or open; when exactly to do any surgery to optimize odds of success; or even whether to do any surgery at all. Not only will AI enable better and more consistent decision-making, but it will also provide more customized counsel to patients regarding risks of specific complications and chances of surgical success defined by personalized criteria.

Surgical planning and intraoperative guidance

For the surgeon, perhaps some of the most technically exciting advances in AI will improve our experience and workflows in our most comfortable space—the operating room. Already, many neurosurgeons have used (knowingly or unknowingly), AI-based tools to automatically register images, plan screw sizes and trajectories, segment white matter, nerve roots, brain tumors and more. In functional neurosurgery, where we have fewer discrete targets, there has been exciting progress in planning deep brain stimulation, laser interstitial thermal therapy and stereotactic electroencephalogram (EEG) electrode trajectories based on data from AI algorithms. In addition to crafting optimal paths to specific anatomic targets, AI can also assist in the sophisticated preoperative reading of EEG to better inform discussions with neurologists. When combined with advances in hardware and robotics, the power of AI software in neuroimaging and neuronavigation is further amplified; read the contributions from Dr Michael Wang and Dr Najib El Tecle for a comprehensive overview. Finally, pushing the boundaries of our technical abilities, AI is powering the growth of the brain–machine interface (BMI) and restoring function—motor, visual, communicative and more—to those who previously had no hope. Here, Dr Vivek Buch writes about the latest updates in functional neurosurgery and neurorestoration.

Health systems and education

Beyond improving care for the single patient, AI will also continue to influence patient care at the health systems level. With the advent of new technologies to rapidly aggregate data from multiple resources—including every corner of patient charts and mountains of billing/coding documents—institutions can work toward improving surgical workflows, as Dr Hani Marcus writes. Though this may initially bore the clinically minded neurosurgeon, one can dream of a system in which cases are booked easily into operating rooms (ORs) that make the most chronological sense with the appropriate equipment on hand; relevant personnel (anesthesia, vendors, etc.) are instantly notified; and coding is automatically optimized to accurately and fully represent a surgeon's efforts. Taking this to the next level, Dr Eric Oermann reviews the use of LLMs and how they should be used to harness the massive power of the modern electronic medical record. To create clean, tabular data as a foundation to improve patient care, it used to take an army of motivated people manually slugging through dense, poorly organized patient records. Today, LLMs can consume terabytes of unstructured data in seconds, and neurosurgeons must appreciate this power to better design novel research questions and understand the bigger impact they can have on patient care. To this end, Dr Percy Liang gives us a deeper background on multimodal foundational models for healthcare. Moreover, we will learn to work with more novel data sources, such as tracking motion of tagged surgical instruments and intraoperative audio/video recordings that capture highs and lows; Dr Daniel Donoho discusses the importance of these concepts. From the lens of education, there also exists ample opportunity for improvement in neurosurgical training, as Dr Roberto Rubio explains in his chapter. And now, with the explosion of LLMs, we can imagine trainees using AI at home to summarize articles, explain figures, create flashcards and review key surgical steps.

With these great promises of AI also come great challenges. At the most fundamental level, any predictive model is only as good as the quality and quantity of data used to train it; Dr John Ratliff discusses the various data sources available in neurosurgery and the significant data needs for deep learning (DL) methodologies. After obtaining high-quality data, it is essential that the data are used properly with guardrails. Most surgeons in practice today were not formally trained in the techniques of data handling for standard ML pipelines including core concepts such as data splitting for training versus validation versus testing, and these do differ from that of traditional statistics. In collaboration with computer scientists and statisticians, we can overcome this hurdle and look to the exciting new horizons for external validation and real-time collaboration across multiple sites, with the advantage of federated learning techniques as discussed by Dr Spyridon Bakas. These ideas will be expanded upon by Dr Victor Staartjes, who teaches about clinically applicable metrics and the necessity of being thoughtful in the design of our research questions and conclusions.

Only if we can harness these explosions of data and computing power may we climb aboard this AI rocketship traveling at unprecedented speed. It is not only neurosurgeons, though, who must keep pace. Because the world of AI has moved so fast, another challenge lies in the relative lack of established FDA regulations for AI. Though this is changing, it is a dynamic arena in which neurosurgeons should have active voices. To take our research discoveries to the bedside, it will be important to smoothly navigate the sharing of health data and algorithms with government and industry partners. Dr Samuel Browd writes about the role of policy on the regulatory landscape, evaluation and translation of AI for neurosurgery.

So, how can neurosurgeons drive relevant technological innovation? Share your clinical frustrations and aspirations with other clinicians, computer scientists and stakeholders. Invite them to the OR to showcase pain points. Learn the basics of their language just as you learned statistics, so that you can have productive conversations. Do not be hesitant to collaborate with other institutions and industry. Share your data, results and algorithms with each other—more than ever before, this is the time to collaborate so we can scale more rapidly and refine our skills.

Undoubtedly, more work is needed to fully understand how neurosurgical care will be reinvented with AI as a backdrop, but we stand at the precipice of an exciting new era. Neurosurgeons aspiring to provide top-notch care will need to know how our omnipresent AI-based tools are derived and how to use them, along with how to critically evaluate new ones and safeguard the integrity of our surgical decision-making—whether it be pre-, intra-, or postoperatively. We hope this book provides a foundation for you to do exactly this.

As journalist Sydney Harris wrote in 1988, "the real danger is not that computers will begin to think like men, but that men will begin to think like computers." No matter how advanced our technology-enabled care becomes, it will be essential to remember our foundational clinical training and maintain our humanity to make the best decisions for our patients. Whether we like it or not, our steamrollers are now planting flowers.

We commend the editors, Dr Anand Veeravagu and Ethan Schonfeld, for their forethought in this textbook on *AI in Neurosurgery* to help us all embrace this new technology as a co-pilot to improve patient diagnosis, treatment and outcomes.

Syed M. Adil, MD and Gerald A. Grant, MD
Department of Neurosurgery
Duke University School of Medicine
Durham, NC

Contributors

Bibhas Amatya
University of Maryland School of Medicine
Baltimore, MD, USA

Ujjwal Baid
Indiana University
Bloomington, IN, USA

Spyridon Bakas
Indiana University
Bloomington, IN, USA

Chetan Bettegowda
Johns Hopkins School of Medicine
Baltimore, MD, USA

Priya Bhanot
Stanford University School of Medicine
Stanford, CA, USA
Mt. Sinai Hospital
New York, NY, USA

Nia Boles
Meharry Medical College
Nashville, TN, USA

Samuel R. Browd
University of Washington
Seattle, WA, USA

Vivek P. Buch
Stanford University School of Medicine
Stanford, CA, USA

Maria José Cavagnaro
Stanford University School of Medicine
Stanford, CA, USA

Andrew K. Chan
Columbia University
New York, NY, USA

Steven D. Chang
Stanford University School of Medicine
Stanford, CA, USA

Rohan Chitale
Vanderbilt University Medical Center
Nashville, TN, USA

Raffaele Da Mutten
University Hospital Zürich
University of Zürich
Zürich, Switzerland

Nader S. Dahdaleh
Northwestern University Feinberg School of Medicine
Chicago, IL, USA

Nehal Doiphode
Stanford University School of Medicine
Stanford, CA, USA
University of Pennsylvania
Philadelphia, PA, USA

Daniel Donoho
Children's National Medical Center
Washington, DC, USA

Christopher Douville
Johns Hopkins School of Medicine
Baltimore, MD, USA

Noah Drewes
Northwestern University Feinberg School of Medicine
Chicago, IL, USA

Najib El Tecle
Northwestern University Feinberg School of Medicine
Chicago, IL, USA

Julian L. Gendreau
Johns Hopkins School of Medicine
Baltimore, MD, USA

Sachin Govind
Northwestern University Feinberg School of Medicine
Chicago, IL, USA

Kritika Gowda
Johns Hopkins University
Baltimore, MD, USA

Heather Grimaudo
Vanderbilt University Medical Center
Nashville, TN, USA

Yassine Guennoun
Stanford University School of Medicine
Stanford University
Stanford, CA, USA

Maria Isabel Barros Guinle
Stanford University School of Medicine
Stanford, CA, USA

Ummey Hani
Stanford University School of Medicine
Stanford, CA, USA

Paul M. Harary
Stanford University School of Medicine
Stanford, CA, USA

Jeremy J. Heit
Stanford University School of Medicine
Stanford, CA, USA

Lara M. Höbner
University Hospital Zürich
University of Zürich
Zürich, Switzerland

Melanie Horowitz
Johns Hopkins School of Medicine
Baltimore, MD, USA

Rishi Jain
Northwestern University Feinberg School of Medicine
Chicago, IL, USA

Thomas Johnstone
Stanford University School of Medicine
Stanford, CA, USA

Danyal Z. Khan
National Hospital for Neurology and Neurosurgery
University College London
London, UK

Arman Koul
Stanford University School of Medicine
Stanford, CA, USA

Jared Lawson
Vanderbilt University
Nashville, TN, USA

Michael Lee
Stanford University School of Medicine
Stanford, CA, USA
University of California
Los Angeles, CA, USA

Simon Levinson
Stanford University School of Medicine
Stanford, CA, USA

Percy Liang
Stanford University School of Medicine
Stanford, CA, USA

Audrey H. Limb
Stanford University School of Medicine
Stanford, CA, USA
Harvard University
Cambridge, MA, USA

Akis Linardos
Indiana University
Bloomington, IN, USA

Michael Longo
Vanderbilt University Medical Center
Nashville, TN, USA

Hani J. Marcus
National Hospital for Neurology and Neurosurgery
University College London
London, UK

Mehul Mittal
Northwestern University Feinberg School of Medicine
Chicago, IL, USA

Michael D. Monterey
University of Miami
and
University of Miami Miller School of Medicine
Miami, FL, USA

Debraj Mukherjee
Johns Hopkins School of Medicine
Baltimore, MD, USA

Atharv Oak
Johns Hopkins School of Medicine
Baltimore, MD, USA

Eric K. Oermann
New York University
New York University Langone Health
New York, NY, USA

Dhiraj Pangal
Stanford University School of Medicine
Stanford, CA, USA

David J. Park
Stanford University School of Medicine
Stanford, CA, USA

Jay J. Park
Stanford University School of Medicine
Stanford, CA, USA
The University of Edinburgh
Edinburgh, UK

Sarthak Pati
Indiana University
Bloomington, IN, USA

Advait Patil
Stanford University School of Medicine
Stanford, CA, USA
Harvard University
Cambridge, MA, USA

Andre A. Payman
University of California
San Francisco, CA, USA

Matthew W. Pease
Indiana University
Bloomington, IN, USA

Dillan Prasad
Northwestern University Feinberg School of Medicine
Chicago, IL, USA

Ritvik Pulya
Johns Hopkins University
Baltimore, MD, USA

Sumedha Rai
New York University
New York, NY, USA

John K. Ratliff
Stanford University School of Medicine
Stanford, CA, USA

Manuel Rebol
Stanford University School of Medicine
Stanford, CA, USA

Luca Regli
University Hospital Zürich
University of Zürich
Zürich, Switzerland

Roberto Rodriguez Rubio
University of California
San Francisco, CA, USA

Carlo Serra
University Hospital Zürich
University of Zürich
Zürich, Switzerland

Aaryan Shah
Stanford University School of Medicine
Stanford, CA, USA

Benjamin C. Sherman
Stanford University School of Medicine
Stanford, CA, USA
Allegheny General Hospital
Pittsburgh, PA, USA

Nabil Simaan
Vanderbilt University
Nashville, TN, USA

Nikhil Sriram
Northwestern University Feinberg School of Medicine
Chicago, IL, USA

Victor E. Staartjes
University Hospital Zürich
University of Zürich
Zürich, Switzerland

Joshua M. Tennyson
Northwestern University Feinberg School of Medicine
Chicago, IL, USA

Henk van Voorst
Stanford University School of Medicine
Stanford, CA, USA

Michael Y. Wang
University of Miami
and
University of Miami Miller School of Medicine
Miami, FL, USA

Eunice Yang
Columbia University
New York, NY, USA

Michihiro Yasunaga
Stanford University School of Medicine
Stanford, CA, USA

Recai Yilmaz
Children's National Medical Center
Washington, DC, USA

Tomasz Jan Zaluska
Stanford University School of Medicine
Stanford, CA, USA

Olivier Zanier
University Hospital Zürich
University of Zürich
Zürich, Switzerland

Abbreviations

3DRA	3D rotational angiography
AANS	American Association of Neurological Surgeons
ACDF	anterior cervical discectomy and fusion
AD	Alzheimer's disease
ADC	apparent diffusion coefficient
ADNI	Alzheimer's Disease Neuroimaging Initiative
AEs	autoencoders
AI	artificial intelligence
AIS	acute ischemic stroke
AI/ML SaMD	Artificial Intelligence and Machine Learning Software
ANN	artificial neural network
AP	average precision
API	application programming interface
APM	automated performance metrics
AR	augmented reality
ASA	American Society of Anesthesiologists
ASI	Adaptive Spine Intelligence
ASPECTS	Alberta Stroke Program Early CT Score
ASR	automated speech recognition
AUC	area under the curve
AUC-PR	area under the precision-recall curve
AUROC	area under the receiver operating characteristic
AVM	arteriovenous malformation
AWS	Amazon Web Services
BBB	blood–brain barrier
BCIs	brain–computer interfaces
BLEU	Bilingual Evaluation Understudy
BMI	body mass index
BraTS	brain tumor segmentation
CapsNet	capsule networks
CAR-T	chimeric antigen receptor T cell
CBV	cerebral blood volume
CDC	Centers for Disease Control and Prevention
CEST	chemical exchange saturation transfer
cf	cell free
cfDNA	cell-free deoxyribonucleic acid
CHARM	Cryosection Histopathology Assessment and Review Machine
CK-MB	Creatine Kinase-Myocardial Band
CLIP	Contrast Language-Images Pre-training
CMU	Carnegie Mellon University
CN	central node
CNNs	convolutional neural networks
CNS	central nervous system
CNVs	copy number variations
COCO	common objects in context
CPT	current procedural terminology
Cryo-EM	cryogenic electron microscopy
CSF	cerebrospinal fluid
CT	computed tomography
CTA	CT angiogram
CTCs	circulating tumor cells
CUSUM	cumulative SUM
CV	computer vision
CWP	connection weight products
DALY	disability adjusted life years
DBS	deep brain stimulation
DCS	dice similarity coefficient
DICOM	Digital Imaging and Communications in Medicine
DIPG	diffuse intrinsic pontine glioma
DL	deep learning
DLR	deep learning reconstruction
DNA	deoxyribonucleic acid

DNN	deep neural network
DRAs	dynamic reference arrays
DSA	digital subtraction angiography
DSC	Sørensen–Dice coefficient
DTI	diffusion tensor imaging
DTW	Dynamic Time Warping
DWI	diffusion-weighted imaging
ECoG	electrocorticography
ECL	Emerald Cloud Lab
ECU	universal cellular embedding
EEG	electroencephalogram
EGFR	epidermal growth factor receptor
EHRs	electronic health records
EMA	European Medicines Agency
EQ-5D	EuroQol 5-Dimension
ET	enhancing tumor
EU	European Union
EVs	extracellular vesicles
EVT	endovascular treatment
FA	fractional anisotropy
FCM	final consensus model
FDA	Food and Drug Administration
FeTS	Federated Tumor Segmentation
FID	Fréchet Inception Distance
FISH	fluorescence *in situ* hybridization
FL	federated learning
FLAIR	fluid-attenuated inversion recovery
FMG	forced myography
fMRI	functional magnetic resonance imaging
GANs	generative adversarial networks
GBM	glioblastoma
GCS	Glasgow Coma Scale
GDP	gross domestic product
GDPR	General Data Protection Regulation
GFAP	glial fibrillary acidic protein
GMLP	Guidelines for good Machine Learning Practice
GNNs	graph neural networks
GPCR	G protein-coupled receptor
GPTs	Generative Pre-trained Transformers
GPT-4	Generative Pre-trained Transformer 4
GPU	graphical processing unit
GWA	genome-wide aneuploidy
HD	Hausdorff distance
HD95	Hausdorff distance 95
HE	hematoma expansion
HIPAA	Health Insurance Portability and Accountability Act
HMI	human–machine interface
HRQoL	health-related quality of life
HTS	high-throughput screening
iAI	intraoperative artificial intelligence
ICD	International Classification of Diseases
ICEMS	Intelligent Continuous Expertise Monitoring System
ICH	intracranial hemorrhage
iCV	intraoperative computer vision
IDH	isocitrate dehydrogenase
IHC	immunohistochemistry
IoT	Internet of Things
IoU	intersection-over-union
IR	infrared
iUS	intraoperative ultrasound
JOA	Japanese Orthopaedic Association
KNN	k-nearest neighbor
KPIs	key performance indicators
KPS	Karnofsy Performance Score
LASSO	least absolute shrinkage and selection operator
LDA	linear discriminant analysis
LGG	low-grade glioma
LIME	local interpretable model-agnostic explanations
LLM	large language models
LP	lumbar puncture
LR	logistic regression
LSTM	long short-term memory
LVO	large vessel occlusions
MAE	mean absolute error
MCID	Minimal Clinically Important Difference
MCI	mild cognitive impairment
MDP	Markov Decision Process
MEG	magnetoencephalography
MGMT	O^6-methylguanine-DNA methyltransferase
MHRA	Medicines and Healthcare Products Regulatory Agency
MI	myocardial infarction
MIAs	membership inference attacks
MIS	minimally invasive surgery
MIMIC	Medical Information Mart for Intensive Care
mJOA	modified scale Japanese Orthopaedic Association

ML	machine learning
MLOps	machine learning operations
MLP	multi-layer perception
MPNSTs	malignant peripheral nerve sheath tumors
MRI	magnetic resonance imaging
MRS	magnetic resonance spectroscopy
MSE	mean squared error
MVD	microvascular decompression
NASS	North American Spine Society
NB	Naïve Bayes
NCCID	National COVID-19 Chest Imaging Database
NCCT	non-contrast CT
NDI	Neck Disability Index; Neurite Density Index
NER	non-enhancing region
NeRFs	neural radiance fields
NGS	next-generation sequencing
NIHSS	National Institutes of Health Stroke Score
NIS	National Inpatient Sample
NLP	natural language processing
NMDA	N-methyl-D-aspartate
NMLTR	neural multitask logistic model
NMR	nuclear magnetic resonance
NPV	negative predictive value
N^2QOD	National Neurosurgery Quality and Outcomes Database
NRS	numeric rating scale
NRS-BP	numeric rating scale–back pain
NRS-LP	numeric rating scale–leg pain
NSQIP	National Surgical Quality Improvement Program
ODI	Oswestry Disability Index
OR	operating room
ORB	oriented FAST and rotated BRIEF
PACS	Picture Archiving and Communication System
PASCAL-VOC	Pattern Analysis, Statistical Modeling and Computational Learning Visual Object Classes
PCA	principal components analysis
PCR	polymerase chain reaction
PET	positron emission tomography
PHI	protected health information
PI-LL	Pelvic Incidence-Lumbar Lordosis
PIM	public initial model
PitNETs	pituitary neuroendocrine tumors
PLL	posterior longitudinal ligament
PLS-DA	partial least-squares discriminant analysis
PMA	pre-market approval
PN	plexiform neurofibroma
POCT	point-of-care test
POV	point-of-view
PPV	positive predictive value
PQ	Panoptic Quality
PR curve	Precision-recall curve
PREMs	patient-reported experience measures
PRIME	Proficiency Index in Microsurgical Education
PROMs	patient-reported outcome measures
PROs	patient-reported outcomes
PSNR	peak signal-to-noise ratio
PVI	peripheral vascular intervention
QOD	Quality Outcomes Database
QoL	quality of life
RA	rheumatoid arthritis
RAAS	Robotic-as-a-Service
RAS	robotically assisted surgery
R-CNN	region-based convolutional neural network
RCTs	randomized controlled trials
ReLUs	rectified linear units
ResNet	residual network
RF	random forest
RL	reinforced learning
RLHF	reinforcement learning with human feedback
RNA	ribonucleic acid
RNNs	recurrent neural networks
RNS	responsive neurostimulation
ROC	receiver operating characteristic
ROUGE	Recall-Oriented Understudy for Gisting Evaluation
RPCA	robust principal components analysis
RSF	random survival forest
SaMD	software as a medical device
SBDD	structure-based drug design
SCAT	spatial convolutional attention inception
SCI	spinal cord injury
sEEG	stereotactic EEG
SEER	Surveillance Epidemiology and End Results
SF-36	Short Form-36
SHAP	SHapley Additive exPlanations

ShEn	Shannon entropy
SMI	surgeon–machine interface
SNR	signal-to-noise ratio
SOCAL	simulated outcomes after carotid artery laceration
SOSpine	simulated outcome for durotomy repair in minimally invasive spine surgery
SPR	surgical phase recognition
SRS-22	Scoliosis Research Society-22
SSIM	Structural Similarity Index
SURF	speeded-up robust features
SVM	support vector machine
SWI	susceptibility-weighted imaging
TBI	traumatic brain injury
TBR	theta/beta ratio
TC	tumor core
TCGA	The Cancer Genome Atlas
TCIA	The Cancer Imaging Archive
TL	transfer learning
TLE-I	temporal lobe epilepsy
TNK	tenecteplase
tPA	tissue plasminogen activator
TPLC	total product lifecycle
TPU	tensor processing unit
t-SNE	t-distributed stochastic neighbor embedding
TWIX	Training with Explanations
UCE	Universal Cellular Embedding
UCH-L1	ubiquitin C-terminal hydrolase L1
UL	unsupervised learning
UMAP	uniform manifold approximation and projection
US	ultrasound
USMLE	United States Medical Licensing Examination
UTIs	urinary tract infections
VAS	Visual Analog Scale
VGG	Visual Geometry Group
ViTs	vision transformers
VMs	vascular malformations
VOA	virtual operative assistant
VP	ventriculoperitoneal
VR	virtual reality
VTE	venous thromboembolism
WGS	whole genome sequencing
WT	whole tumor
XAI	explainable AI

1

Neurons to Networks: Introducing the Role of Artificial Intelligence in Modern Neurosurgery

ETHAN SCHONFELD AND ANAND VEERAVAGU

INTRODUCTION

At the time of this textbook's conception, artificial intelligence (AI) displayed a substantial ability in neurosurgery to optimize patient selection and surgical parameters. While it was clear that these technologies were mainly in a phase of preclinical investigation, early clinical and intraoperative applications suggested that the translation of AI technology to neurosurgery was already well underway. Patient-specific rod design and predictive algorithms for screw trajectory planning were being incorporated into spinal fusions.[1,2] Machine learning (ML)-enhanced neuronavigation systems were associated with reduced radiation exposure compared to prior generations.[3] In the cranial setting, AI systems were being developed for the operating room (OR) to identify residual tumor accounting for brain shift with intraoperative ultrasound (US).[4] Yet, the vast majority of AI development remained confined to preclinical studies, evidencing the opportunity for the technology to improve almost every facet of the delivery of neurosurgical care to our patients. However, in addition to the many areas for AI to improve neurosurgery, several major hurdles remained such as the lack of clinically applicable evaluation metrics and a limited integration of neurosurgical expertise into model development. This textbook was conceived to address these challenges by equipping neurosurgeons with the foundational knowledge necessary to develop, responsibly translate and evaluate AI technologies for clinical practice.

Since that time, the pace of AI development has accelerated dramatically. Within only a few years, proof of concept studies have demonstrated fully autonomous performance of complex procedures such as cholecystectomy in *ex vivo* settings.[5] In parallel, large language models (LLMs) have progressed from knowledge-based systems to systems capable of structured and complex reasoning. Non-reasoning knowledge-based models already impressively performed on medical tasks, for example, Generative Pre-trained Transformer 4 (GPT-4) was capable of correctly diagnosing 57% of complex cases.[6] However, the introduction of reasoning capability in models has resulted in order of magnitude improvements on difficult tasks. In International Math Olympiad problems, the earliest reasoning models achieved an 83% solved rate compared to the 13% rate achieved by GPT-4.[7] The introduction of reasoning capabilities enabled AI systems to advance beyond question-answering tasks, with the emergence of agentic systems. Agentic systems are characterized by the ability to autonomously execute complex, multistep workflows over extended time horizons. These systems can plan, generate, execute and iteratively refine code within real computational environments, in some cases completing full project lifecycles, marking a transition from AI as a passive tool to an active participant in complex technical and clinical problem-solving.

DOI: 10.1201/9781003471165-1

This rapid pace of development has exposed a fundamental limitation of traditional academic evaluation: the inability to assess technologies evolving on timescales shorter than the publication cycle. As a result, models evaluated in the medical literature are often already outdated, limiting the durability and clinical relevance of reported findings.[8] This "evaluation lag" is further compounded by inconsistent use of real-world clinical data and insufficient consideration of bias, fairness and deployment constraints in medical model evaluation.[9] In light of these limitations, it is increasingly important that clinicians develop a foundational understanding of AI systems to critically evaluate emerging technologies and directly engage in their development and implementation.

Although the capability and real-world translation of agentic systems have been demonstrated in domains such as software engineering, the underlying capabilities of reasoning, iteration and autonomous task execution are directly relevant to medicine. As agentic systems seek to become active participants in complex medical tasks, one major difference between software engineering and medicine becomes apparent: medicine largely exists as an out-of-distribution domain. While basic knowledge required for models to perform well on United States Medical Licensing Examination (USMLE) tests and neurosurgical written boards[10–12] does exist on the internet and is part of the training of these models, real-world clinical reasoning is embedded within complex, high-dimensional and multimodal data in electronic health records (EHRs). Agentic systems can provide immense benefit to medicine and neurosurgery. However, to achieve such benefit will require integration with these data sources, alongside careful consideration of generalizability, safety and interpretability. Despite the rapid evolution of AI since this textbook's conception, the core challenges remain and have become increasingly urgent. These include the development of clinically meaningful evaluation frameworks, the curation of high-quality and generalizable datasets and the active involvement of neurosurgeons in guiding AI development. Beyond these concerns, the rapid evolution of AI systems necessitates careful attention to issues of regulatory oversight and accountability, as well as whether traditional clinical trial frameworks are appropriate for evaluating continuously evolving and adaptive AI systems. Addressing these challenges will be essential to the safe and effective integration of AI into neurosurgical practice and will serve as a central focus of this textbook.

REFERENCES

1. Ou-Yang D, Burger EL, Kleck CJ. Preoperative planning in complex deformities and use of patient-specific UNiD™ instrumentation. *Global Spine J* 2022; 12(2_suppl): 40S–44S. https://doi.org/10.1177/21925682211055096
2. Patel AV, White CA, Schwartz JT, et al. Emerging technologies in the treatment of adult spinal deformity. *Neurospine* 2021; 18(3): 417–27. https://doi.org/10.14245/ns.2142412.206
3. Dorilio J, Utah N, Dowe C, et al. Comparing the efficacy of radiation free machine-vision image-guided surgery with traditional 2-dimensional fluoroscopy: A randomized, single-center study. *HSS J* 2021; 17(3): 274–80. https://doi.org/10.1177/15563316211029837
4. Saß B, Zivkovic D, Pojskic M, et al. Navigated intraoperative 3D ultrasound in glioblastoma surgery: Analysis of imaging features and impact on extent of resection. *Front Neurosci* 2022; 16. https://doi.org/10.3389/fnins.2022.883584
5. Kim JW (Brian), Chen JT, Hansen P, et al. SRT-H: A hierarchical framework for autonomous surgery via language-conditioned imitation learning. *Sci Robot* 2025; 10(104): eadt5254. https://doi.org/10.1126/scirobotics.adt5254
6. Eriksen AV, Möller S, Ryg J. Use of GPT-4 to diagnose complex clinical cases. *NEJM AI* 2024; 1(1): AIp2300031. https://doi.org/10.1056/AIp2300031
7. GPT-4o-vs-o1 complete model comparison guide. *Galileo AI* September 5, 2025. https://galileo.ai/blog/gpt-4o-vs-o1-openai-model-comparison-guide (Accessed May 2026).
8. Hond A de, Leeuwenberg T, Bartels R, et al. From text to treatment: The crucial role of validation for generative large language models in health care. *Lancet Digit Health* 2024; 6(7): e441–e3. https://doi.org/10.1016/S2589-7500(24)00111-0
9. Bedi S, Liu Y, Orr-Ewing L, et al. Testing and evaluation of health care applications of

large language models: A systematic review. *JAMA* 2025; 333(4): 319–28. https://doi.org/10.1001/jama.2024.21700

10. Bicknell BT, Butler D, Whalen S, et al. ChatGPT-4 omni performance in USMLE disciplines and clinical skills: Comparative analysis. *JMIR Med Educ* 2024; 10: e63430. https://doi.org/10.2196/63430
11. Hopkins BS, Nguyen VN, Dallas J, et al. ChatGPT versus the neurosurgical written boards: A comparative analysis of artificial intelligence/machine learning performance on neurosurgical board–style questions. *J Neurosurg* 2023; 139(3): 904–11. https://doi.org/10.3171/2023.2.JNS23419
12. Ali R, Tang OY, Connolly ID, et al. Performance of ChatGPT and GPT-4 on neurosurgery written board examinations. *Neurosurgery* 2023; 93(6): 1353–65. https://doi.org/10.1227/neu.0000000000002632

2

Multimodal Foundation Models for Healthcare

MICHIHIRO YASUNAGA AND PERCY LIANG

AI is undergoing a paradigm shift with the rise of large models such as Gemini and GPT-4 that are trained on broad data at scale and can be adapted to a wide range of downstream tasks.[1–3] These models are called foundation models.[1] For example, foundation models such as Gemini were trained on a massive collection of text and image data using tasks such as next-word prediction and, as a result, the models learn to comprehend and generate textual and visual content. Concretely, when the model is queried (prompted) with "Please write a radiology report based on this X-ray image," the model is able to generate the response accordingly.

Healthcare and biomedicine are an enormous application area in society; for instance, the expenditures account for 17% of gross domestic product (GDP) in the United States.[4–7] Healthcare focuses on the delivery of care to patients via diagnosis, treatment and health administration, and biomedical research focuses on the scientific understanding of disease and the discovery of new therapies.[8,9] Both healthcare and biomedical research demand significant expenses, time and comprehensive medical knowledge.[10,11]

We envision that foundation models can be a central storage of medical knowledge that is trained on diverse sources and modalities of data in medicine[12–14] (**Figure 2.1**, left), and they can be queried or updated interactively by medical professionals (healthcare providers and biomedical researchers access published findings and upload new publications) and queried by the public.[15] As foundation models have strong adaptation capabilities through techniques like fine-tuning and prompting,[16–18] they can be efficiently adapted to various individual tasks in healthcare and biomedicine. For example, they can be adapted as a question answering app used by patients[19–22] and as a clinical trial matching system,[23–25] accessed by researchers and patients (**Figure 2.1**, right).

In this way, foundation models can be a central interface that supports various interactions between data, tasks and people in healthcare and biomedicine, thereby advancing the efficiency and accuracy of healthcare/biomedical applications.[26,27] Indeed, an increasing number of foundation models are developed recently for healthcare and biomedicine—for instance, Med-Gemini[28] and MedAlign[29] for healthcare and medical language processing, and AlphaFold,[30] ESMFold,[31] Evo[32] and BioDiscoveryAgent[33] for protein/gene modeling, which can be useful for scientific discovery (*see* "Opportunities in Healthcare" and "Opportunities in Biomedicine."

At the same time, healthcare and biomedical applications pose unique challenges that motivate further research in foundation models, such as integrating multimodal data in healthcare/biomedicine[34,35] and observing ethical and legal regulations in medicine (privacy, safety and explainability) (*see* "Challenges and Future Research in Foundation Models."[36,37]

DOI: 10.1201/9781003471165-2

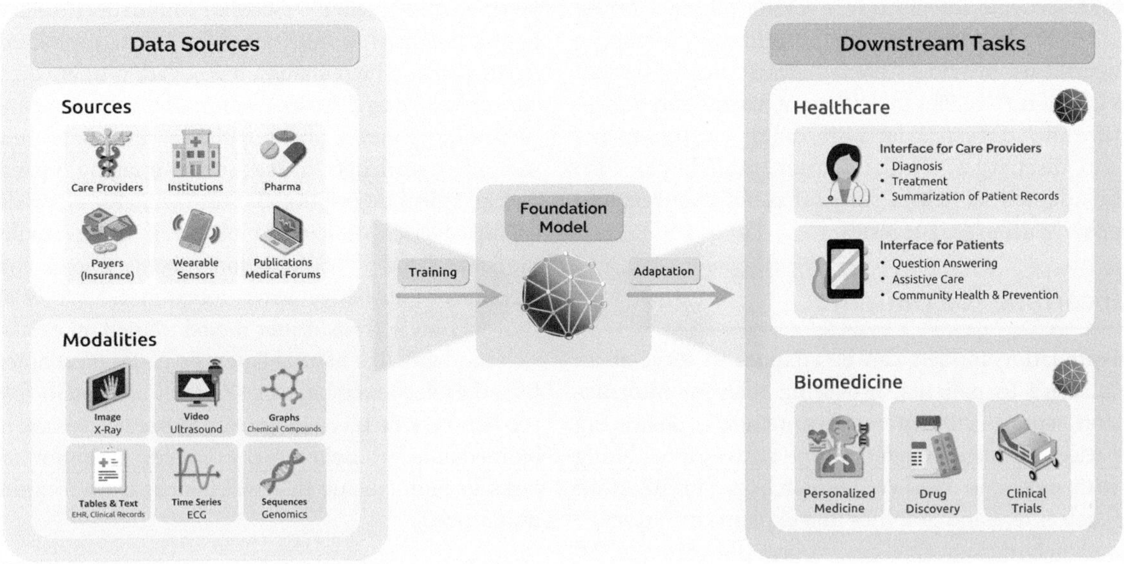

Figure 2.1 Foundation models in healthcare and biomedicine. We visualize an interactive framework where foundation models enable various tasks across healthcare and biomedicine when trained on multimodal data generated by various sources in the healthcare ecosystem. The first box – top left lists several sources of data, including care providers, payers, institutions (universities, non-profits and governments), pharma, wearables and medical publications and forums. The second box – bottom left shows several data modalities generated by the data sources. They include images (e.g. chest X-rays), videos (e.g. ultrasounds), graphs of chemical compounds, tables for electronic health records (EHRs), text such as clinical notes, time series such as ECGs and genetic data. The middle and fourth boxes on the right visualize a foundation model trained on such data and then applied to healthcare and biomedicine downstream tasks listed in the right-hand box. This process can generate new data that will further improve the foundation model, hence the bidirectional relation between the foundation models and the tasks.

OPPORTUNITIES IN HEALTHCARE

Foundation models may improve the delivery of care to patients through healthcare providers and hospitals. Currently, healthcare costs increase every year,[6,7] and studies estimate that 30% of healthcare spending may be wasteful due to administrative inefficiency and preventable medical errors.[38] Moreover, as the demand for healthcare increases, society faces a serious shortage in healthcare providers.[39] This inefficiency and shortage in healthcare necessitate the development of fast and accurate interfaces for healthcare providers and patients, such as automated aid systems for diagnosis/treatment, summarization of patient records and answering of patient questions.[40–42] In particular, in urgent medical scenarios such as the outbreak of COVID-19 and emergent patient care, fast diagnosis and screening such as automatic analysis of chest X-ray images, as well as automated question-answering for patients and the public for symptom checking, care and disease prevention are vital to reduce the spread of diseases and allocate healthcare resources for critical patients, saving more lives.[43] As foundation models have a strong capability to serve as an integrated knowledge reservoir, they can be queried and adapted to various individual tasks in healthcare. Below are examples of important tasks in healthcare that would benefit from foundation models.

Interface for healthcare providers

Foundation models can improve the efficiency and accuracy of care by providers. Healthcare providers spend unnecessary time editing electronic health records (EHRs),[38] and preventable medical errors such as hospital readmissions and surgical errors cause waste in healthcare.[44,45] Foundation models can be adapted as an efficient and accurate interface into EHRs (clinical notes, lab value histories and imaging files),[46–48] helping healthcare providers create summaries of patient visitation,[49] retrieving relevant cases and literature and suggesting lab tests, diagnosis, treatments and discharges.[50,51] Foundation models can also be adapted to help a surgical robot monitor and achieve accurate surgeries.[52–54]

Interface for patients

Foundation models can be adapted to serve as an interface to patients, providing relevant information about clinical appointments,[55] answering patient questions related to preventive care,[56] along with relevant medical explanatory information (such as text and graphics that explain conditions)[57] and helping assistive care robots for patients.[58,59] Foundation models can also serve as an interface with the general public to answer questions related to public health and pandemic prevention.[60,61] At the same time, we note that the interface must guarantee factual accuracy to ensure public trust in medical advice.[62]

OPPORTUNITIES IN BIOMEDICINE

Foundation models may facilitate biomedical research such as discovery of drugs and understanding of diseases, which ultimately translates to improved healthcare solutions.[63] Currently, biomedical discovery requires significant human resources, experimental time and financial costs. For instance, drug development involves a complex process, from basic drug research of protein target identification and potent molecule discovery to clinical development and trials to the final drug approval, which typically takes over 10 years and costs more than $1 billion.[64] Facilitating and accelerating biomedical discovery using existing data and published findings is an imperative problem in biomedicine.[10] In particular, a novel disease outbreak such as COVID-19 costs millions of lives and trillions of dollars;[43,65] if we can speed up drug development for new diseases, that would be very helpful. Foundation models can be particularly helpful for biomedical discovery in two aspects. First, foundation models have a strong generative capability such as coherent text generation in GPT-4. This can help generative tasks in biomedical research and drug discovery such as generating experimental protocols in clinical trials and designing effective drug molecules given existing data.[24,66] Second, foundation models have a potential to integrate diverse data modalities in medicine, which enables investigating biomedical concepts such as diseases from multiple scales (using molecule-, patient- and population-level data) and multiple knowledge sources (using imaging, textual and chemical descriptions). This facilitates biomedical discoveries difficult to obtain if using single-modality data.[67–74] Foundation models also enable transfer of knowledge across modalities.[75] Wu et al. showed how a Transformer model trained on a data-rich modality like natural language could be adapted for other sequence-based tasks such as protein fold prediction, which is a long-studied predictive task in biomedicine.[30,75] Below are examples of important tasks in biomedicine that will benefit from foundation models.

Drug discovery

To discover a drug or a therapeutic that treats a disease, researchers must first identify a target (proteins, genes, RNA causally implicated in the disease) and must then search for molecules (chemical compounds, antibodies) that bind to the target and treat the disease. Typically, identifying the appropriate target and generating a corresponding molecule requires years of expensive wet lab experiments.[76–78] Foundation models' generativity can improve the search space and efficiency, which not only reduces the amount of experiments but also helps to discover new and better drugs.[79–82] Moreover, the simultaneous solution of related drug discovery problems (such as target identification, efficacy prediction, side effect prediction and others) by a single foundation model may improve the solutions to each of them.[83–86] As an example, one area where foundation models have shown significant potential for impacting therapeutic design is the modeling of proteins using language models. Successful applications range from predicting viral mutations that can escape a vaccine-induced immune response to predicting protein docking potential for better design of therapeutic antibodies.[87–91]

Personalized medicine

Personalized medicine aims to select the optimal treatment for individual patients based on their health history, genetics, imaging and other personal measurements.[92,93] For instance, given a set of drugs and a patient genome, foundation models may help predict which drug is likeliest to treat the patient with minimal side effects.[94–98] Foundation models are uniquely powerful in their ability to integrate multimodal patient data ranging from the EHR[99] to medical imaging[100,101] to drug and molecular measurements to make an optimal prediction.[73,102]

Clinical trials

Clinical trials study efficacy and safety of treatment or drug candidates. Conventional clinical trials are inefficient and costly: 80% of trials fail due to inability to show efficacy and safety or due to problems with patient matching.[103,104] Foundation models can help in the following: predicting potential failures and design promising clinical trial protocols, including patient eligibility criteria, based on existing studies; and automating matching of eligible patients based on patients' individual profiles, which are multimodal data including EHRs, gene sequence, etc.[24]

CHALLENGES AND FUTURE RESEARCH IN FOUNDATION MODELS

While there are potential opportunities for foundation models to help, healthcare/biomedical applications also pose unique challenges that motivate further research in foundation models.

Multimodality

Medical data are highly multimodal. They can have various data types (text, image, video, database, molecule),[105] scales (molecule, gene, cell, tissue, patient, population),[69,73] and styles (professional and lay language).[106,107] Existing foundation models are developed for each modality (for example, text,[108] image,[109] gene,[110] protein[30]) or for a few select modalities like images and text,[111] and do not jointly learn from diverse modalities. To learn the intermodality and cross-modality information from these diverse multimodal medical data, we need to investigate both feature-level and semantic-level fusion strategies in the training of foundation models. If done effectively, this has a potential to unify biomedical knowledge and facilitate discoveries.

Explainability

Explainability—providing evidence and logical steps for decision-making—is crucial in healthcare and biomedicine,[112–114] and is made obligatory under the General Data Protection Regulation (GDPR). For instance, in diagnosis and clinical trials, patient symptoms and temporal relevance must be explained as evidence. This helps the resolution of potential disagreement between the system and human experts. Explainability is also needed for informed consent in healthcare.[115] However, current foundation models' training objectives do not include explainability, requiring future research in this direction.[116] Incorporation of knowledge graphs may be a step to further improve model explainability.[117–119]

Legal and ethical regulations

Healthcare applications must observe legal and ethical regulations with guarantees, such as patient safety, privacy and fairness.[120–122] For instance, regarding safety, predictions made by foundation models must be factually accurate with established medical knowledge, and must quantify uncertainty or choose to defer to an expert when uncertain.[123,124] For privacy, the use of patient health records must observe the privacy laws, such as Health Insurance Portability and Accountability Act, 1996 (HIPAA) in the case of the US.[125] Federated learning is one potential solution to keeping the raw, sensitive data private in the training of foundation models.[126] For fairness, researchers will need to be mindful of common pitfalls or otherwise risk exacerbating existing social inequalities.[127–129] They must ensure that the training and evaluation data for foundation models is sufficiently representative of different sexes, races, ethnicities and socioeconomic backgrounds; an area where medical datasets and clinical trials have had a long history of bias.[130,131] Research is also needed to debias and regularize models to ensure fairness when representative data are scarce.[132] Foundation model developers also need to consult with ethics and law researchers, and observe regulations in the specific circumstances (e.g. country, region) where they are deployed.

Extrapolation

The process of biomedical discovery involves extrapolation. For instance, it requires quick adaptation to new experimental settings like new assays and target diseases, and new technologies like high-resolution microscopy or imaging techniques.[133,134] The ability to leverage existing datasets and extrapolate to new settings is a key machine learning (ML) challenge in biomedicine.[135,136] While the current foundation models like GPT-4 exhibits some extrapolation behaviors, such as generating new text or predictions that were not seen before, its mechanism is unclear and still in its infancy. Further research is needed for improving the extrapolation capability of foundation models, especially when considering the diverse range of data modalities and tasks that are inherent to healthcare and biomedicine but not commonly studied in current GPT-4 and related models.[105]

ACKNOWLEDGMENTS

This manuscript is an extended version of our original paper (§3.1 Biomedicine and Healthcare Application).[1] We thank all the original authors of the paper.

REFERENCES

1. Bommasani R, Hudson DA, Adeli E, et al. On the opportunities and risks of foundation models. *arXiv:2108.07258*, 2021.
2. Achiam J, Adler S, Agarwal S, et al. GPT-4 Technical Report. *arXiv:2303.08774*, 2023.
3. Gemini Team Google, Anil R, Borgeaud S, et al. Gemini: A family of highly capable multimodal models. *arXiv:2312.11805*, 2023.
4. Swensen SJ, Kaplan GS, Meyer GS, et al. Controlling healthcare costs by removing waste: What American doctors can do now. *BMJ Qual Saf* 2011; 20(6): 534–7.
5. van Hartskamp M, Consoli S, Verhaegh W, et al. Artificial intelligence in clinical health care applications: Viewpoint. *Interact J Med Res* 2019; 8(2): e12100.
6. Keehan SP, Cuckler GA, Poisal JA, et al. National health expenditure projections, 2019–28: Expected rebound in prices drives rising spending growth: National health expenditure projections for the period 2019–2028. *Health Aff (Millwood)* 2020; 39(4): 704–14.
7. Hartman M, Martin AB, Whittle L, et al. National health care spending in 2022: Growth similar to prepandemic rates: National health care spending growth in 2022 similar to prepandemic rates. *Health Aff (Millwood)* 2024; 43(1): 6–17.
8. National Research Council, Committee to Study the National Needs for Biomedical, and Clinical Research Personnel. *Research Training in the Biomedical, Behavioral, and Clinical Research Sciences*. Washington DC: National Academies Press; 2011.
9. Faulkner A, Nicholson M. *Data-Centric Safety: Challenges, Approaches, and Incident Investigation*. London: Elsevier; 2020, 387.
10. Yu K-H, Beam AL, Kohane IS. Artificial intelligence in healthcare. *Nat Bomed Eng* 2018; 2(10): 719–31.
11. Korngiebel DM, Mooney SD. Considering the possibilities and pitfalls of generative pre-trained transformer 3 (GPT-3) in healthcare delivery. *NPJ Digit Med* 2021; 4(1): 93.
12. Krumholz HM, Terry SF, Waldstreicher J. Data acquisition, curation, and use for a continuously learning health system. *JAMA* 2016; 316(16): 1669–70.
13. Soltanian-Zadeh H. Multimodal analysis in biomedicine. In: El-Baz AS, Suri JS (eds). *Big Data in Multimodal Medical Imaging*. Boca Raton: CRC Press; 2020, pp. 193–203.
14. Suresh A, Udendhran R, Vimal S (eds). *Deep Neural Networks for Multimodal Imaging and Biomedical Applications*. Hershey: IGI Global; 2020.
15. Ionescu D. Deep learning algorithms and big health care data in clinical natural language processing. *Linguist Philos Investig* 2020; (19): 86–92.
16. Brown TB, Mann B, Ryder N, et al. Language models are few-shot learners. *arXiv:2005.14165*, 2020.
17. Wei J, Bosma M, Zhao VY, et al. Finetuned language models are zero-shot learners. *arXiv:2109.01652*, 2021.
18. Ouyang L, Wu J, Jiang X, et al. Training language models to follow instructions with human feedback. *NeurIPS* 2022; 5: 27730–44.
19. Klasnja P, Pratt W. Healthcare in the pocket: Mapping the space of mobile-phone health interventions. *J Biomed Inform* 2012; 45(1): 184–98.

20. Zhu M, Aman Ahuja A, Wei W, Reddy CK. A hierarchical attention retrieval model for healthcare question answering. *The World Wide Web Conference*, 2019; 2472–82.
21. Daniel JE, Brink W, Eloff R, Copley C. Towards automating healthcare question answering in a noisy multilingual low-resource setting. In: *Proceedings of the 57th Annual Meeting of the Association for Computational Linguistics*, 2019; pp. 948–53.
22. Liu Y, Chowdhury S, Zhang C, et al. Interpretable multi-step reasoning with knowledge extraction on complex healthcare question answering. *arXiv:2008.02434*, 2020.
23. Ni Y, Kennebeck S, Dexheimer JW, et al. Automated clinical trial eligibility prescreening: Increasing the efficiency of patient identification for clinical trials in the emergency department. *J Am Med Inform Assoc* 2015; 22(1): 166–78.
24. Harrer S, Shah P, Antony B, Hu J. Artificial intelligence for clinical trial design. *Trends Pharmacol Sci* 2019; 40(8): 577–91.
25. Beck JT, Rammage M, Jackson GP, et al. Artificial intelligence tool for optimizing eligibility screening for clinical trials in a large community cancer center. *JCO Clin Cancer Inform* 2020; 4: 50–59.
26. Elbattah M, Arnaud É, Gignon M, Dequen G. The role of text analytics in healthcare: A review of recent developments and applications. *HEALTHINF*, 2021; 825–32.
27. Moor M, Banerjee O, Abad ZSH, et al. Foundation models for generalist medical artificial intelligence. *Nature* 2023; 616(7956): 259–65.
28. Saab K, Tu T, Weng W-H, et al. Capabilities of gemini models in medicine. *arXiv:2404.18416*, 2024.
29. Fleming SL, Lozano A, Haberkorn WJ, et al. Medalign: A clinician-generated dataset for instruction following with electronic medical records. *Proc AAAI Conf Artif Intell* 2024; 38(20): 22021–30.
30. Jumper J, Evans R, Pritzel A, et al. High accuracy protein structure prediction using deep learning. *Fourteenth Critical Assessment of Techniques for Protein Structure Prediction (Abstract Book)* 2020; 22.
31. Lin Z, Akin H, Rao R, et al. Language models of protein sequences at the scale of evolution enable accurate structure prediction. *bioRxiv*, 2022.
32. Nguyen E, Poli M, Durrant MG, et al. Sequence modeling and design from molecular to genome scale with Evo. *Science* 2024; 386(6723): eado9336.
33. Roohani Y, Vora J, Huang Q, et al. Biodiscoveryagent: An AI agent for designing genetic perturbation experiments. *arXiv:2405.17631*, 2024.
34. Miura Y, Zhang Y, Tsai EB, et al. Improving factual completeness and consistency of image-to-text radiology report generation. *NAACL*, 2021.
35. Fenglin Liu, Shen Ge, Xian Wu. Competence-based multimodal curriculum learning for medical report generation. *ACL Anthology*, 2021.
36. Guan J. Artificial intelligence in healthcare and medicine: Promises, ethical challenges and governance. *Chin Med Sci J* 2019; 34(2): 76–83.
37. Xu J, Yang P, Xue S, et al. Translating cancer genomics into precision medicine with artificial intelligence: Applications, challenges and future perspectives. *Hum Genet* 2019; 138(2): 109–24.
38. Kocher RP. Reducing administrative waste in the US health care system. *JAMA* 2021; 325(5): 427–8.
39. Kirch DG, Petelle K. Addressing the physician shortage: The peril of ignoring demography. *JAMA* 2017; 317(19): 1947–8.
40. Davenport T, Kalakota R. The potential for artificial intelligence in healthcare. *Future Healthc J* 2019; 6(2): 94–8.
41. Allen Nie A, Zehnder A, Page RL, et al. Deeptag: Inferring diagnoses from veterinary clinical notes. *NPJ Digit Med* 2018; 1(1): 1–8.
42. Wang Y, Li J, Naumann T, et al. Domain-specific pretraining for vertical search: Case study on biomedical literature. *ACM SIGKDD Conference on Knowledge Discovery and Data Mining (KDD)*, 2021.
43. Lalmuanawma S, Hussain J, Chhakchhuak L. Applications of machine learning and artificial intelligence for COVID-19 (SARS-CoV-2) pandemic: A review. *Chaos Solitons Fractals* 2020; 139: 110059.

44. Shrank WH, Rogstad TL, Parekh N. Waste in the US health care system: Estimated costs and potential for savings. *JAMA* 2019; 322(15): 1501–9.
45. Shah NA, Jue J, Mackey TK. Surgical data recording technology: A solution to address medical errors? *Ann Surg* 2020; 271(3): 431–3.
46. Li K, Rao S, Solares JRA, et al. BEHRT: Transformer for electronic health records. *Sci Rep* 2020; 10(1): 1–12.
47. Steinberg E, Jung K, A Fries JA, et al. Language models are an effective representation learning technique for electronic health record data. *J Biomed Inform* 2021; 113: 103637.
48. Percha B. Modern clinical text mining: A guide and review. *Annu Rev Biomed Data Sci* 2021; 4: 165–87.
49. Krishna K, Khosla S, Bigham JP, Lipton ZC. Generating soap notes from doctor-patient conversations. *arXiv:2005.01795*, 2020.
50. Zhang Y, Nie A, Zehnder A, et al. Vettag: Improving automated veterinary diagnosis coding via large-scale language modeling. *NPJ Digit Med* 2019; 2(1): 1–8.
51. Laila Rasmy, Yang Xiang, Ziqian Xie, et al. Med-bert: Pretrained contextualized embeddings on large-scale structured electronic health records for disease prediction. *NPJ Digit Med* 2021; 4(1): 1–13.
52. Diana M, Marescaux J. Robotic surgery. *J Br Surg* 2015; 102(2): e15–e28.
53. Agrigoroaie RM, Tapus A. Developing a healthcare robot with personalized behaviors and social skills for the elderly. *2016 11th ACM/IEEE International Conference on Human-Robot Interaction (HRI)*, 2016; 589–90.
54. Yu C, Liu J, Nemati S. Reinforcement learning in healthcare: A survey. *arXiv:1908.08796*, 2019.
55. Bates M. Health care chatbots are here to help. *IEEE Pulse* 2019; 10(3): 12–14.
56. Demner-Fushman D, Mrabet Y, Abacha AB. Consumer health information and question answering: Helping consumers find answers to their healthrelated information needs. *J Am Med Inform Assoc* 2020; 27(2): 194–201.
57. Chaix B, Bibault J-E, Pienkowski A, et al. When chatbots meet patients: One-year prospective study of conversations between patients with breast cancer and a chatbot. *JMIR Cancer* 2019; 5(1): e12856.
58. Jeong S, Dos Santos K, Graca S, et al. Designing a socially assistive robot for pediatric care. *Proceedings of the 14th International Conference on Interaction Design and Children*, 2015; 387–90.
59. Abdi J, Al-Hindawi A, Ng T, Vizcaychipi MP. Scoping review on the use of socially assistive robot technology in elderly care. *BMJ Open* 2018; 8(2): e018815.
60. Bharti U, Bajaj D, Batra H, et al. Medbot: Conversational artificial intelligence powered Chatbot for delivering tele-health after COVID-19. *2020 5th International Conference on Communication and Electronics Systems (ICCES)*, 2020; 870–5.
61. Herriman M, Meer E, Rosin R, et al. Asked and answered: Building a chatbot to address covid-19-related concerns. *NEJM Catalyst Innovations in Care Delivery*, 2020.
62. Kreps SE, Kriner DL. Model uncertainty, political contestation, and public trust in science: Evidence from the covid-19 pandemic. *Sci Adv* 2020; 6(43): eabd4563.
63. Hanney SR, Castle-Clarke S, Grant J, et al. How long does biomedical research take? Studying the time taken between biomedical and health research and its translation into products, policy, and practice. *Health Res Policy Syst* 2015; 13(1): 1–18.
64. Wouters OJ, McKee M, Luyten J. Estimated research and development investment needed to bring a new medicine to market, 2009–2018. *JAMA* 2020; 323(9): 844–53.
65. McKibbin W, Fernando R. The economic impact of covid–19. In: Baldwin R, Weder di Mauro B (eds). *Economics in the Time of COVID-19.* London: CEPR Press; 2020, pp. 45–51.
66. Kadurin A, Nikolenko S, Khrabrov K, et al. druGAN: An advanced generative adversarial autoencoder model for de novo generation of new molecules with desired molecular properties in silico. *Mol Pharm* 2017; 14(9): 3098–104.

67. Lanckriet GRG, De Bie T, Cristianini N, et al. A statistical framework for genomic data fusion. *Bioinformatics* 2004; 20(16): 2626–35.
68. Aerts S, Lambrechts D, Maity S, et al. Gene prioritization through genomic data fusion. *Nat Biotechnol* 2006; 24(5): 537–44.
69. Kong J, Cooper LAD, Wang F, et al. Integrative, multimodal analysis of glioblastoma using TCGA molecular data, pathology images, and clinical outcomes. *IEEE Trans Biomed Eng* 2011; 58(12): 3469–74.
70. Ribeiro RT, Marinho RT, Sanches JM. Classification and staging of chronic liver disease from multimodal data. *IEEE Trans Biomed Eng* 2012; 60(5): 1336–44.
71. Wang W, Yang S, Zhang X, Li J. Drug repositioning by integrating target information through a heterogeneous network model. *Bioinformatics* 2014; 30(20): 2923–30.
72. Wang X, Xing EP, Schaid DJ. Kernel methods for large-scale genomic data analysis. *Brief Bioinform* 2015; 16(2): 183–92.
73. Ruiz C, Zitnik M, Leskovec J. Identification of disease treatment mechanisms through the multiscale interactome. *Nat Commun* 2021; 12(1): 1796.
74. Wu KE, Yost KE, Chang HY, Zou J. Babel enables cross-modality translation between multiomic profiles at single-cell resolution. *Proc Natl Acad Sci USA* 2021; 118(15): e2023070118.
75. Lu K, Grover A, Abbeel P, Mordatch I. Pretrained transformers as universal computation engines. *arXiv:2103.05247v2*, 2021.
76. Hughes JP, Rees S, Kalindjian SB, Philpott KL. Principles of early drug discovery. *Br J Pharmacol* 2011; 162(6): 1239–49.
77. Schenone M, Dančík V, Wagner BK, Clemons PA. Target identification and mechanism of action in chemical biology and drug discovery. *Nat Chem Biol* 2013; 9(4): 232–40.
78. Schneider G. Automating drug discovery. *Nat Rev Drug Discov* 2018; 17(2): 97–113.
79. Jin W, Barzilay R, Jaakkola T. Junction tree variational autoencoder for molecular graph generation. *arXiv:1802.04364v4*, 2018.
80. You J, Liu B, Ying R, et al. Graph convolutional policy network for goal-directed molecular graph generation, 2018. Available from: https://papers.neurips.cc/paper_files/paper/2018/file/d60678e8f2ba9c540798ebbde31177e8-Paper.pdf (Accessed April 2026).
81. Walters WP, Barzilay R. Applications of deep learning in molecule generation and molecular property prediction. *Acc Chem Res* 2020; 54(2): 263–70.
82. Stokes JM, Yang K, Swanson K, et al. A deep learning approach to antibiotic discovery. *Cell* 2020; 180(4): 688–702.
83. Ramsundar B, Kearnes SM, Riley P, et al. Massively multitask networks for drug discovery. *arXiv:1502.02072v1*, 2015.
84. Camacho DM, Collins KM, Powers RK, et al. Next-generation machine learning for biological networks. *Cell* 2018; 173(7): 1581–92.
85. Duran-Frigola M, Pauls E, Guitart-Pla O, et al. Extending the small-molecule similarity principle to all levels of biology with the Chemical Checker. *Nat Biotechnol* 2020; 38(9): 1087–96.
86. Huang K, Fu T, Gao W, et al. Therapeutics data commons: Machine learning datasets and tasks for therapeutics. *arXiv:2102.09548*, 2021.
87. Bepler T, Berger B. Learning the protein language: Evolution, structure, and function. *Cell Syst* 2021; 2(6): 654–69.
88. Hie B, Zhong ED, Berger B, Bryson B. Learning the language of viral evolution and escape. *Science* 2021; 371(6526): 284–8.
89. Tsaban T, Varga JK, Avraham O, et al. Harnessing protein folding neural networks for peptide-protein docking. *Nat Commun* 2022; 13(1): 176.
90. Wu Z, Johnston KE, Arnold FH, Yang KK. Protein sequence design with deep generative models. *Curr Opin Chem Biol* 2021; 65: 18–27.
91. Rives A, Meier J, Sercu T, et al. Biological structure and function emerge from scaling unsupervised learning to 250 million protein sequences. *Proc Natl Acad Sci USA* 2021; 118(15): e2016239118.
92. Collins FS, Varmus H. A new initiative on precision medicine. *N Engl J Med* 2015; 372(9): 793–5.
93. Ashley EA. Towards precision medicine. *Nat Rev Genet* 2016; 17(9): 507–22.

94. Whirl-Carrillo M, McDonagh EM, Hebert JM, et al. Pharmacogenomics knowledge for personalized medicine. *Clin Pharmacol Ther* 2012; 92(4): 414–17.
95. Tatonetti NP, Patrick PY, Daneshjou R, Altman RB. Datadriven prediction of drug effects and interactions. *Sci Transl Med* 2012; 4(125): 125ra31.
96. Gerstung M, Papaemmanuil E, Martincorena I, et al. Precision oncology for acute myeloid leukemia using a knowledge bank approach. *Nat Genet* 2017; 49(3): 332–40.
97. Grinfeld J, Nangalia J, Baxter EJ, et al. Classification and personalized prognosis in myeloproliferative neoplasms. *N Engl J Med* 2018; 379(15): 1416–30.
98. Adam G, Rampášek L, Safikhani Z, et al. Machine learning approaches to drug response prediction: Challenges and recent progress. *NPJ Precis Oncol* 2020; 4(1): 1–10.
99. Rajkomar A, Oren E, Chen K, et al. Scalable and accurate deep learning with electronic health records. *NPJ Digit Med* 2018; 1(1): 1–10.
100. Bera K, Schalper KA, Rimm DL, et al. Artificial intelligence in digital pathology—new tools for diagnosis and precision oncology. *Nat Rev Clin Oncol* 2019; 16(11): 703–15.
101. Ouyang D, He B, Ghorbani A, et al. Video-based AI for beat-to-beat assessment of cardiac function. *Nature* 2020; 580(7802): 252–6.
102. Gottlieb A, Stein GY, Ruppin E, Sharan R. PREDICT: A method for inferring novel drug indications with application to personalized medicine. *Mol Syst Biol* 2011; 7(1): 496.
103. Ali Z, Zibert JR, Thomsen SF. Virtual clinical trials: Perspectives in dermatology. *Dermatology* 2020; 236(4): 375–82.
104. Liu R, Rizzo S, Whipple S, et al. Evaluating eligibility criteria of oncology trials using real-world data and AI. *Nature* 2021; 592(7855): 629–33.
105. Tu T, Azizi S, Driess S, et al. Towards generalist biomedical AI. *NEJM AI* 2024; 1(3): AIoa2300138.
106. Lavertu A, Altman RB. Redmed: Extending drug lexicons for social media applications. *J Biomed Inform* 2019; 99: 103307.
107. Li I, Yasunaga M, Nuzumlalı MY, et al. A neural topic-attention model for medical term abbreviation disambiguation. *arXiv:1910.14076v1*, 2019.
108. Yasunaga M, Leskovec J, Liang P. Linkbert: Pretraining language models with document links. *arXiv:2203.15827v1*, 2022.
109. Chaitanya K, Erdil E, Karani N, Konukoglu E. Contrastive learning of global and local features for medical image segmentation with limited annotations. *arXiv:2006.10511v2*, 2020.
110. Ji Y, Zhou Z, Liu H, Davuluri RV. DNABERT: Pre-trained bidirectional encoder representations from transformers model for dna-language in genome. *Bioinformatics* 2021; 37(15): 2112–20.
111. Moor M, Huang Q, Wu S, et al. Med-flamingo: A multimodal medical few-shot learner. *arXiv:2307.15189v1*, 2023.
112. Holzinger A, Langs G, Denk H, et al. Causability and explainability of artificial intelligence in medicine. *WIREs Data Min Knowl Discov* 2019; 9(4): e1312.
113. Albahri AS, Duhaim AM, Fadhel MA, et al. A systematic review of trustworthy and explainable artificial intelligence in healthcare: Assessment of quality, bias risk, and data fusion. *Inf Fusion* 2023; 96: 156–91.
114. Sindiramutty SR, Tee WJ, Balakrishnan S, et al. Explainable AI in healthcare application. In: Ghonge MM, Pradeep N, Jhanjhi NZ, et al. (eds). *Advances in Explainable AI Applications for Smart Cities*. IGI Global; 2024, pp. 123–76.
115. Amann J, Blasimme A, Vayena E, et al. Explainability for artificial intelligence in healthcare: A multidisciplinary perspective. *BMC Med Inform Decis Mak* 2020; 20(1): 1–9.
116. Linardatos P, Papastefanopoulos V, Kotsiantis S. Explainable AI: A review of machine learning interpretability methods. *Entropy* 2021; 23(1): 18.
117. Roberts A, Raffel C, Shazeer N. How much knowledge can you pack into the parameters of a language model? *arXiv:2002.08910v4*, 2020.
118. Xu J, Kim S, Song M, et al. Building a pubmed knowledge graph. *Sci Data* 2020; 7(1):1–15.
119. Jin Q, Yuan Z, Xiong G, et al. Biomedical question answering: A comprehensive review. *arXiv:2102.05281*, 2021.

120. Naik N, Hameed BM, Shetty DK, et al. Legal and ethical consideration in artificial intelligence in healthcare: Who takes responsibility? *Front Surg* 2022; 9: 266.
121. Alam MN, Kaur M, Kabir MdS. Explainable ai in healthcare: Enhancing transparency and trust upon legal and ethical consideration. *Int Res J Eng Technol* 2023; 10(6): 1–9.
122. Gerke S, Minssen T, Cohen G. Ethical and legal challenges of artificial intelligence-driven healthcare. In: Bohr A, Memarzadeh K (eds). *Artificial Intelligence in Healthcare*. San Diego: Elsevier; 2020, pp. 295–336.
123. Challen R, Denny J, Pitt M, et al. Artificial intelligence, bias and clinical safety. *BMJ Qual Saf* 2019; 28(3): 231–7.
124. Mozannar H, Sontag D. Consistent estimators for learning to defer to an expert. *arXiv:2006.01862v3*, 2020.
125. Accountability Act. Health insurance portability and accountability act of 1996. Public Law 104–191, 1996.
126. Chamikara MAP, Bertok P, Khalil I, et al. Privacy preserving distributed machine learning with federated learning. *Comput Commun* 2021; 171: 112–25.
127. Chen IY, Szolovits P, Ghassemi M. Can AI help reduce disparities in general medical and mental health care? *AMA J Ethics* 2019; 21(2): 167–79.
128. Wiens J, Saria S, Sendak M, et al. Do no harm: A roadmap for responsible machine learning for health care. *Nat Med* 2019; 25(9): 1337–40.
129. Chen IY, Joshi S, Ghassemi M. Treating health disparities with artificial intelligence. *Nat Med* 2020; 26(1): 16–17.
130. Martinez-Martin N, Luo Z, Kaushal A, et al. Ethical issues in using ambient intelligence in health-care settings. *Lancet Digit Health* 2020; 3(2): E115–23.
131. Kaushal A, Altman R, Langlotz C. Geographic distribution of us cohorts used to train deep learning algorithms. *JAMA* 2020; 324(12): 1212–13.
132. Zhao Q, Adeli E, KM Pohl. Training confounder-free deep learning models for medical applications. *Nat Commun* 2020; 11(1): 6010.
133. Jaroch K, Jaroch A, Bojko B. Cell cultures in drug discovery and development: The need of reliable in vitro-in vivo extrapolation for pharmacodynamics and pharmacokinetics assessment. *J Pharm Biomed Anal* 2018; 147: 297–312.
134. Benam KH, Gilchrist S, Kleensang A, et al. Exploring new technologies in biomedical research. *Drug Discov Today* 2019; 24(6): 1242–7.
135. Snell J, Swersky K, Zemel RS. Prototypical networks for few-shot learning. *arXiv:1703.05175*, 2017.
136. Ma J, Fong SH, Luo Y, et al. Few-shot learning creates predictive models of drug response that translate from high-throughput screens to individual patients. *Nat Cancer* 2021; 2(2): 233–44.

3

From Data to Decisions: AI-Driven Outcome Prediction in Spine Surgery

EUNICE YANG AND ANDREW K. CHAN

Spine surgery is expanding faster than the frameworks surgeons use to navigate it. As the field expands to meet the needs of an evolving patient population, surgeons will face increasingly complex decisions in case selection and procedure choice. In this chapter, we examine the potential of artificial intelligence (AI) as an innovative tool to predict surgical outcomes and navigate these challenges in spine surgery.

INTRODUCTION

Understanding the scope of modern spine surgery is the first step needed to highlight critical areas of need for predictive models. Spinal fusion is currently one of the most frequently performed surgeries in the country, with a projected doubling in single-level instrumentation cases from 2024 to 2050, driven in part by a rise in degenerative spinal disease.[1] This highlights a central problem in the field—that our current healthcare structures may not be well equipped for a significant rise in cases and associated costs. Within this context, AI has matured as a promising tool to alleviate burden on healthcare systems and enhance clinical decision-making. Current work is exploring the capacity of AI tools to predict surgical outcomes which, in an ideal world, could help surgeons meet the demands of modern practice by triaging high-risk patients and forecasting which patients are ideal surgical candidates.

KEY OUTCOMES IN SPINE SURGERY

Before starting to construct an AI model, we must first define what actually constitutes a successful surgery. What outcomes should a model predict? On a fundamental level, models may aim to characterize patient safety, with mortality, adverse events and other major complications serving as critical benchmarks of surgical quality. These core metrics are intrinsically linked to key performance indicators (KPIs) like readmission, reoperation and length of stay. Such analysis is straightforward because these outcomes are direct and quantifiable but, in the modern era of spine surgery, they inadequately capture the full measure of surgical success. Patient-reported outcomes (PROs) have thus become particularly valuable tools to assess targeted domains following an operation and capture the daily impact of surgery, as quantified through validated instruments known as patient-reported outcome measures (PROMs). These measures capture a wide range of patient experiences and provide unique insight into lived recovery that may not be apparent through traditional clinical or radiographic assessment.

While PROMs are inherently subjective and can be developed or modified to address specific research questions, their true power lies in standardization, allowing meaningful comparison of patient experiences across studies and institutions. Although a 2016 review identified over 200 unique

DOI: 10.1201/9781003471165-3

spine-related PROMs in orthopedic literature over a decade,[2] the field has largely consolidated around a core set of validated, widely adopted instruments that enable robust cross-study comparison. In "Patient-Reported Outcomes in Performance Measurement," Dr Cella and colleagues describe a framework to categorize PROs into five categories: functional status, symptoms and symptom burden, health behaviors, health-related quality of life (HRQoL) and the patient's healthcare experience.[3] These domains are largely applicable within spine surgery, though we will broaden "functional status" to "physical function / health status."

Metrics of physical function / health status allow us to quantify specific physical limitations and daily activity restrictions, which are often the primary impediments addressed by spine surgery. The Oswestry Disability Index (ODI) is the most widely used PROM by lumbar spine surgeons and assesses the level of lower back pain-related disability.[4] For conditions of the cervical spine, the Neck Disability Index (NDI) is a comparable measurement of neck pain-related disability on activities of daily living.[5] These PROMs can also be condition-specific, such as the Japanese Orthopaedic Association (JOA) used to assess the severity of cervical myelopathy and the modified scale (mJOA) designed for Western patients.[6,7] The domain of symptom burden is similarly critical in spine surgery, often representing the primary complaints that drive patients to seek care. Most commonly, pain intensity is measured through the Visual Analog Scale (VAS) or Numeric Rating Scale (NRS) measures.[8] Notably, VAS was the most frequently utilized PROM among five prominent spine journals from 2004 to 2013.[2]

Complementing these measures are robust tools quantifying subjective aspects of the surgical journey from overall well-being to patient satisfaction. The Short Form-36 (SF-36) is a widely used HRQoL instrument assessing physical functioning, role limitations, social functioning, and mental health.[9] The EuroQol 5-Dimension (EQ-5D) is another common tool for measuring health status that can generate utility scores for economic analyses.[10] Some QoL PROMs are designed for specific conditions, such as the Scoliosis Research Society-22 Questionnaire (SRS-22), initially created for patients with adolescent idiopathic scoliosis but now frequently used across deformity outcome assessment.[11] Health behavior measures are utilized less frequently, though medication use, particularly opioid consumption, has become a more critical element of post-surgical evaluation. Finally, patient-reported experience measures, sometimes termed PREMs, can help evaluate the alignment between expectations and outcomes. The North American Spine Society (NASS) Satisfaction Index provides a standardized assessment on a 4-point scale ranging from "The treatment met my expectations" to "I am the same or worse than before treatment."[12]

The inherent subjectivity of PROs does present a key challenge in standardization and interpretation that should be considered prior to development of predictive models. The history of the ODI serves as one of many cautionary tales in this regard. Following its original publication in 1980, there have been several "approved" updates to the index.[13] However, other researchers and clinicians have created new variants of the ODI to address perceived limitations or adapt to specific patient populations. While these modifications are often well-intentioned, the resulting proliferation of non-validated versions has, at times, obfuscated the scientific literature, making it more difficult to compare results across studies and synthesize evidence effectively.[14] This challenge is not specific to the ODI metric and is further compounded by the continuous introduction of novel PRO instruments. Despite rigorous development, many may never achieve widespread adoption or validation, raising questions about the pragmatic value of creating new measures rather than properly refining and standardizing existing ones.

For those needing strictly objective outcomes, radiographic and physical measurements are additional assets in our toolbox. For instance, in spinal deformity surgery, postoperative evaluation of achievement of sagittal alignment via parameters such as sagittal vertical axis, pelvic tilt and pelvic incidence–lumbar lordosis mismatch are predictive of surgical benefit. However, these radiographic measurements warrant careful interpretation, as they may not directly reflect clinical status, and their correlation with outcomes can even diminish over time.[15] Ultimately, perfect alignment may not matter if the patient is debilitated and in constant pain. Physical tests can also be performed in clinic, with options including the timed-up-and-go, six-minute walk, and hand grip strength.[16–18] However, these tests provide an assessment of singular points in time and may be confounded by factors such as patient motivation, comorbidities and environmental conditions.

Increasingly in the digital age, wearables are being assessed for their capability to provide objective, continuous functional assessment of patients. Data regarding activity tracking, gait analysis and sleep patterns can elucidate digital biomarkers, offering insights into patient function beyond the constraints of periodic clinical visits.[19,20] There is also movement towards objective measurements of biological status by using multi-omic biomarkers.[21] As these technologies evolve and validation studies accumulate, digital and biological phenotyping may help bridge the gap between subjective PROs and traditional objective measures, thereby increasing the validity of data flowing through AI tools.

CURRENT LANDSCAPE OF SPINE MODELS

The creation of a predictive model that can accurately forecast these surgical outcomes from a patient's baseline demographic and clinical features has been a longstanding goal of spine surgeons. We have long used conventional statistical methods like regression modeling to forecast surgical results and identify predictive clinical features. However, these approaches are limited when handling complex, nonlinear relationships in data. Modern ML approaches can overcome these limitations, fundamentally shifting our ability to process large-scale clinical data.

The classic outcome prediction task in medicine is a quintessential supervised learning problem. We take structured data like demographics and baseline functional assessments, where each variable is clearly defined and systematically categorized. Our goal is to leverage a collection of baseline characteristics to predict clinical outcomes, which might be continuous (i.e. length of hospital stays), ordinal (i.e. NASS Satisfaction), or binary (i.e. presence or absence of complications). For an AI algorithm to succeed at this task, it must learn on a labeled set of patients, such that the patient's independent variables are matched to the intended outcome.

Depending on the complexity of the prediction task, the amount of data required to train a model may be substantial. As a result, many researchers have relied upon the large-scale clinical databases and national registries that traditionally served a complementary role to "gold standard" randomized controlled trials. These repositories, which include insurance claim databases, national quality registries and electronic healthcare record (EHR) databases vary significantly in their scope, collection methods and available outcomes.

The National Inpatient Sample (NIS) and the National Surgical Quality Improvement Program (NSQIP) are the largest administrative and quality databases, respectively. However, because these databases are built primarily on procedural and billing codes, they are limited in clinical granularity and vulnerable to the well-documented flaws of administrative coding.[22,23] Coding practices are primarily influenced by reimbursement priorities, which may vary significantly across institutions, and therefore do not always provide accurate reflections of a patient's diagnosis, comorbidities or complications.[24] Beyond coding inaccuracy, the size and design of these databases can also lead to inconsistent analytic practices in the literature, with one review of over 1000 NIS-based publications from 2015 to 2016 finding that 85% failed to adhere to at least one required methodological practice, and 62% failed to adhere to two or more.[25] With full recognition of these limitations, administrative datasets are best used as a first step for exploration of national trends and hypothesis generation, whereas clinically meaningful AI models may ultimately require data with superior clinical detail.

More recently, efforts have emerged in spine surgery to create largescale multicenter databases that can be used to follow PROs longitudinally, such as the Quality Outcomes Database (QOD) and the International Spine Study Group which both boast prospectively collected, multicenter data.[26,27] Unlike administrative datasets, these registries are carefully curated by clinicians and research teams (e.g. QOD Spine CORe™)[28–50] from the medical record to capture targeted variables related to disease severity, operative details and standardized PROs. Beyond increasing accuracy and clinical granularity, the design of these registries enables a high level of longitudinal follow-up, with PROs now even being collected at the 5-year mark, far beyond the reach of administrative sources.[48] Such features make these registries uniquely valuable for developing and validating AI models centered on outcome prediction. However, they remain resource-intensive and logistically complex to maintain, especially across multiple sites, so researchers often rely on smaller, single-institution datasets as a more practical source of high-quality clinical data.

Many models developed for spine surgery are created for one of two primary clinical use cases: risk assessment and treatment efficacy forecasting. Early development of AI models in spine surgery largely centered around risk assessment because of the critical nature of patient safety and the ready accessibility of such outcomes in large claims databases. Many of these studies served as a proof-of-concept of the capability of ML and deep learning approaches to make reasonably accurate predictions (**Table 3.1**). Several early studies focused on the prediction of intraoperative and/or postoperative complications, showing that deep learning techniques could accurately predict rare complications in moderately sized study samples. In 2018, Arvind et al. analyzed anterior cervical discectomy and fusion (ACDF) patients from the NSQIP database and found that an artificial Neural Network (NN) outperformed logical regression, support vector machine (SVM) and random forest (RF) models on the prediction of venous thromboembolism (VTE), wound complications and mortality.[51] The artificial NN consistently demonstrated the highest area under the curve (AUC) across outcomes ranging from 0.518 to 0.979, including against a clinical benchmark of ASA physical status classification. The difference in performance was most stark for mortality, where the AUC of the NN was 0.979 and of the ASA classification was 0.346. A subsequent study from Wang et al. in 2021 on single-level ACDF patients from the NSQIP found that an artificial NN significantly outperformed the ASA and Charlson Comorbidity Index stratification metrics, with an AUC of 0.74 versus 0.66 and 0.60, respectively.[52] Some research groups have expanded beyond conventional complication metrics to predict which patients may require perioperative interventions, with Durand et al. using tree-based models to predict perioperative blood transfusions in adult spinal deformity patients and Veeramani et al. modeling unplanned intubations during ACDF cases.[53,54]

There has also been a focus on measures of resource utilization, which can serve as proxies for medical complexity and healthcare costs. Shahrestani et al. were able to train nonlinear k-nearest neighbor (KNN) classification models on the QOD lumbar spondylolisthesis dataset to identify patients at risk of extended length of stay, defined as the top quartile within the dataset (4.0 days).[55] Two models were constructed, one with and one without the patient's arthrodesis status as an input feature. Both reached an AUC of 0.998 and thus showed high predictive value for the predicted outcome, though the model that was fusion agnostic showed slightly higher accuracy, specificity and positive predictive value (PPV). Unplanned readmissions can also be modeled, as shown by work from Hopkins et al. on a cohort of posterior lumbar fusion patients from the NSQIP database. Here, a 7-layer deep neural network was able to predict 30-day readmissions with a mean AUC of 0.812, far outperforming the mean AUC of 0.717 from the baseline regression model.[56] ML models can similarly be used to simulate discharge planning as per Karnuta et al.'s prediction of discharge disposition following dorsal and lumbar fusion. The Naïve Bayes algorithm trained on data from the New York Statewide Planning and Research Cooperative System was able to predict discharge to home with an AUC of 0.906.[57] Interestingly, a separate study from Goyal et al. on patients in the NSQIP receiving cervical or lumbar fusion found that ML classification algorithms were better able to predict non-home discharge (AUC 0.85–0.877) unplanned 30-day readmission (AUC 0.63–0.66).[58] This variance in predictive performance highlights the importance of careful model selection and evaluation, as some postoperative events may be more challenging for a model to interpret than others. Altogether development of risk-prediction tools will build up a safety net that can screen for high-risk patients and possible complications. Accurate stratification of patient risk could additionally inform optimization before surgery and even guide decisions about surgical approach (e.g. choosing minimally invasive techniques or staged procedures) or postoperative management.

On the other hand, treatment efficacy forecasting typically aims to predict long-term outcomes and provide more multifaceted identification of ideal surgical candidates (**Table 3.2**). This can be inherently more challenging, given that PROs are often more complex than binary complications and capture multiple domains of a patient's health status. Additionally, there are often data limitations from the PRO collection process requiring active patient participation over extended follow-up periods.[22] In a study by Park et al. on the QOD cervical spondylotic

Table 3.1 Selected risk prediction models in spine surgery using multicenter data

Author, year	Dataset, no. patients	Pathology/Procedure	Model	Prediction task	Best AUC
Scheer et al.[70] 2016	Multicenter 510 patients	Adult spinal deformity	DT	Proximal junctional failure or clinically significant proximal junctional kyphosis	0.89
Scheer et al.[71] 2017	ISSG 557 patients	Adult spinal deformity	DT	Intraoperative or perioperative complication	0.89
Arvind et al.[51] 2018	NSQIP 20,879 patients	ACDF	LR, SVM, RF, ANN	Cardiac complications, VTE, wound complications, mortality	0.518–0.979
Durand et al.[53] 2018	ACS NSQIP 1029 patients	Adult spinal deformity	DT, RF	Intra-/postoperative blood transfusion	0.85
Goyal et al.[58] 2019	NSQIP 59,145 patients	Cervical or lumbar spinal fusion	GLM, RF, GB, LDA, Naïve Bayes, ANN	Discharge to nonhome facility, unplanned readmission	0.66–0.87
Hopkins et al.[56] 2019	NSQIP 23,264 patients	Posterior lumbar fusion	Deep neural network	Hospital readmission	0.812
Karnuta et al.[57] 2020	New York Statewide Planning and Research Cooperative System 38,070 patients	Dorsal and lumbar fusion for nondeformity indications	Naïve Bayes	LOS, discharge disposition, total inpatient payments	0.880–0.941
Wang et al.[52] 2021	NSQIP 12,492 patients	ACDF	LR, ANN	1-week complications	0.757

Author, year	Dataset, no. patients	Pathology/Procedure	Model	Prediction task	Best AUC
Chan et al.[72] 2022	NIS 653,815 patients	Spinal fusion	LR (with CMS hierarchical condition category risk adjustment)	Death, nonroutine discharge, LOS, total charges, perioperative complication	0.725–0.843
Shahrestani et al.[55] 2023	QOD 544 patients	Lumbar spondylolisthesis	KNN	LOS above top quartile of 4.0 days	0.998
Veeramani et al.[54] 2023	NSQIP 54,502 patients	ACDF	LR, DT, RF, GB, XGB, NN	Unplanned intubation	0.766
Shahrestani et al.[73] 2024	Nationwide Readmissions Database 750,183 patients	Spinal fusion	Generalized linear mixed-effects	Mortality, nonroutine discharge, top-quartile cost, top-quartile length of stay, 30-day readmission	0.831–0.910

LR: Logistic Regression; DT: Decision Tree; RF: Random Forest; SVM: Support Vector Machine; GB: Gradient Boosting; XGB: Extreme Gradient Boosting; LDA: Linear Discriminant Analysis; NN: Neural Network; ANN: Artificial Neural Network.

Table 3.2 Selected treatment efficacy forecasting models in spine surgery using multicenter data

Author	Dataset	Pathology/ Procedure	Model	Prediction Task	Best AUC
Oh et al.[74]	ISSG 234 patients	Adult spinal deformity	DT	2-year ODI MCID	0.96
Scheer et al.[75]	ISSG 198 patients	Adult spinal deformity	DT	2-year ODI MCID	0.94
Ames et al.[76]	ISSG, ESSG 570 patients	Adult spinal deformity	GLM, GB, RF, XGB	1- and 2-year ODI, SRS22r and SF-36v2	MAE: 8–15%
Merali et al.[77]	AO Spine 757 patients	Degenerative cervical myelopathy	LR, RF, SVM, DT, ANN	6-, 12- and 24-month SF-6D MCID	0.65–0.7
Khan et al.[78]	AO Spine 757 patients	Cervical spondylotic myelopathy	LR, SVM, Naïve Bayes, GB	1-year mJOA	0.834
Mummaneni et al.[79]	QOD 502 patients	Lumbar spondylolisthesis	LR	2-year NASS satisfaction	N/A
Berg et al.[59]	Prospective multicenter 22,707 cases	Lumbar disc herniation	LR, RF, LDA, MLP, GB, XGB	12-month improvement in ODI, NRS-BP, NRS-LP	C-stat: 0.77–0.84
Park et al.[33]	QOD 535 patients	Cervical spondylotic myelopathy	LR, SVM, DT, RF, Naïve Bayes, KNN, MLP	3- and 24-month MCID VAS-neck pain	0.762–0.773

LR: Logistic Regression; DT: Decision Tree; RF: Random Forest; SVM: Support Vector Machine; GB: Gradient Boosting; XGB: Extreme Gradient Boosting; LDA: Linear Discriminant Analysis; NN: Neural Network; ANN: Artificial Neural Network.

myelopathy dataset, a survey of ML algorithms ultimately showed that logistic regression was the most predictive model of minimal clinically important difference (MCID) for neck pain at 3 and 24 months (AUC 0.762, 0.773).[34] However, for 3-month outcomes, a multi-layer perceptron demonstrated superior recall, and an SVM showed the highest specificity. These results demonstrate that predicting long-term PROs remains challenging and that different ML approaches may be better suited for specific clinical prediction tasks. Another study by Berg et al. on the Norwegian Registry for Spine Surgery, which features a higher volume of 22,707 lumbar disc herniation cases as of May 2021, also surveyed a range of ML models on the prediction of 1-year improvement in ODI, numeric rating scale–back pain (NRS-BP) and numeric rating scale–leg pain (NRS-LP).[59] The XGBoost model consistently demonstrated the strongest performance on a *C* statistic metric across ODI (0.83), NRS-BP (0.78), and NRS-LP (0.76), where >0.7 is typically considered reasonable and >0.8 considered strong discriminative ability. Internal-external cross-validation demonstrated strong performance across geographic regions and hospital type, with $C > 0.81$ for ODI. These findings highlight both the promise and ongoing limitations of ML prediction of long-term surgical efficacy, with existing studies largely predicting to the 1- or 2-year mark. Continued development of novel algorithmic approaches may further improve our ability to forecast treatment outcomes.

Commercial surgical systems are now beginning to integrate predictive modeling into routine clinical practice. One example is Medtronic's UNiD Adaptive Spine Intelligence (ASI), which the company describes as "using data science and AI" to enable "spine surgeons [to] provide predictable and reproducible outcomes for patients with spinal deformity."[60] The system is targeted towards deformity surgery, to improve patient outcomes by combining AI-driven preoperative planning for spinopelvic parameters and the manufacturing of patient-specific rods. An early study of 60 patients treated with UNiD rods found that the cohort was 2.6 times more likely to achieve a normal pelvic incidence–lumbar lordosis mismatch compared to historical cohorts in the literature.[61] Another review of 16 cases at 1-year follow-up found specifically that the UNiD system's predictive modeling halved the mean error in forecasting thoracic kyphosis (from approximately 13.2 to 6.6 degrees) and improved pelvic tilt prediction accuracy as well.[62]

Other companies have also developed AI-enabled surgical planning platforms, including Carlsmed's Aprevo Technology, which is marketed as an "end-to-end integrated platform" that similarly combines surgical planning with custom implants.[63] Although there is limited literature on the exact accuracy of long-term alignment predictions, a retrospective study of 217 deformity patients who received Aprevo implants reported that intervertebral lordosis was achieved within 5 degrees of the preoperative plan across 299 levels, with follow-up ranging from 6 weeks to 12 months.[64] Carlsmed has additionally highlighted their proprietary Aprevo Implant Registry, which currently includes data from over 300 patients across 16 centers. Collectively, platforms such as those developed by Medtronic and Carlsmed suggest the potential for more reliable alignment outcomes and lower rates of mechanical complications. As companies continue to aggregate de-identified data from these surgical systems, the predictive algorithms are also expected to evolve iteratively, though the proprietary nature of such datasets limits independent validation.

The increasing availability of wearables has also sparked a recent search for digital biomarkers that are predictive of surgical outcomes. Findings remain limited, and the few existing studies have shown mixed results. In preliminary data from the SpineTrak study,[20] which fitted 198 patients undergoing elective spinal surgery with Apple Watch devices, 95% of neurosurgeons surveyed by the study found that the device's reports "helped them understand their patients' recovery." However, there was a reported "poor correlation" between the watch data and recorded PROMs, which included SF-36, EQ-5D, VAS-Pain and ODI/NDI. A recently published study by Greenberg et al. used Fitbit devices to monitor 133 lumbar surgery patients, which extracted minute-level step counts, heart rate and sleep measurements that were then consolidated into clinically meaningful predictors.[19] In subsequent modeling of a Quality of Recovery-15 metric, a model built on these Fitbit markers outperformed a logical regression model trained on traditional patient-reported measures with an AUC of 0.69 versus 0.57. While these early studies show promise for digital biomarkers in postoperative monitoring, more research is needed to validate their clinical utility and determine optimal approaches for integrating wearable data with traditional outcome measures.

CHALLENGES AND FUTURE DIRECTIONS

There is active discussion surrounding the challenges of integrating AI into medicine. Rajpurkar et al. highlight technical issues, regulation, and ethical concerns as predominant concerns.[65] Notably, there remain many unanswered questions surrounding the "black box" nature of AI models. If an outcome prediction model has strong accuracy but no transparency, how much utility does it have to a surgeon engaging a patient in shared decision-making? Surgeons should certainly be skeptical of AI systems when they appear to challenge established clinical expertise without providing clear logic or reasoning. This resistance is not merely a matter of professional pride—it reflects legitimate concerns about ensuring patient safety during complex clinical decisions. Frameworks for explainable AI must be developed alongside the advancement of model performance.

Numerous technical hurdles remain before widespread clinical implementation of these models. Perhaps the most imminent is simply that existing models must improve significantly in their predictive power, a process bottlenecked by the availability of clinical data. The colloquial term "garbage in, garbage out" is relevant here, meaning that any AI model will only be as good as the training data it is fed. This is a problem for models trained on national administrative databases, which may boast an impressive quantity of data, but suffer from the questionable reliability of ICD codes subject to coding inaccuracies and documentation errors.[66] On the other hand, registries like the QOD require substantial institutional labor to ensure trustworthy collection of PROs with a rigorous level of follow-up.[26]

The advent of large language modeling (LLM) has opened a new frontier in outcome prediction to address some of those weaknesses. Rather than being reliant on the structural data that most spine-tailored models are built on, LLMs can extract and interpret meaningful information from unstructured text, including patient EHRs. ClinicalBERT was one of the first transformer models trained on a large corpus of clinical notes, specifically the MIMIC-III dataset, and was able to outperform existing baselines on the prediction of 30-day hospital readmission.[67] This has been followed by models trained exclusively on clinical text, including entire institutional EHRs, with parameters scaling into the hundreds of millions or billions.[68,69] These models have improved upon traditional benchmarks on prediction tasks, including 30-day readmission, in-hospital mortality and length of stay. Generalist foundation models can be flexibly applied across specialty domains and should be further explored within the specific context of spine surgery. Furthermore, expansion from risk prediction to PRO forecasting represents a natural evolution of these models' capabilities. Rather than focusing solely on adverse events, these models could potentially utilize the rich contextual information in clinical documentation to predict functional outcomes, pain scores and QoL measures.

CONCLUSION

The development of AI-driven outcome prediction within spine surgery stands at an exciting yet critical juncture. As explored, these tools have demonstrated promising capabilities in risk assessment and even long-term PRO forecasting. However, significant hurdles remain before widespread clinical implementation becomes feasible. Data quality and availability, particularly of PROs, continue to be limiting factors, while the "black box" nature of many AI models raises legitimate concerns about transparency and clinical trust. Yet, the future holds intriguing possibilities. As we move toward more sophisticated models, perhaps integrated directly with EHRs and enriched by digital biomarkers from wearable devices, we may see these tools evolve from simple prediction engines to comprehensive clinical decision support systems. The ultimate goal is to harness the power of AI, not to replace the clinical judgment of spine surgeons, but to augment their expertise in an increasingly complex healthcare landscape.

REFERENCES

1. Mani K, Kleinbart E, Goldman SN, et al. Projections of single-level and multilevel spinal instrumentation procedure volume and associated costs for Medicare patients to 2050. *J Am Acad Orthop Surg Glob Res Rev* 2024; 8(5): e24.00053.
2. Guzman JZ, Cutler HS, Connolly J, et al. Patient-reported outcome instruments in spine surgery. *Spine (Phila PA 1976)* 2016; 41(5): 429–37.
3. Cella D, Hahn E, Jensen S, et al. *Patient-Reported Outcomes in Performance Measurement.* Research Triangle Park: RTI Press; 2015.
4. Fairbank JC, Couper J, Davies JB, O'Brien JP. The Oswestry low back pain disability questionnaire. *Physiotherapy* 1980; 66(8): 271–3.
5. Vernon H, Mior S. The Neck Disability Index: A study of reliability and validity. *J Manip Physiol Ther* 1991; 14(7): 409–15.
6. Hirabayashi K, Miyakawa J, Satomi K, et al. Operative results and postoperative progression of ossification among patients with ossification of cervical posterior longitudinal ligament. *Spine (Phila PA 1976)* 1981; 6(4): 354–64.
7. Benzel EC, Lancon J, Kesterson L, Hadden T. Cervical laminectomy and dentate ligament section for cervical spondylotic myelopathy. *J Spinal Disord* 1991; 4(3): 286–95.
8. Shafshak TS, Elnemr R. The visual analogue scale versus numerical rating scale in measuring pain severity and predicting disability in low back pain. *J Clin Rheumatol* 2021; 27(7): 282–5.
9. Grevitt M, Khazim R, Webb J, et al. The short form-36 health survey questionnaire in spine surgery. *J Bone Jt Surg* 1997; 79(1): 48–52.
10. Devlin NJ, Brooks R. EQ-5D and the EuroQol Group: Past, present and future. *Appl Heal Econ Heal Polic* 2017; 15(2): 127–37.

11. Berven S, Deviren V, Demir-Deviren S, et al. Studies in the modified Scoliosis Research Society Outcomes Instrument in adults: Validation, reliability, and discriminatory capacity. *Spine (Phila PA 1976)* 2003; 28(18): 2164–9.
12. Daltroy LH, CatsBaril WL, Katz JN, et al. The North American Spine Society lumbar spine outcome assessment instrument. *Spine (Phila PA 1976)* 1996; 21(6): 741–9.
13. Fairbank JCT, Pynsent PB. The Oswestry Disability Index. *Spine (Phila PA 1976)* 2000; 25(22): 2940–52.
14. Fairbank JCT. Why are there different versions of the Oswestry Disability Index? *J Neurosurg Spine* 2014; 20(1): 83–6.
15. Hsieh MK, Kao FC, Chen WJ, et al. The influence of spinopelvic parameters on adjacent-segment degeneration after short spinal fusion for degenerative spondylolisthesis. *J Neurosurg Spine* 2018; 29(4): 407–13.
16. Gautschi OP, Corniola MV, Schaller K, et al. The need for an objective outcome measurement in spine surgery—The timed-up-and-go test. *Spine J* 2014; 14(10): 2521–2.
17. Enright PL. The six-minute walk test. *Respir Care* 2003; 48(8): 783–5.
18. Savino E, Martini E, Lauretani F, et al. Handgrip strength predicts persistent walking recovery after hip fracture surgery. *Am J Med* 2013; 126(12): 1068–75.e1.
19. Greenberg JK, Frumkin M, Xu Z, et al. Preoperative mobile health data improve predictions of recovery from lumbar spine surgery. *Neurosurgery* 2024; 95(3): 617–26.
20. Tang M, Leung C, Malacon K, et al. 189. SpineTrak: The first randomized controlled trial using the Apple Watch to objectively track spine surgical patients. *Spine J* 2023; 23(9): S97.
21. Choy W, Azad TD, Scheer JK, et al. Biomarkers in adult spinal deformity surgery. *Semin Spine Surg* 2023; 35(4): 101058.
22. Johnson EK, Nelson CP. Values and pitfalls of the use of administrative databases for outcomes assessment. *J Urol* 2013; 190(1): 17–18.
23. Golinvaux NS, Bohl DD, Basques BA, et al. Limitations of administrative databases in spine research: A study in obesity. *Spine J* 2014; 14(12): 2923–8.
24. Yoshihara H, Yoneoka D. Understanding the statistics and limitations of large database analyses. *Spine (Phila PA 1976)* 2014; 39(16): 1311–12.
25. Khera R, Angraal S, Couch T, et al. Adherence to methodological standards in research using the national inpatient sample. *JAMA* 2017; 318(20): 2011–18.
26. Asher AL, Haid RW, Stroink AR, et al. Research using the Quality Outcomes Database: Accomplishments and future steps toward higher-quality real-world evidence. *J Neurosurg* 2023; 139(6): 1757–75.
27. Chan AK, Eastlack RK, Fessler RG, et al. Two- and three-year outcomes of minimally invasive and hybrid correction of adult spinal deformity. *J Neurosurg Spine* 2022; 36(4): 595–608.
28. Chan AK, Shaffrey CI, Gottfried ON, et al. Cervical spondylotic myelopathy with severe axial neck pain: Is anterior or posterior approach better? *J Neurosurg Spine* 2023; 38: 42–55.
29. Yang E, Howell H, Mummaneni PV, et al. Defining cervical spondylotic myelopathy surgical endotypes using comorbidity clustering: A Quality Outcomes Database cervical spondylotic myelopathy study. *Neurosurg Focus* 2025; 59(1): E4.
30. Yang E, Mummaneni PV, Chou D, et al. What factors predict the best outcomes for older patients operated on for grade I degenerative lumbar spondylolisthesis? A machine learning analysis from the Quality Outcomes Database. *J Neurosurg Spine* 2026; 44(3): 399–410.
31. Yang E, Mummaneni PV, Chou D, et al. Cervical laminoplasty versus laminectomy and posterior cervical fusion for cervical myelopathy: Propensity-matched analysis of 24-month outcomes from the Quality Outcomes Database. *J Neurosurg Spine* 2023; 39(5): 671–81.
32. Chan AK, Shaffrey CI, Park C, et al. Do comorbid self-reported depression and anxiety influence outcomes following surgery for cervical spondylotic myelopathy? *J Neurosurg Spine* 2023; 39(1): 11–27.
33. Park C, Shaffrey CI, Than KD, et al. What factors influence surgical decision-making in anterior versus posterior surgery for cervical myelopathy? A QOD analysis. *J Neurosurg Spine* 2023; 40(2): 206–15.

34. Park C, Mummaneni PV, Gottfried ON, et al. Which supervised machine learning algorithm can best predict achievement of minimum clinically important difference in neck pain after surgery in patients with cervical myelopathy? A QOD study. *Neurosurg Focus* 2023; 54(6): E5.
35. Yang E, Mummaneni PV, Chou D, et al. Is upper extremity or lower extremity function more important for patient satisfaction? An analysis of 24-month outcomes from the QOD Cervical Spondylotic Myelopathy Cohort. *Clin Spine Surg* 2024; 37(4): 188–97.
36. Englander Z, Ambati VS, Yang E, et al. How much do patients benefit in quality of life after surgery for cervical spondylotic myelopathy? A Spine CORe™ analysis of QOD data. *Neurosurg Focus* 2026; 60(5): E2.
37. Chan AK, Bisson EF, Bydon M, et al. Obese patients benefit, but do not fare as well as nonobese patients, following lumbar spondylolisthesis surgery: An analysis of the quality outcomes database. *Neurosurgery* 2018; 86: 80–7.
38. Chan AK, Bisson EF, Bydon M, et al. Women fare best following surgery for degenerative lumbar spondylolisthesis: A comparison of the most and least satisfied patients utilizing data from the Quality Outcomes Database. *Neurosurg Focus* 2018; 44(1): E3.
39. Chan AK, Bisson EF, Bydon M, et al. A comparison of minimally invasive transforaminal lumbar interbody fusion and decompression alone for degenerative lumbar spondylolisthesis. *Neurosurg Focus* 2019; 46: E13.
40. Chan AK, Bisson EF, Bydon M, et al. Laminectomy alone versus fusion for grade 1 lumbar spondylolisthesis in 426 patients from the prospective Quality Outcomes Database. *J Neurosurg Spine* 2019; 30: 234–41.
41. Chan AK, Bisson EF, Fu KM, et al. Sexual dysfunction: Prevalence and prognosis in patients operated for degenerative lumbar spondylolisthesis. *Neurosurgery* 2019; 87: 200–10.
42. Chan AK, Bisson EF, Bydon M, et al. A comparison of minimally invasive and open transforaminal lumbar interbody fusion for grade 1 degenerative lumbar spondylolisthesis: An analysis of the prospective quality outcomes database. *Neurosurgery* 2020; 87: 555–62.
43. Chan AK, Bisson EF, Bydon M, et al. Predictors of the best outcomes following minimally invasive surgery for grade 1 degenerative lumbar spondylolisthesis. *Neurosurgery* 2020; 87: 1130–8.
44. Chan AK, Patel AB, Bisson EF, et al. "July Effect" revisited: July surgeries at residency training programs are associated with equivalent long-term clinical outcomes following lumbar spondylolisthesis surgery. *Spine (Phila PA 1976)* 2020; 46: 836–43.
45. Chan AK, Wozny TA, Bisson EF, et al. Classifying patients operated for spondylolisthesis: A K-means clustering analysis of clinical presentation phenotypes. *Neurosurgery* 2021; 89: 1033–41.
46. Chan AK, Mummaneni PV, Burke JF, et al. Does reduction of the Meyerding grade correlate with outcomes in patients undergoing decompression and fusion for grade I degenerative lumbar spondylolisthesis? *J Neurosurg Spine* 2021; 36(2): 177–84.
47. Chan AK, Letchuman V, Mummaneni PV, et al. Inferior clinical outcomes for patients with medicaid insurance after surgery for degenerative lumbar spondylolisthesis: A prospective registry analysis of 608 patients. *World Neurosurg* 2022; 164: e1024–33.
48. Chan AK, Bydon M, Bisson EF, et al. Minimally invasive versus open transforaminal lumbar interbody fusion for grade I lumbar spondylolisthesis: 5-year follow-up from the prospective multicenter Quality Outcomes Database registry. *Neurosurg Focus* 2023; 54: E2.
49. Yang E, Schonfeld E, Boyett D, et al. Does back pain catastrophizing influence 60-month surgical outcomes for patients with degenerative lumbar spondylolisthesis? A Quality Outcomes Database study. *J Neurosurg Spine* 2025; 43(5): 529–39.
50. Chan AK, Ambati VS, Upadhyayula P, et al. Five-year follow-up after minimally invasive transforaminal lumbar interbody fusion versus decompression alone for grade 1 spondylolisthesis: Are there any differences in outcomes? *J Neurosurg Spine* 2025; 43(5): 547–56.
51. Arvind V, Kim JS, Oermann EK, et al. Predicting surgical complications in adult patients undergoing anterior cervical discectomy and fusion using machine learning. *Neurospine* 2018; 15(4): 329–37.

52. Wang KY, Suresh KV, Puvanesarajah V, et al. Using predictive modeling and machine learning to identify patients appropriate for outpatient anterior cervical fusion and discectomy. *Spine (Phila PA 1976)* 2021; 46(10): 665–70.
53. Durand WM, DePasse JM, Daniels AH. Predictive modeling for blood transfusion after adult spinal deformity surgery. *Spine (Phila PA 1976)* 2018; 43(15): 1058–66.
54. Veeramani A, Zhang AS, Blackburn AZ, et al. An artificial intelligence approach to predicting unplanned intubation following anterior cervical discectomy and fusion. *Glob Spine J* 2023; 13(7): 1849–55.
55. Shahrestani S, Chan AK, Bisson EF, et al. Developing nonlinear k-nearest neighbors classification algorithms to identify patients at high risk of increased length of hospital stay following spine surgery. *Neurosurg Focus* 2023; 54(6): E7.
56. Hopkins BS, Yamaguchi JT, Garcia R, et al. Using machine learning to predict 30-day readmissions after posterior lumbar fusion: An NSQIP study involving 23,264 patients. *J Neurosurg Spine* 2020; 32(3): 399–406.
57. Karnuta JM, Golubovsky JL, Haeberle HS, et al. Can a machine learning model accurately predict patient resource utilization following lumbar spinal fusion? *Spine J* 2020; 20(3): 329–36.
58. Goyal A, Ngufor C, Kerezoudis P, et al. Can machine learning algorithms accurately predict discharge to nonhome facility and early unplanned readmissions following spinal fusion? Analysis of a national surgical registry: Presented at the 2019 AANS/CNS Section on Disorders of the Spine and Peripheral Nerves. *J Neurosurg Spine* 2019; 31(4): 568–78.
59. Berg B, Gorosito MA, Fjeld O, et al. Machine learning models for predicting disability and pain following lumbar disc herniation surgery. *JAMA Netw Open* 2024; 7(2): e2355024.
60. Medtronic. UNiD™ adaptive spine intelligence. Available from: https://www.medtronic.com/en-us/healthcare-professionals/products/spinal-orthopedic/complex-spine/fixation-systems/unid-adaptive-spine-intelligence.html (Accessed April 2026).
61. Solla F, Barrey CY, Burger E, et al. Patient-specific rods for surgical correction of sagittal imbalance in adults. *Clin Spine Surg* 2018; 32(2): 80–6.
62. Ou-Yang D, Burger EL, Kleck CJ. Pre-operative planning in complex deformities and use of patient-specific UNiD™ instrumentation. *Glob Spine J* 2022; 12(2_suppl): 40S–44S.
63. Carlsmed. Aprevo® Technology Platform. Available from: https://carlsmed.com/aprevo-technology-platform/ (Accessed April 2026).
64. Sadrameli SS, Blaskiewicz DJ, Asghar J, et al. Predictability in achieving target intervertebral lordosis using personalized interbody implants. *Int J Spine Surg* 2024; 18(S1): S16–23.
65. Rajpurkar P, Chen E, Banerjee O, Topol EJ. AI in health and medicine. *Nat Med* 2022; 28(1): 31–8.
66. Gologorsky Y, Knightly JJ, Chi JH, Groff MW. The Nationwide Inpatient Sample database does not accurately reflect surgical indications for fusion: Clinical article. *J Neurosurg Spine* 2014; 21(6): 984–93.
67. Huang K, Altosaar J, Ranganath R. Clinical BERT: Modeling clinical notes and predicting hospital readmission. Available from: http://arxiv.org/abs/1904.05342 (Accessed April 2026).
68. Yang X, Chen A, PourNejatian N, et al. A large language model for electronic health records. *NPJ Digit Med* 2022; 5(1): 194.
69. Jiang LY, Liu XC, Nejatian NP, et al. Health system-scale language models are all-purpose prediction engines. *Nature* 2023; 619(7969): 357–62.
70. Scheer JK, Osorio JA, Smith JS, et al. Development of validated computer-based preoperative predictive model for proximal junction failure (PJF) or clinically significant PJK with 86% accuracy based on 510 ASD patients with 2-year follow-up. *Spine (Phila PA 1976)* 2016; 41(22): E1328–35.
71. Scheer JK, Smith JS, Schwab F, et al. Development of a preoperative predictive model for major complications following adult spinal deformity surgery. *J Neurosurg Spine* 2017; 26(6): 736–43.

72. Chan AK, Shahrestani S, Ballatori AM, et al. Is the Centers for Medicare & Medicaid Services hierarchical condition category risk adjustment model satisfactory for quantifying risk after spine surgery? *Neurosurgery* 2022; 91(1): 123–31.
73. Shahrestani S, Reardon T, Brown NJ, et al. Developing mixed-effects models to compare the predictive ability of various comorbidity indices in a contemporary cohort of patients undergoing lumbar fusion. *Neurosurgery* 2024; 94(4): 711–20.
74. Oh T, Scheer JK, Smith JS, et al. Potential of predictive computer models for preoperative patient selection to enhance overall quality-adjusted life years gained at 2-year follow-up: A simulation in 234 patients with adult spinal deformity. *Neurosurg Focus* 2017; 43(6): E2.
75. Scheer JK, Osorio JA, Smith JS, et al. Development of a preoperative predictive model for reaching the Oswestry Disability Index minimal clinically important difference for adult spinal deformity patients. *Spine Deform* 2018; 6(5): 593–9.
76. Ames CP, Smith JS, Pellisé F, et al. Development of deployable predictive models for minimal clinically important difference achievement across the commonly used health-related quality of life instruments in adult spinal deformity surgery. *Spine (Phila PA 1976)* 2019; 44(16): 1144–53.
77. Merali ZG, Witiw CD, Badhiwala JH, et al. Using a machine learning approach to predict outcome after surgery for degenerative cervical myelopathy. *PLoS ONE* 2019; 14(4): e0215133.
78. Khan O, Badhiwala JH, Akbar MA, Fehlings MG. Prediction of worse functional status after surgery for degenerative cervical myelopathy: A machine learning approach. *Neurosurgery* 2020; 88(3): 584–91.
79. Mummaneni PV, Bydon M, Alvi MA, et al. Predictive model for long-term patient satisfaction after surgery for grade I degenerative lumbar spondylolisthesis: Insights from the Quality Outcomes Database. *Neurosurg Focus* 2019; 46(5): E12.

4

Outcome Prediction in Brain Surgery

JULIAN L. GENDREAU, BIBHAS AMATYA, RITVIK PULYA, KRITIKA GOWDA, MELANIE HOROWITZ AND DEBRAJ MUKHERJEE

INTRODUCTION

The use of machine learning (ML) for outcome prediction in brain surgery is a growing field of clinical interest. In the most general sense, outcome prediction benefits the healthcare system on many levels, aiding in perioperative clinical decision-making and long-term precision patient prognostication and assisting in making the delivery of patient care easier.[1] While there has been significant development in this field over the past 20 years, outcome prediction in brain surgery generally incorporates quantitative clinical data along with imaging to create models for the purpose of predicting patient outcomes.

In particular, the most predicted outcomes include overall survival, progression-free survival and perioperative outcomes such as 30-day readmission and nonroutine discharges.[2] Some common models are composed of logistic regression (LR), support vector machines (SVMs), random forest (RF) models and convolutional neural networks[3] with different models having higher accuracies for different types of input data.

This chapter summarizes key advancements and examples of ML algorithms used for outcome prediction in brain surgery.

GLIOMA

Novel ML algorithms are showing promise to predict patient survival using individualized clinical variables. These models are often deployed as online and public-accessible calculators that allow for easy clinician access. Senders et al. retrospectively reviewed the Surveillance Epidemiology and End Results (SEER) database for all patients treated for glioblastoma (range of C-indexes for survival models 0.66–0.70).[4] They found that an accelerated failure time model was superior at predicting survival outcomes when compared to traditional statistical methods. The authors made the algorithm available to the public as a web-based survival calculator, which can be used by anyone to obtain individualized survival predictions based on individualized clinical data. Other online web-based ML models have also been created for predicting perioperative outcomes such as extended length of stay, nonroutine discharges and high hospital costs (range of c-indexes for referenced models 0.68–0.82).[5–8]

In addition to using clinical data variables for glioma outcome prediction, MRI and other methods of advanced imaging play an essential role in attempting to predict early recurrences in glioma. Notably, Kim et al. investigated the peritumoral non-enhancing region (NER), after noticing its frequent incomplete removal during surgical resection.[9] They found an association with the imaging features of the NER with disease recurrence. After examining 83 consecutive glioblastoma patients, they utilized contrast-enhanced T1-weighted images, fluid-attenuated inversion recovery (FLAIR) images, fractional anisotropy (FA), and normalized cerebral blood volume (CBV) maps to extract radiomic features.[9] They found that both FA and CBV radiomics in the NER can predict 6-month progression and overall survival (c-index 0.79).[9]

DOI: 10.1201/9781003471165-4

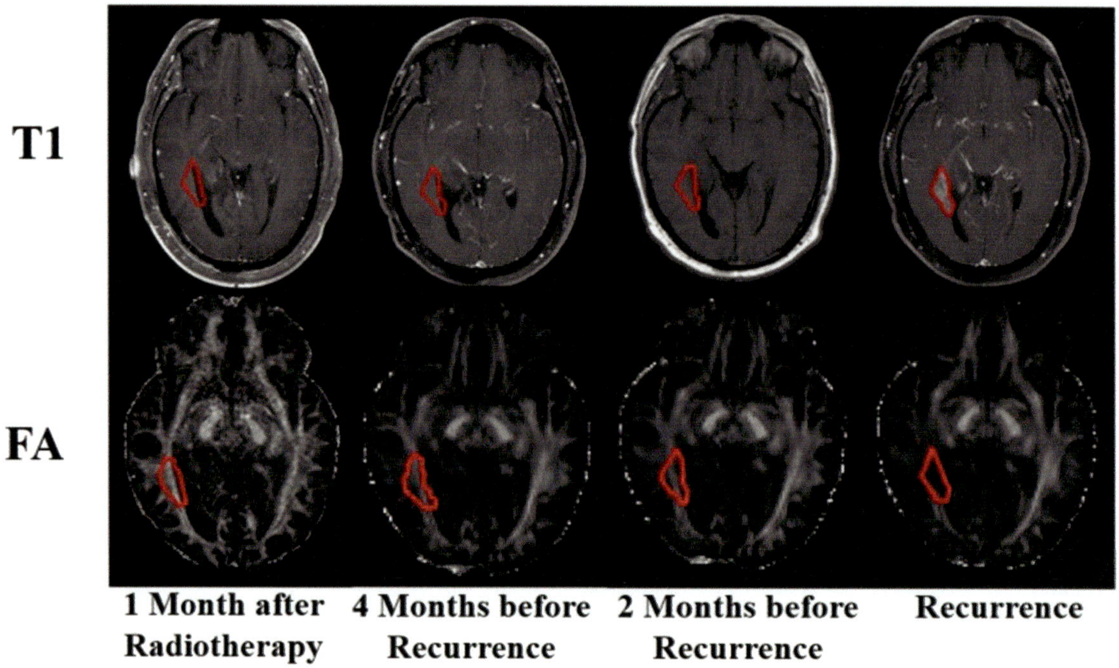

Figure 4.1 Serial T1 and fractional anisotropy images of a representative patient. Red outlines indicate the location of the recurrent tumor. (This figure is adapted and unaltered from Jin et al.[10])

An additional study by Jin et al. found that the FA and Neurite Density Index (NDI) may be reduced 2 months before glioblastoma recurrence and can serve as a non-contrast MR-based biomarker (**Figure 4.1**).[10]

Furthermore, supplementing imaging modalities with clinical features can have an additional predictive value compared to clinical features alone. Mazurowski et al. investigated the effectiveness of combining MRI features with clinical parameters to predict 1-year survival in patients with glioblastoma. They found that adding tumor functional grade, necrosis grade, edema grade and enhancement grade led to an increase in model accuracy (C-index 0.69 vs 0.58).[11] Many of these prognostication models that incorporate both imaging and clinical variables are almost ready for translation, however, they are limited in generalizability. Most models use one institutional dataset for training, and future models should incorporate multicenter data from many different geographic locations. Additionally, C-indexes should be optimized in future models that have larger datasets and include more input variables.

Other notable studies using imaging and ML for glioblastoma prognostication can be found in **Table 4.1**.[12–16]

Other ML developments include the ability to predict successful glioblastoma resectability from preoperative imaging[17] and the ability to differentiate glioblastoma from primary central nervous system (CNS) lymphoma with the use of neural network models.[18] Ritschel et al. developed an ML model that utilizes contrast-enhanced ultrasound (US) to accurately detect glioblastoma resection margins.[19] Many programs are also available for tumor segmentation and to detect changes in size of the tumor over time.[20] Nasrallah et al. developed a Cryosection Histopathology Assessment and Review Machine (CHARM) that has the ability to distinguish IDH-mutant tumors from wild-type tumors with an area under the curve (AUC) rating of 0.79.[21] This system utilizes frozen section specimens from the operating room. They can additionally identify malignant cells with an AUC of 0.98.[21] Furthermore, Vermeulen et al. developed an intraoperative rapid nanopore sequencer for histologic analysis of all CNS tumors including glioma. It can assess methylation profiles and provide an accurate diagnosis in 40 minutes.[22]

Table 4.1 Characteristics of machine learning studies using advanced imaging techniques in brain surgery

Author	Types of imaging	Features	Accuracy
Kim et al.[9]	MRI	FA, CBV, Clinical variables	0.87
Jin et al.[10]	DTI, T1 MRI	FA, NDI	–
Mazurowski et al.[11]	MRI	Major axis length, minor axis length, tumor location, side of lesion center, eloquent brain, enhancement quality, proportion enhancing, proportion necrosis, cysts, multifocal or multicentric, T1/FLAIR ratio, thickness of enhancing margin, definition of the enhancing margin, definition of the nonenhancing margin, proportion of edema, edema crosses midline, hemorrhage, diffusion characteristics, pial invasion, ependymal invasion, cortical involvement, deep white matter invasion, tumor crosses midline, enhancing tumor crosses midline, satellites, and calvarial remodeling	0.69
Stadlbauer et al.[12]	Axial FLAIR, MRI T1 with contrast, DWI, GESE-DSC, qBOLD	Oxygen metabolism, tissue hypoxia, neovascularization and microvascular architecture	0.879
Zhou et al.[13]	T1 MRI contrast enhanced, T2-FLAIR sequences	Histogram, shape and texture features	0.92
Choi et al.[14]	T2 MRI, FLAIR MRI, T1 MRI with contrast	71 Radiomic features	0.71
Wijethilake et al.[15]	MRI FLAIR, MRI T1 with contrast	Radiomic features and genomic data	Accuracy: 91.6%
Macyszyn et al.[16]	T1 MRI, T1 MRI with contrast, T2 MRI, T2 FLAIR MRI, DTI, DSC-MRI, GRE-EPI	FA, radial diffusivity, axial diffusivity, trace, rCBV, peak height, percentage signal recovery, other radiomic features from segmentation	0.84 for > 18 months

CBV: Cerebral Blood Volume; DSC: Dynamic Susceptibility Contrast; DTI: Diffusion Tensor Imaging; DWI: Diffusion-Weighted Imaging; EPI: Echo-Planar Imaging; FA: Fractional Anisotropy; FLAIR: Fluid Attenuated Inversion Recovery; GESE: Gradient Echo-Spin Echo; GRE: Gradient Echo Imaging; MRI: Magnetic Resonance Imaging; NDI: Neuron Density Index; rCBV: relative Cerebral Blood Volume; qBOLD: Blood Oxygenation Level Dependent.

MENINGIOMA

Tumor grade prediction

One study has provided evidence that artificial neural networks (ANNs) can be used to accurately predict the tumor grade of meningiomas.[23] Khayat Kashani et al. aimed to predict meningioma tumor grade by utilizing an ANN with preoperative blood markers, tumor location and demographic characteristics as inputs. They found that higher levels of monocytes and neutrophil counts were associated with higher grade of meningioma. Through the utilization of this ANN model, the authors were able to achieve an 83% accuracy in predicting tumor grade overall.[23]

In addition to cell counts, Moreau et al. developed and validated models that can predict survival

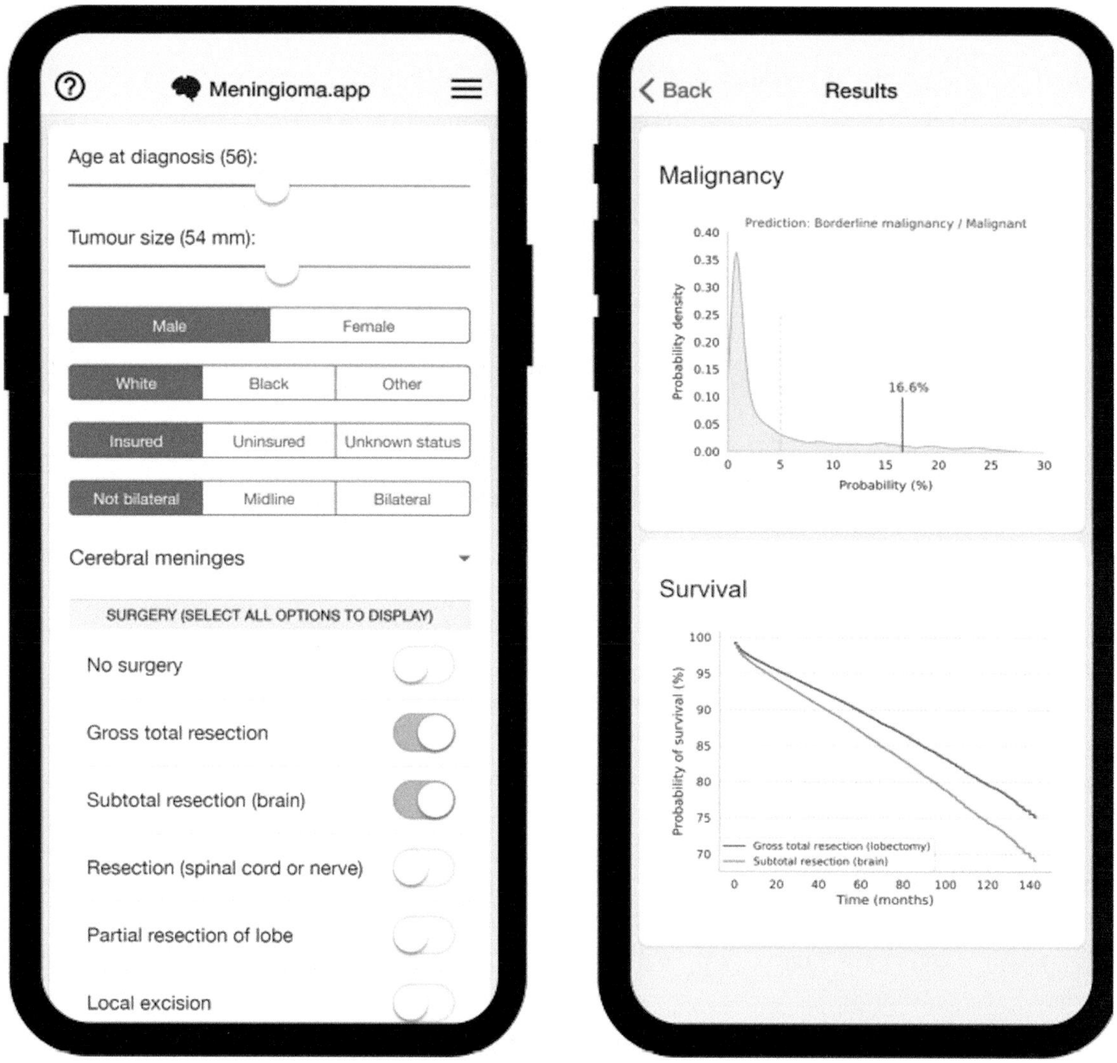

Figure 4.2 Example of predicted malignancy and survival curves for an insured 56-year-old White man with a unilateral 54mm wide meningioma localizing to the cerebral meninges. (This figure is adapted and unaltered from Moreau et al.[24])

of meningioma cases using clinical variables such as tumor size, location and surgical procedure. The model was incorporated into a user-friendly mobile application called Meningioma.app, offering individual-specific predictions for clinical outcomes (**Figure 4.2**).[24]

Several other web applications are available for predicting outcomes after meningioma surgery such as predicting the likelihood of extended length of stay, nonroutine discharge disposition, 90-day hospital readmission and local recurrence.[25–28]

PITUITARY ADENOMA

A study by Hollon et al. found that an LR model with elastic net regularization best predicted post-surgical outcomes in patients undergoing pituitary adenoma surgery.[29] It is able to predict outcomes such as the likelihood of having diabetes insipidus with an accuracy of 87%.[29] They found the most important predictive variables in this patient sample were age, body mass index (BMI), sodium abnormalities and Cushing's disease.[30] They found that this algorithm was much more accurate than imaging scoring systems that have traditionally been used to predict outcomes after surgery. Additionally, McKevitt et al. developed a k-nearest neighbor (KNN) model that was able to predict remission of functional pituitary disease after surgery with an accuracy of 75.6%.[30]

BRAIN METASTASES

Hulsbergen et al. developed an LR ML model that was able to predict 6-month survival after resection of brain metastases with an AUC of 0.71.[31] Additionally, several studies have evaluated ML algorithms for detecting treatment response and local failure in patients with brain metastases undergoing radiosurgery. A systematic review of these studies performed by Habibi et al. in 2024 found a total of 17 studies assessing ML algorithms of patients undergoing stereotactic radiosurgery for brain metastases.[32] They found a pooled estimate of 0.93 (95% CI: 0.76–0.98) for sensitivity of detecting local failure.[32]

VESTIBULAR SCHWANNOMA

For patients undergoing vestibular schwannoma surgery, cranial nerve injury can be a significant complication. Heman-Ackah et al. developed an ML model for predicting facial nerve injury from a retrospective review of multiple centers with an accuracy of 84% when validated in a smaller prospective dataset.[33] The most common contributing predictors in this model were age, BMI, case length and tumor dimension. Additionally, Cha et al. were able to develop a deep neural network (DNN) model that had an accuracy of 90% when predicting hearing preservation after vestibular schwannoma surgery.[34]

CHORDOMA

Patients with chordoma often undergo surgical resection and suffer from highly recurrent disease postoperatively making prognostication difficult in this patient population. Peng et al. used ML algorithms to account for the nonlinear relationships in chordoma patient data.[35] Using the SEER database to gather chordoma data, this research team developed three ML models, DeepSurv, neural multitask logistic model (NMLTR), and random survival forest (RSF), and compared them to the CoxPH model.[35] The results indicated that the ML DNN model (DeepSurv) significantly outperformed the CoxPH model in predicting survival with the final DeepSurv model having a 10-year AUC of 0.88.[35]

EPILEPSY SURGERY

Surgery can sometimes offer benefit in patients with refractory epilepsy. An important related aim is identifying *a priori* which patients might benefit most from surgery. A study by the Montreal Neurological Institute found that ML could differentiate between mesiotemporal structures in a way that was not previously possible by global measurements.[36] They were then able to classify patients into four types of hippocampal atrophy including bilateral asymmetric atrophy (temporal lobe epilepsy [TLE]-I), ipsilateral mesiotemporal atrophy (TLE-II), bilateral symmetric atrophy in all structures (TLE-III) or increased hippocampal volume (TLE-IV).[36] Through a class-wise analysis, they found that TLE-II patients had the highest seizure-free rates after a successful surgery.[36]

ARTERIOVENOUS MALFORMATION

The Department of Radiology at Beaumont Hospital conducted a study to identify factors influencing cerebral arteriovenous malformation (AVM) outcomes treated with endovascular embolization, one of the more popular forms of treating this disease.[37] Through this study, they were also able to compare ML techniques to conventional statistical analyses in predicting successful embolization rates.[37]

In this study, most patients treated for brain AVMs were treated at the time of intracranial hemorrhage, with a spontaneous hemorrhage or procedural-related hemorrhage occurring in the follow-up period.[37] Many complications were found in these patients, such as ischemic stroke and symptomatic hemorrhage, and they found that ML was able to show superior accuracy (97.5%) in predicting these outcomes when compared to traditional statistics.[37] The ML model identified the absence of nidal fistulae as the most critical predictor factor for predicting mortality in AVM.[37]

Of course, endovascular embolization is not the only way AVMs are treated, as radiosurgery is also commonly used.[38] While scoring systems are already used to predict a patient's outcome after

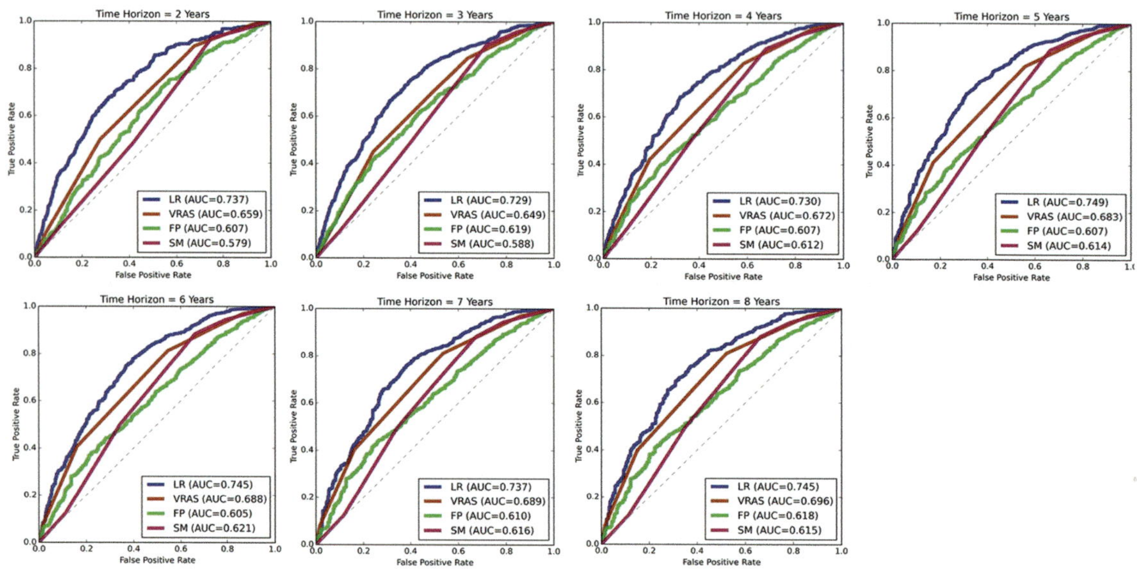

Figure 4.3 Receiver operator curves for four predictive models of arteriovenous malformation outcomes after radiosurgery at all assessed follow-up time points on the testing. (This figure is adapted and unaltered from Oermann et al.[38])

AVM radiosurgery, several limitations are presented that warrant exploring alternative approaches.[38] The Icahn School of Medicine at Mount Sinai hoped to address this issue. They explored ML as a possible approach to predicting individual patient outcomes after AVM radiosurgery while assessing the predictive capability of already existing grading systems.[38] The study used a large multicenter dataset of AVM patients explicitly treated with radiosurgery (1810 patients), and an ML-based prognostic model was applied to identify the potential predictive factors and construct models for an outcome prediction. Their developed predictive model, utilizing LR, had an AUC of 0.74 across all time-thresholds (**Figure 4.3**).[38]

FUNCTIONAL NEUROSURGERY

There are few studies that investigate the use of ML in functional neurosurgery outcomes. Valsky et al. have developed an ML algorithm that identifies when a deep brain stimulation lead is improperly placed in the subthalamic nucleus when treating patients with Parkinson's disease.[39] Additionally, Kostoglou et al. devised a system that can predict postoperative motor improvement in Parkinson's disease after deep brain stimulation of the subthalamic nucleus.[40]

TRAUMATIC BRAIN INJURY

Subdural, epidural and intraparenchymal hemorrhage

A recent systematic review by Courville et al. found that ML models have been employed for prediction of mortality, hypotension and functional outcomes in patients with traumatic brain injury (TBI).[41] They found that the most common algorithms used in ML for TBI patients include SVM, ANNs, RF models and Naïve Bayes models. Patients who had lower Glasgow Coma Scale (GCS) upon admission, were older in age and had abnormal glucose levels were more likely to have worse outcomes following TBI.[41] In patients with epidural hematoma, Karabacak et al. describe an ML model that predicted in-hospital mortality, non-home discharges, prolonged length of stay and major complications.[42] With respect to predicting intraparenchymal hemorrhage progression, Mao et al. developed a least absolute shrinkage and selection operator (LASSO) regression model that can predict in-hospital mortality inclusive of patients undergoing surgical intervention.[43] The external validation of this calculator had an AUC of 0.91.[43] In subdural hematoma patients, Fuse et al. describe an SVM model that demonstrates an accuracy of 92% in predicting unfavorable outcomes after burr hole evacuation.[44]

SURGICAL PLANNING AND SKILLS

Many other studies investigate the use of ML to assist surgeons in the operating room. Dundar et al. utilized an ML algorithm and structural cranial model to detect optimal incision points and trajectories for tumor resection.[45] Han et al. began testing a novel ML neuronavigation system that intraoperatively updates patient imaging as tumor is debulked, which would traditionally cause inaccurate displacement of imaging during surgery due to brain shift.[46] Hu et al. discovered ML algorithms that allow for removal of tumor residual by robotic ablation after the larger portion of the tumor is removed.[47] Additionally, Marcus et al. proposes algorithms to find the optimal trajectories for brain biopsies with computer assistance.[48] Furthermore, Fazlollahi et al. describe using artificial intelligence (AI) to teach medical students surgical skills and directly compare this type of feedback to expert instruction alone. They found that AI resulted in superior learning via a randomized controlled trial.[49]

LARGE LANGUAGE MODELS

In 2024, AtlasGPT was launched, which was the first LLM for the neurosurgical literature. Partnered with the Journal of Neurosurgery Publishing Group, AtlasGPT allows neurosurgeons to access a comprehensive database of peer-reviewed articles and research findings for assisting in clinical decision support related to brain surgery.[50]

Clinical integration: Incorporating machine learning models into patient care

For providers considering whether to incorporate the use of ML models into patient care, there are several attributes of a model to consider. First, models should ideally be trained on a large amount of accurate patient data. They should also be trained on data generalizable to the population being treated. Therefore, providers in the United States should look to incorporate a model that has accurate training data from multiple different sites in the United States so the outcome can be generalizable. Second, the model should have a selected algorithm where the data analyst has tested multiple different algorithm types to deliver a high rate of prediction accuracy. Third, the model should have a high predictive accuracy typically described as a C-index or C-statistic. This is also known as an area under the curve (AUC) in some studies.[51] A C-statistic of 0.5 typically indicates a level of accuracy consistent with random occurrence, while a c-statistic of 1.0 indicates a model is truly perfect at predicting an outcome.[51] Typically, a model with a C-statistic of >0.70 is considered decent while a model with a C-statistic >0.90 is considered excellent.[51] Models that have adequate training data, models that have generalizable data and models that have high C-statistic values could be considered for translation into patient care practices. Of all the current models discussed in this chapter, the model provided by Senders et al. provides an excellent tool to predict survival outcomes in glioblastoma patients while utilizing an easy-to-use online user interface available to providers.[4]

Food and Drug Administration-approved models

It is important to note, however, that there are currently no Food and Drug Administration (FDA)-approved algorithms for predicting outcomes in brain tumor patients using ML. Therefore, physicians should use caution when integrating these predictive algorithms into clinical practice. There are FDA-approved models to assist with automatic detection and segmentation of tumors using ML. These algorithms, however, are not designed to replace a physician, but they are designed to assist in the process of treatment. A model by VBrain (Vysioneer Inc., Cambridge, MA, USA) uses deep learning to assist in brain tumor contouring for stereotactic radiosurgery.[52] Cirrus Brain Mapping Software (Sora Neuroscience, Minneapolis, MN, USA) uses AI-based software to rapidly map essential brain functions using resting state-fMRI, making surgical resection near eloquent areas easier for neurosurgeons.[53] In the future, algorithms for predicting outcomes after brain tumor surgery will ideally be developed and approved by the FDA for use by clinicians.

CONCLUSION

As ML becomes an emerging field in all industries including the field of medicine, it is actively being incorporated into some clinical practices. There is current evidence that it can offer unparalleled precision in predicting patient outcomes at an accuracy superior to traditional statistics. Future advancements include fine tuning models to continuously improve accuracy while also testing generalizability in an effort to make models useful across a wide range of patient populations within cranial neurosurgery. Ultimately, we will need models that obtain FDA approval before widespread adoption of ML models that predict outcomes in brain tumor patients.

REFERENCES

1. Harris AHS. Path from predictive analytics to improved patient outcomes. *Ann Surg* 2017; 265(3): 461–3.
2. Levine N, DeMonte F. Functional outcome in the neurosurgical patient and its impact on quality of life. *Skull Base* 2010; 20(01): 19–22.
3. Tewarie IA, Senders JT, Kremer S, et al. Survival prediction of glioblastoma patients—Are we there yet? A systematic review of prognostic modeling for glioblastoma and its clinical potential. *Neurosurg Rev* 2021; 44(4): 2047–57.
4. Senders JT, Staples P, Mehrtash A, et al. An online calculator for the prediction of survival in glioblastoma patients using classical statistics and machine learning. *Neurosurgery* 2020; 86(2): 184–92.
5. Du P, Yang X, Shen L, et al. Nomogram model for predicting the prognosis of high-grade glioma in adults receiving standard treatment: A retrospective cohort study. *J Clin Med* 2022; 12(1): 196.
6. Wei R, Zhao C, Li J, et al. Online calculator to predict early mortality in patient with surgically treated recurrent lower-grade glioma. *BMC Cancer* 2022; 22(1): 114.
7. Huq S, Khalafallah AM, Patel P, et al. Predictive model and online calculator for discharge disposition in brain tumor patients. *World Neurosurg* 2021; 146: 786–98.
8. Nair SK, Chakravarti S, Jimenez AE, et al. Novel predictive models for high-value care outcomes following glioblastoma resection. *World Neurosurg* 2022; 161: 572–9.
9. Kim JY, Yoon MJ, Park JE, et al. Radiomics in peritumoral non-enhancing regions: Fractional anisotropy and cerebral blood volume improve prediction of local progression and overall survival in patients with glioblastoma. *Neuroradiology* 2019; 61(11): 1261–72.
10. Jin Y, Randall JW, Elhalawani H, et al. Detection of glioblastoma subclinical recurrence using serial diffusion tensor imaging. *Cancers* 2020; 12(3): 568.
11. Mazurowski MA, Desjardins A, Malof JM. Imaging descriptors improve the predictive power of survival models for glioblastoma patients. *Neuro Oncol* 2013; 15(10): 1389–94.
12. Stadlbauer A, Nikolic K, Oberndorfer S, et al. Machine learning-based prediction of glioma *IDH* gene mutation status using physio-metabolic MRI of oxygen metabolism and neovascularization (a bicenter study). *Cancers (Basel)* 2024; 16(6): 1102.
13. Zhou H, Chang K, Bai HX, et al. Machine learning reveals multimodal MRI patterns predictive of isocitrate dehydrogenase and 1p/19q status in diffuse low- and high-grade gliomas. *J Neurooncol* 2019; 142: 299–307.
14. Choi YS, Ahn SS, Chang JH, et al. Machine learning and radiomic phenotyping of lower grade gliomas: Improving survival prediction. *Eur Radiol* 2020; 30: 3834–42.
15. Wijethilake N, Islam M, Ren H. Radiogenomics model for overall survival prediction of glioblastoma. *Med Biol Eng Comput* 2020; 58: 1767–77.
16. Macyszyn L, Akbari H, Pisapia JM, et al. Imaging patterns predict patient survival and molecular subtype in glioblastoma via machine learning techniques. *Neuro Oncol* 2016; 18: 417–25.
17. Marcus AP, Marcus HJ, Camp SJ, et al. Improved prediction of surgical resectability in patients with glioblastoma using an artificial neural network. *Sci Rep* 2020; 10: 1–9.
18. McAvoy M, Prieto PC, Kaczmarzyk JR, et al. Classification of glioblastoma versus primary central nervous system lymphoma using convolutional neural networks. *Sci Rep* 2021; 11: 15219.

19. Ritschel K, Pechlivanis I, Winter S. Brain tumor classification on intraoperative contrast-enhanced ultrasound. *Int J Comput Assist Radiol Surg* 2015; 10: 531–40.
20. Tustison NJ, Shrinidhi KL, Wintermark M, et al. Optimal symmetric multimodal templates and concatenated random forests for supervised brain tumor segmentation (simplified) with ANTsR. *Neuroinformatics* 2015; 13: 209–25.
21. Nasrallah MP, Zhao J, Tsai CC, et al. Machine learning for cryosection pathology predicts the 2021 WHO classification of glioma. *Med* 2023; 4(8): 526–40.
22. Vermeulen C, Pagès-Gallego M, Kester L, et al. Ultra-fast deep-learned CNS tumour classification during surgery. *Nature* 2023; 622(7984): 842–9.
23. Khayat Kashani HR, Azhari S, Nayebaghayee H, et al. Prediction value of preoperative findings on meningioma grading using artificial neural network. *Clin Neurol Neurosurg* 2020; 196: 105947.
24. Moreau JT, Hankinson TC, Baillet S, et al. Individual-patient prediction of meningioma malignancy and survival using the Surveillance, Epidemiology, and End Results database. *NPJ Digit Med* 2020; 3: 12.
25. Cai L, Yang Z, Song D, et al. Nomogram model for predicting the overall survival of patients with meningiomas: A retrospective cohort study. *World Neurosurg* 2023; 171: 309–22.
26. Jimenez AE, Chakravarti S, Liu S, et al. predicting high-value care outcomes after surgery for non-skull base meningiomas. *World Neurosurg* 2022; 159: 130–8.
27. Wang Y, Wang X, Yu T, et al. Epidemiology and survival of patients with spinal meningiomas: A large retrospective cohort study. *Int J Surg* 2024; 110(2): 921–33.
28. Gennatas ED, Wu A, Braunstein SE, et al. Preoperative and postoperative prediction of long-term meningioma outcomes. *PLoS One* 2018; 13(9): 0204161.
29. Hollon TC, Parikh A, Pandian B, et al. A machine learning approach to predict early outcomes after pituitary adenoma surgery. *Neurosurg Focus* 2018; 45(5): E8.
30. McKevitt C, Gabriel E, Marenco-Hillembrand L, et al. Supervised machine learning to validate a novel scoring system for the prediction of disease remission of functional pituitary adenomas following transsphenoidal surgery. *Sci Rep* 2023; 13(1): 15409.
31. Hulsbergen AFC, Lo YT, Awakimjan I, et al. survival prediction after neurosurgical resection of brain metastases: A machine learning approach. *Neurosurgery* 2022; 91(3): 381–8.
32. Habibi MA, Rashidi F, Habibzadeh A, et al. Prediction of the treatment response and local failure of patients with brain metastasis treated with stereotactic radiosurgery using machine learning: A systematic review and meta-analysis. *Neurosurg Rev* 2024; 47(1): 199.
33. Heman-Ackah SM, Blue R, Quimby AE, et al. A multi-institutional machine learning algorithm for prognosticating facial nerve injury following microsurgical resection of vestibular schwannoma. *Sci Rep* 2024; 14(1): 12963.
34. Cha D, Shin SH, Kim SH, et al. Machine learning approach for prediction of hearing preservation in vestibular schwannoma surgery. *Sci Rep* 2020; 10(1): 7136.
35. Peng C, Xie X, Knoedler S, et al. Predicting overall survival in chordoma patients using machine learning models: A web-app application. *J Orthop Surg Res* 2023; 18(1): 652.
36. Munsell BC, Wee CY, Keller SS, et al. Evaluation of machine learning algorithms for treatment outcome prediction in patients with epilepsy based on structural connectome data. *Neuroimage* 2015; 118: 219–30.
37. Asadi H, Kok HK, Looby S, et al. Outcomes and complications after endovascular treatment of brain arteriovenous malformations: A prognostication attempt using artificial intelligence. *World Neurosurg* 2016; 96: 562–9.
38. Oermann EK, Rubinsteyn A, Ding D, et al. Using a machine learning approach to predict outcomes after radiosurgery for cerebral arteriovenous malformations. *Sci Rep* 2016; 6(1): 21161.
39. Valsky D, Marmor-Levin O, Deffains M, et al. Stop! Border ahead: Automatic detection of subthalamic exit during deep brain stimulation surgery. *Mov Disord* 2017; 32: 70–9.

40. Kostoglou K, Michmizos KP, Stathis P, et al. Classification and prediction of clinical improvement in deep brain stimulation from intraoperative microelectrode recordings. *IEEE Trans Biomed Eng* 2017; 64(5): 1123–30.
41. Courville E, Kazim SF, Vellek J, et al. Machine learning algorithms for predicting outcomes of traumatic brain injury: A systematic review and meta-analysis. *Surg Neurol Int* 2023; 14: 262.
42. Karabacak M, Margetis K. Prognosis at your fingertips: A machine learning-based web application for outcome prediction in acute traumatic epidural hematoma. *J Neurotrauma* 2024; 41(1–2): 147–60.
43. Mao B, Ling L, Pan Y, et al. Machine learning for the prediction of in-hospital mortality in patients with spontaneous intracerebral hemorrhage in intensive care unit. *Sci Rep* 2024; 14(1): 14195.
44. Fuse Y, Nagashima Y, Nishiwaki H, et al. Development of machine learning models for predicting unfavorable functional outcomes from preoperative data in patients with chronic subdural hematomas. *Sci Rep* 2023; 13(1): 16997.
45. Dundar TT, Yurtsever I, Pehlivanoglu MK, et al. Machine learning-based surgical planning for neurosurgery: Artificial intelligent approaches to the cranium. *Front Surg* 2022; 9: 863633.
46. Han R, Jones CK, Lee J, et al. Deformable MR-CT image registration using an unsupervised, dual-channel network for neurosurgical guidance. *Med Image Anal* 2022; 75: 102292.
47. Hu D, Gong Y, Hannaford B, et al. Path planning for semi-automated simulated robotic neurosurgery. *Rep US* 2015; 2015: 2639–45.
48. Marcus HJ, Vakharia VN, Sparks R, et al. Computer-assisted versus manual planning for stereotactic brain biopsy: A retrospective comparative pilot study. *Oper Neurosurg* 2020; 18: 417–22.
49. Fazlollahi AM, Bakhaidar M, Alsayegh A, et al. Effect of artificial intelligence tutoring vs expert instruction on learning simulated surgical skills among medical students: A randomized clinical trial. *JAMA Netw Open* 2022; 5(2): 2149008.
50. Hopkins B, Carter B, Lord J. AtlasGPT: Dawn of a new era in neurosurgery for intelligent care augmentation, operative planning and performance. *J Neurosurg* 2024; 140(5): 1211–14.
51. Pencina MJ, D'Agostino RB Sr. Evaluating discrimination of risk prediction models: The C statistic. *JAMA* 2015; 314(10): 1063–4.
52. Wang JY, Qu V, Hui C, et al. Stratified assessment of an FDA-cleared deep learning algorithm for automated detection and contouring of metastatic brain tumors in stereotactic radiosurgery. *Radiat Oncol* 2023; 18(1): 61.
53. WashU Medicine. Neurosurgery News. AI-based brain-mapping software receives FDA market authorization, 2025. Available from: https://neurosurgery.wustl.edu/ai-based-brain-mapping-software-receives-fda-market-authorization// (Accessed April 2026).

5

Outcome Prediction in Neurosurgery: Liquid Biopsy and the Role of Machine Learning

ATHARV OAK, CHETAN BETTEGOWDA AND CHRISTOPHER DOUVILLE

OVERVIEW OF LIQUID BIOPSY

Traditional approaches for detecting and monitoring disease often involve the use of invasive biopsies to sample the affected organ. Liquid biopsy is a safer and less invasive diagnostic approach that analyzes bodily fluids such as blood, cerebrospinal fluid (CSF), urine and saliva, to obtain information regarding disease states.

The concept of liquid biopsy is based on the principle that diseased tissues release various molecules, including deoxyribonucleic acid (DNA), ribonucleic acid (RNA), proteins and extracellular vesicles into the bloodstream or other bodily fluids. These circulating biomarkers provide information about genetic alterations and biochemical changes associated with the underlying disease. Biomarkers can be analyzed to detect, characterize and monitor progression of various diseases.

The most studied biomarkers in liquid biopsy include the following.

Cell-free DNA

Apoptotic and necrotic cells can release DNA fragments into bodily fluids, which is referred to as cell-free (cf) DNA. cfDNA represents a mixture of DNA from normal and diseased tissues, providing information about both physiologic and pathologic disease processes.

Blood is the most used bodily fluid. Centrifugation separates plasma from the cellular component, after which, another centrifugation step removes all cellular debris. Other bodily fluids are similarly pre-processed to remove cellular components.

Various kits can be used to extract cfDNA, which involve some combination of silica-based size-exclusion columns, magnetic bead-based DNA purification, or DNA extraction using organic solvent preparations. Fragments typically 50–200 bp are obtained. Sequencing libraries are prepared using this DNA in the standard fashion, with end repair, adapter ligation, polymerase chain reaction (PCR) amplification and then DNA purification from the PCR reaction. These libraries are sequenced using next-generation sequencing (NGS) approaches. The NGS DNA reads (often tens of millions) can be analyzed to identify genetic aberrations such as mutations, copy number variations and other DNA base-level changes such as methylation which are commonly associated with cancer.[1] More recently, short interspersed nuclear elements have also been used to distinguish cancerous from noncancerous cell signatures in liquid biopsy.[2]

DOI: 10.1201/9781003471165-5

MicroRNAs (miRNAs)

MicroRNAs are small non-coding RNA molecules involved in post-transcriptional regulation of gene expression. miRNA dysregulation is implicated in several disease states such as nervous system disorders (Alzheimer's, epilepsy, Parkinson's), cancers and cardiovascular disease.[3]

Cell-free miRNA preparation is done with bodily fluid preparation like that of cfDNA isolation. RNA extraction is often performed with commercial kits that use organic solvents or silica-based size-exclusion methods, with removal of potential contaminants that could interfere with downstream RNA processing (proteins, salts, etc.). RNA is quantified and quality is assessed, followed by library preparation with adapter ligation, followed by reverse transcription which generates cDNA libraries. The rest of the library preparation is like that of cfDNA.

Proteins and metabolites

In addition to nucleic acids, proteins and metabolites present in bodily fluids can also serve as biomarkers for disease states. Proteomic and metabolomic analyses of bodily fluids can reveal disease-specific protein mutations and expression variants, metabolic changes and dysregulated signaling pathways.[4]

Initial pre-processing of samples is similar to that mentioned above.

For proteins, high-abundance proteins (such as albumin and immunoglobulins) are depleted to prevent masking of low-abundance proteins; this is performed using commercially available columns. Proteins are then precipitated using organic solvents or acids to concentrate and purify them. Proteins are then denatured and reduced, followed by alkylation of free cysteines to prevent reformation of disulfide bonds. The sample can then be desalted to remove salts and other contaminants that interfere with downstream analysis. Enzymes such as trypsin are then used to digest the proteins and the peptides are analyzed by mass spectrometry.

For metabolites, proteins are removed using organic solvents and centrifugation to pellet protein, followed by metabolite extraction based on polarity or other specific chemical properties. Metabolites can be profiled using mass spectrometry or nuclear magnetic resonance (NMR).

Extracellular vesicles

Cells release small, membrane-bound vesicles into the extracellular space. Vesicles can carry proteins, nucleic acids, lipids and other metabolites. Extracellular vesicles (EVs) are important for intercellular (and sometimes intracellular) signaling. Analysis of EVs can reveal molecules associated with aberrant signaling mechanisms or disease-specific metabolic pathways.[5]

Bodily fluids are initially processed as above. EVs can be isolated/enriched via techniques such as differential centrifugation, density gradient centrifugation, immunoaffinity capture (with antibodies specific to EV surface markers) and size-exclusion chromatography. The rest of the processing is handled as described above depending on the type of analyte (DNA, miRNA, protein, metabolites) of interest.

Circulating tumor cells

Circulating tumor cells (CTCs) represent a cancer-specific approach that can detect cells that have detached from a primary tumor and entered the bloodstream. CTCs can be isolated, and their biochemical properties, heterogeneity and drug sensitivity studied.[6] Body fluids are pre-processed by centrifugation and the buffy coat layer containing leukocytes and CTCs is preserved for further analysis. Enrichment of CTCs can involve positive selection (targeting CTC markers) or negative selection (selective depletion of non-CTCs). Immunoaffinity-based methods are often used to select for CTC markers such as EpCAM or cytokeratins with depletion of leukocytes with leukocyte-specific markers. CTC characterization includes immunochemistry, fluorescence in situ hybridization (FISH) and molecular analysis of CTC analytes. Downstream analysis often involves single-cell approaches.

CHALLENGES WITH ANALYSIS OF LIQUID BIOPSY DATA

There are several technical challenges associated with analysis of liquid biopsy data.

First, liquid biopsy analytes are often present in very low concentrations in bodily fluids and their detection may require highly sensitive methods and development of new approaches. Low concentrations can result in non-specific enrichment at a level higher than the low true signal, resulting in poor signal-to-noise ratios (SNRs). ML can also be used in denoising. Specifically, denoising autoencoders and variational autoencoders can learn latent representations from liquid biopsy datasets that separate biological signals from noise. Further, low-rank and sparse decomposition methods such as robust principal components analysis (RPCA) can be used to separate true signal from background variation.

Second, liquid biopsy ML performance is highly dependent on data generation and processing methods. Sample collection parameters (types of tubes, time to processing, storage parameters) and analytical parameters (extraction kits used, sequencing platform, read length and depth) can introduce systematic differences that the model may unintentionally learn as predictive signals; this can limit external validity. Some strategies to mitigate this include normalization approaches, batch correction methods for when data is pooled, and assessing discrimination and calibration of developed models across data generation sites. Further, federated and distributed learning approaches can be used for multicenter training while preserving privacy and minimizing batch effects.

Third, tumor-derived biomarkers are often heterogenous due to the complexity of the tumor and its microenvironment. Tumor subclones and their cellular environment can be associated with different types of biomarkers, making identification of appropriate targets difficult. Further, tumors can evolve over time and a liquid biopsy at a single timepoint only provides insight into tumor behavior at that time.

Fourth, different liquid biopsy methods (cfDNA, CTCs, miRNAs, protein, etc.) are often applied to the same sample, resulting in multiomic data. Integrating these data types to obtain a comprehensive view of the disease and identify unique molecular signatures requires sophisticated computational approaches. Further, these methods are supplemented by orthogonal methods such as imaging, tissue biopsy, etc. that need to be correlated with liquid biopsy data. This analytical challenge, in our opinion, is currently amenable to the application of novel ML techniques.

ROLE OF MACHINE LEARNING IN LIQUID BIOPSY

The use of ML techniques has opened new avenues to analyze complex genomics, proteomics and metabolomics data obtained from liquid biopsies. ML algorithms, ranging from traditional classifiers to advanced deep learning models, have already shown promise in obtaining insights from liquid biopsy datasets across a variety of medical disciplines as described below. We refer the reader to the plethora of online resources for a primer on ML.

Oncology is one of the most common applications of liquid biopsy. In oncology, ML has been used to analyze cfDNA, CTCs and EVs for cancer detection, prognostication and treatment selection. In breast cancer, SVM classifiers have been used to distinguish between benign and malignant tumors based on circulating cfDNA.[7] Recurrent neural networks (RNNs) have been used to detect and characterize CTCs in blood samples from patients with metastatic prostate cancer as a non-invasive means of disease monitoring.[8]

Beyond oncology, ML techniques have been used in liquid biopsy in other medical fields. In infectious diseases, XGBoost has been used to analyze metabolomic markers to identify pathogenic organisms in septic patients.[9] In neurology, ML has been used for microRNA analysis in CSF samples to detect neurodegenerative diseases such as Alzheimer's disease.[10] In psychiatry, ML analysis of microRNA in saliva has been used for the forecasting of alcohol dependency.[11] In rheumatology, ML has been used to identify features of serum bone biomarkers that distinguish rheumatoid arthritis (RA) patients from psoriatic arthritis, systemic sclerosis and healthy controls.[12]

FUTURE GENERAL ROLE OF ML IN NEUROSURGICAL LIQUID BIOPSY

Labeling of generated liquid biopsy datasets is key to allow for the data to be fully analyzed and for conclusions to be drawn using ML approaches. It is essential to define ground truth for each patient sample with the most specific labels based on expert diagnosis, including WHO diagnosis, IDH mutation status, presence of other key mutations, etc. Labels should also have a temporal assignment relative to key milestones such as diagnosis, surgery, chemotherapy or radiation cycles, as well as interval imaging, to allow for longitudinal time-to-event analyses. Similarly, outcomes and their timing should also be noted, such as progression-free survival, overall survival and treatment toxicities. The methods of labeling the data and establishing timelines should be standardized across institutions that report and share this data. Separate discovery, training, validation and testing sets should be used to prevent overfitting of ML models.

Various ML approaches will be used to answer questions in liquid biopsy for neurosurgical conditions.

ML classification algorithms such as SVMs, Random Forests (RFs) and Neural Networks can be trained on labeled liquid biopsy datasets from previous studies to learn differences between tumor-derived markers and non-tumor derived components in bodily fluids. These models can learn subtle relationships associated with the pathology of interest that cannot be identified with more elementary techniques such as LR. Ensemble learning methods such as XGBoost and AdaBoost can combine output from multiple models to improve accuracy.

Deep learning models such as autoencoders and Convolutional Neural Networks (CNNs) are suited to integration and analysis of multi-omics data with identification of complex molecular signatures. These models can also handle multimodal input, integrating liquid biopsy data with other clinical information to understand the disease better. This other clinical information can include laboratory tests and imaging (pathology, radiology).

Unsupervised learning methods such as k-means and hierarchical clustering can be used for clustering to identify subgroups of patients with inter-subgroup variations in biomarker profiles and responses to treatment. Unsupervised learning methods like principal components analysis (PCA), t-Distributed Stochastic Neighbor Embedding (t-SNE) or Uniform Manifold Approximation and Projection (UMAP) can be used for dimensionality reduction in the initial process of analyzing high-dimensional multi-omics data.

Supervised learning can be used for classification (stroke yes/no identification given clinical data input) and regression (to predict continuous outcomes such as stroke severity and percent neurologic impairment as well as recovery timelines).

Time-series analysis in liquid biopsy has not been significantly explored. RNNs and long short-term memory (LSTM) models can analyze time series data from serial liquid biopsies and track disease progression and treatment response. Reinforcement learning (a form of trial-error learning) can be used to develop optimal treatment plans for patients given a set of input clinical parameters such as imaging, liquid biopsy data, etc. These techniques can be broadly applied to all neurosurgical conditions.

The use of ML in liquid biopsy for neurosurgical conditions is a relatively new development. We discuss liquid biopsy approaches and the role for ML in neurosurgical subspecialties as noted below.

NEUROSURGICAL ONCOLOGY

Background

Neurosurgical oncology represents the majority usage, by far, of liquid biopsy techniques in the neurosurgical field. CNS tumors are a heterogenous group of tumors that vary in anatomic location, biochemical characterization and clinical management.[13] CNS tumors can involve primary tumors of the brain and spinal cord as well as intracranial metastases. Brain tumors often present with nonspecific symptoms such as persistent headaches or memory changes and may thus not be discovered using the current standard of care until the tumor is sufficiently advanced. Current approaches to CNS tumor detection involve pathologic tissue analysis obtained from traditional invasive biopsies as tumor characterization and monitoring by imaging is often limited in diagnostic power.[14] Biopsies only represent a sample of the tumor and may not reflect details regarding tumor heterogeneity and the complex tumor microenvironment.

Current state of liquid biopsy

Liquid biopsy has thus recently emerged as an adjunct to traditional biopsy methods. Liquid biopsy allows monitoring of tumors located in critical or inaccessible areas and provides information in a manner more representative of the heterogenous tumor. For brain tumor diagnosis, peripheral blood and CSF are the most commonly used bodily fluids. A few examples are provided below.

GLIOBLASTOMA MULTIFORME

One study identified CTCs with epidermal growth factor receptor (*EGFR*) gene amplifications from peripheral blood of 20 out of 141 patients with glioblastoma multiforme (GBM); this suggested that hematogenous spread was an intrinsic feature of

GBM biology, contrary to dogma.[15] Another study demonstrated that tumor cfDNA can be identified in CSF from a lumbar puncture (LP) even though the cfDNA concentrations were lower than that of CSF adjacent to the tumor. In >60% of samples, CSF from LP was sufficient to molecularly characterize the tumors based on IDH and TERT promoter mutations, *EGFR* amplification, *CDKN2A/B* deletion and O^6-methylguanine-DNA methyltransferase (MGMT) methylation, enabling GBM identification as well as other glioma subtypes.[16] Several diagnostic miRNAs as well as prognostication miRNAs for GBM have been identified.[17,18,19]

MEDULLOBLASTOMA

Several miRNA signatures have been identified in EVs from medulloblastoma patient CSF.[20,21,22] cfDNA has also been used for characterization and monitoring of medulloblastoma, covering mutations such as *TMC8*:p.S315N, *BMP5*:p.R321, *MIB1*:p.M468I.[23]

MENINGIOMA

One study identified cfDNA methylation signatures in plasma samples of meningioma patients.[24] First, they demonstrated that they could use differentially methylated probes to identify meningioma cases separate from other CNS conditions. They also built a classifier to identify meningioma samples from non-meningioma samples, with accuracy ranging from 68.4% to 84.9%. They also identified molecular signatures associated with high versus low risk of recurrence tumors and created a prognostic meningioma liquid biopsy score to predict recurrence versus no recurrence with an accuracy of 87.7%.

PITUITARY ADENOMA

Methylation patterns for pituitary adenoma obtained from cfDNA in blood have been reported.[25] miRNA patterns are also being increasingly studied.[26]

BRAINSTEM GLIOMAS

Stereotactic biopsy and resection of these tumors carries significant risks. One study utilized CSF samples either intraoperatively, from ventriculoperitoneal (VP) shunt or LP and deep-sequenced cfDNA.[27] In approximately 90% of cases, they were able to identify at least half of the genetic tumor alterations from tissue biopsy in the CSF; in 83% of cases, they were able to identify all the primary tumor alterations. They also noted that the sensitivity of plasma cfDNA detection was less than that of CSF detection. Another study showed a strong correlation between *H3F3A* K27M copies in CSF of children with diffuse intrinsic pontine glioma (DIPG) and high-grade glioma (better correlation with CSF reservoirs adjacent to tumor) and the contrast-enhancing cross-sectional tumor area.[28] Further, *H3F3A* K27M copies were temporarily raised in the CSF following a successful radiation treatment regimen, suggesting a potential application to disease surveillance.

BRAIN METASTASES

One study cultured, genotyped and characterized brain metastatic potential of breast cancer CTCs.[29] Through culture and injection into nude mice, they identified a signature EpCAM-/HER2+/EGFR+/HPSE+/Notch1+ with high brain metastatic potential. Other studies have looked at the optimal bodily fluid to sample with one prospective study showing high reliability for CSF-derived cfDNA than plasma-derived cfDNA for prognosticating, monitoring treatment response and studying tumor evolution of brain metastases.[30]

Finally, we note that a recent study (under review) utilizes a modified library preparation protocol with targeted nanopore sequencing efforts to sequence ~5000 pre-selected CpG sites within an hour and classify brain tumor types.[31] This approach could be used to identify tumor type from CSF (lumbar puncture) or in real-time during a tumor biopsy to determine if tumor resection /debulking would be appropriate.

Role of machine learning in liquid biopsy

One of the main challenges of liquid biopsy data involves interpretation of the high dimensional dataset obtained from various multi-omics approaches.[32] ML can be used to analyze and identify patterns from high dimensional datasets. So far, the majority of ML-related work has been done for gliomas, with the potential to expand into other tumor types.

GLIOMA

Glioma-derived cfDNA is usually difficult to detect in bodily fluids due to low cfDNA amounts. One study looked at matched tumor and liquid biopsy samples and identified that tumor-derived cfDNA fragments were shorter than non-mutant cfDNA fragments in CSF, plasma and urine samples of glioma patients.[33] They then classified the cfDNA fragments into bins and used the fragmentation patterns to train an RF model to distinguish non-glioma from glioma samples with a median AUC of 0.91 (range 0.76–1). While the study was small and the model will require validation with an independent dataset, it suggests that fragmentation patterns can be utilized to develop ML models for liquid biopsy.

Another study used information from infrared (IR) spectroscopy speaks of plasma samples to train a partial least-squares discriminant analysis (PLS-DA) model to predict high- and low-grade gliomas separately from non-cancer control patients with high sensitivity and specificity.[34] Yet another study identified miRNA signatures in tumor-educated platelets using particle swarm optimization-driven SVM optimization, a method inspired by bees that use a collection of particles moving through solution space to represent potential parameters of the model that can together provide input regarding parameter optimization.[35]

ML in liquid biopsy is also helpful in sellar tumors, such as rare sellar tumors or non-neoplastic diseases that can be misdiagnosed as Pituitary Neuroendocrine tumors (PitNETs). One study used an RF classifier to identify methylation patterns specific to PitNETs in plasma samples, enabling differentiation from other tumors and sellar lesions.[25]

Future direction for machine learning approaches in liquid biopsy

One aspect is continued development of algorithms that can effectively recognize molecular signatures in multi-omic liquid biopsy data for early detection. ML algorithms can also be used for analysis of longitudinal liquid biopsy data to guide real-time data adjustments depending on signatures of efficacy and treatment resistance.

Another aspect involves improved subtyping and molecular characterization. While ML methods have been developed for gliomas and can differentiate between low-versus high-grade glioma, ongoing development of larger datasets and training of ML models will allow for better subtype classification by liquid biopsy. This will provide personalized prognostic information.

Tumor signatures identified by ML can also be used to guide new therapeutic targets. Therapeutic development after signature identification, however, will also depend on a continuously improving understanding of tumor biology and target druggability.

With the increasing use of newer therapies such as chimeric antigen receptor T cell (CAR-T) for tumor targeting, liquid biopsy can be used to track the progress of the treatment. Tumors may shed antigens in response to CAR-T targeting and express new ones. ML models can be trained on copy number profiles and methylation signatures to detect when an antigen target is being downregulated while also detecting expressed neoantigens that can be targeted. Temporal models can be used to evaluate the change in tumor antigen expression across several sample collections.

Finally, ML for liquid biopsy presents a way to process and integrate raw liquid biopsy data into larger diagnostic, treatment and prognostication models that include demographic factors, laboratory measurements and data from non-invasive imaging.

As datasets expand, model development will have to emphasize generalizability across institutions, robust calibration and inference from serial liquid biopsy samples to allow for monitoring of disease progression, treatment resistance and inform additional therapeutic approaches.

SPINAL TUMORS

One study was able to identify specific mutations in cfDNA from spinal chordomas in blood and showed a high concordance of these mutations with genomic analysis of the chordoma biopsy.[36] These mutations were shown to be potentially associated with response to chemotherapy and potential for recurrence. Another study with four patients showed potential feasibility for liquid biopsy in diagnosis and prognostication of primary intramedullary astrocytoma.[37]

PERIPHERAL NERVE SHEATH TUMORS

One study looked at the role of liquid biopsy in transformation from benign plexiform neurofibroma (PN) to malignant peripheral nerve sheath tumors (MPNSTs) in patients with NF1.[38] They used ultra-low-pass whole genome sequencing

(WGS) of plasma cfDNA. A classifier relying solely on plasma cfDNA tumor fraction to differentiate MPNST versus PN achieved a receiver operating characteristic (ROC) of 0.83. There was also a significantly different distribution of cfDNA fragment sizes in MPNST versus PN. They demonstrated the utility of plasma cfDNA to monitor disease progression as well as minimal residual disease post-therapy. Another study which compared healthy individuals to those with PN and MPNST found significant differences in genome-wide aneuploidy (GWA) scores of plasma cfDNA between the groups and differences in sub-chromosomal copy number variations (CNVs).[39] Incorporating GAS and sub-chromosomal CNVs yielded a sensitivity of 50% and a high specificity of 97% in identifying MPNST.

Given the relative rarity of spinal tumors compared to intracranial tumors, liquid biopsy and the role for ML in spinal tumors has not been well studied. This remains an open area of active investigation.

NEUROTRAUMA: TRAUMATIC BRAIN INJURY AND SPINAL CORD INJURY

Background

There are approximately 2 million cases of traumatic brain injury (TBI) annually and the Centers for Disease Control and Prevention (CDC) reported that approximately 5.3 million Americans live with long-term effects of TBI.[40] TBI is very heterogenous and includes penetrating injury, hematomas, diffuse injury and concussions. While some markers of brain injury have been identified in preclinical models, a lack of understanding of CNS biomarkers due to heterogeneity, in addition to poor translatability of preclinical models, has prevented development of efficacious drugs.[41] The development of biomarkers from liquid biopsy approaches will enable a better molecular understanding of TBI and improve diagnosis, especially for cases of mild TBI when neuroimaging may be inconclusive. Current biomarker candidates include the glial calcium binding protein S100-B (astrocyte injury), ubiquitin hydrolase UCH-L1 (neuron cell body injury), glial intermediate filament protein GFAP, IL-6 (microglia activation) and the myelin protein MBP.[41,42] A recently published point-of-care test (POCT) used glial fibrillary acidic protein (GFAP) and ubiquitin C-terminal hydrolase L1 (UCH-L1) from plasma to diagnose TBI.[43] The test achieved a sensitivity of 0.958 and specificity of 0.404 when compared to imaging as a gold standard. Liquid biopsy can also be used in TBI to identify secondary injury mechanisms such as inflammation and oxidative stress that can contribute to poor recovery or decline after the initial TBI.

Spinal cord injury (SCI) can cause debilitating deficits with an estimated 18,000 new cases of traumatic SCI each year.[44] SCI can also be non-traumatic in conditions such as myelopathy and infection. The current standard of care for SCI involves neurological examination and MRI. Neurological examinations have significant interprovider variability and MRI readings are often more qualitative than quantitative.[45,46] Rapid intervention in cases of suspected SCI is key to preserving function. Liquid biopsy for SCI can provide a more objective assessment and may be particularly helpful in low-resource settings with limited or minimal imaging capability.

Current state of liquid biopsy

Most current SCI liquid biopsy approaches focus on Protein and RNA.[47]

PROTEIN

Several preclinical studies of SCI exist and have identified proteins such as S100-B, UCH-L1, GFAP, MBP and the matrix metalloproteinases MMP-8/9.[48,49] In clinical investigations, several biomarkers such as neurofilament proteins, GFAP and S100-B have been studied.[50,51] These markers are similar to those discussed for TBI above.

RNA

Transcriptomic signatures have been identified in peripheral leukocytes associated with severity and prognosis.[52] There has been particular focus on two types of RNA. The first is lncRNA, a form of non-protein coding RNA that can serve a variety of regulatory roles within a cell. Various lncRNAs are involved in genetic networks that have been implicated in the molecular pathophysiology of SCI.[53,54] Clinical studies of lncRNAs in SCI remain an active area of research. miRNAs have also been shown to be associated with severity and prognosis of SCI.[55,56] One clinical study identified miRNAs associated with SCI severity in CSF of patients.[57]

Future direction for machine learning approaches in liquid biopsy

There are already several studies, as mentioned above, of biomarker identification in CSF and plasma of patients with TBI and SCI. However, many of the abovementioned markers are not specific with there being several common markers between TBI and SCI. Further, these markers also overlap with non-neurotrauma conditions. For example, S100B is associated with melanoma outcomes and GFAP with Alzheimer's.[58,59] ML methods are not commonly used for TBI and SCI liquid biopsy, but they are likely to become more common as datasets become larger and enable training of better models. A key role of ML will likely be to identify TBI and SCI-specific signatures. ML methods will be increasingly used to condense high-dimensional liquid biopsy data into highly specific and predictive markers for TBI and SCI.

The other goals of ML will be similar to that of ML in neuro-oncology. ML will allow better diagnostic classification and prognostication of TBI/SCI as well as real-time monitoring of treatment effect. Molecular signatures identified by ML may also provide better insight into the pathophysiology of TBI/SCI.

VASCULAR

Background

The largest application of liquid biopsy in vascular neurosurgery is the prompt diagnosis and management of acute ischemic strokes (AIS).

ACUTE ISCHEMIC STROKE

AIS is the most common type of stroke. There is a short time-window for effective treatment of AIS with recombinant tissue plasminogen activator (tPA) or TNK (Tenecteplase). While CT can often identify hemorrhagic strokes easily, the sensitivity of CT is significantly less for AIS. Unfortunately, only ~7% of patients with AIS are diagnosed in time to be eligible for tPA.[60] While the mainstay of AIS diagnosis involves neuroimaging, an effective blood test could enable better stratification of patients and prompt treatment of suspected AIS.[61]

Current state of liquid biopsy

Biomarkers of glial activation in AIS include S100B, GFAP and MBP.[62,63] Markers of neuronal injury include N-methyl-D-aspartate (NMDA) receptor peptide and neuron-specific enolase, a neuronal glycolytic enzyme.[64,65] There are other markers pertaining to inflammation and coagulation including CRP, IL-6, D-dimer, etc., which are not specific on their own. More recently, biomarker panels such as (IGFBP-3, TNF-R1, FasL, S100B, Hsc70, Apolipoprotein CIII and NCAM) have been developed with AUC of 0.75 for distinguishing real stroke versus stroke mimics and distinguishing AIS from hemorrhagic stroke.[66] Finally, some circulating cfDNA biomarkers have been proposed for prediction of short-term outcomes following tPA and/or mechanical thrombectomy.[67,68]

Future directions for machine learning approaches in liquid biopsy

Most stroke biomarkers that have been identified are proteins, as discussed above, and have significant overlap with other conditions involving neuronal injury. Future work will largely focus on the development of highly specific stroke biomarkers (equivalent to the use of Troponin and Creatine Kinase-Myocardial Band [CK-MB] for MI). Specific biomarkers are more likely to involve changes at the cellular level in response to ischemia and hypoxia and are more likely to be detected as cell-free nucleic acid as cells die. To date, there has been minimal investigation into mRNA or cfDNA biomarkers for stroke detection. Work at high-volume centers involving collection of blood samples and other tissues will provide insights into biological mechanisms underlying the cellular response to AIS and will generate large multi-omic and spatial transcriptomic datasets amenable to analysis and pattern recognition by ML. ML methods can enable development of specific stroke biomarkers by condensing high-dimensional multi-omics input. Unsupervised learning can also be used to discover clusters of patients or biomarkers who may be predisposed to poor functional outcomes or who may benefit from different approaches to treatment.

Once biomarkers are identified, ML will also enable integration of multimodal input (patient histories and symptoms, CT imaging and blood biomarker values) for point-of-care stroke detection. Similar multimodal models will also prove useful for prognostication of functional recovery (which will consider factors like administration of tPA or TNK, TICI score post-MT, etc).

REFERENCES

1. Bronkhorst AJ, Ungerer V, Holdenrieder S. The emerging role of cell-free DNA as a molecular marker for cancer management. *Biomol Detect Quantif* 2019; 17: 100087.
2. Douville C, Curtis S, Summers M, et al. Seq-ing the SINEs of central nervous system tumors in cerebrospinal fluid. *Cell Rep Med* 2023; 4(8): 101148.
3. Condrat CE, Thompson DC, Barbu MG, et al. miRNAs as biomarkers in disease: Latest findings regarding their role in diagnosis and prognosis. *Cells* 2020; 9(2): 276.
4. Issaq HJ, Veenstra TD (eds). *Proteomic and Metabolomic Approaches to Biomarker Discovery*. San Diego: Elsevier; 2020.
5. Ciferri MC, Quarto R, Tasso R. Extracellular vesicles as biomarkers and therapeutic tools: From pre-clinical to clinical applications. *Biology* 2021; 10(5): 359.
6. Lin D, Shen L, Luo M, et al. Circulating tumor cells: Biology and clinical significance. *Signal Transduct Target Ther* 2021; 6(1): 404.
7. Gawad C, Koh W, Quake SR. Single-cell genome sequencing: Current state of the science. *Nat Rev Genet* 2016; 17(3): 175–88.
8. Lu YT, Zhao L, Shen Q, et al. NanoVelcro rare-cell assays for detection and characterization of circulating tumor cells. *Adv Drug Deliv Rev* 2018; 125: 78–93.
9. Zheng L, Lin F, Zhu C, et al. Machine learning algorithms identify pathogen-specific biomarkers of clinical and metabolomic characteristics in septic patients with bacterial infections. *Biomed Res Int* 2020; 2020: 6950576.
10. Lusardi TA, Phillips JI, Wiedrick JT, et al. MicroRNAs in human cerebrospinal fluid as biomarkers for Alzheimer's disease. *J Alzheimers Dis* 2017; 55(3): 1223–33.
11. Rosato AJ, Chen X, Tanaka Y, et al. Salivary microRNAs identified by small RNA sequencing and machine learning as potential biomarkers of alcohol dependence. *Epigenomics* 2019; 11(7): 739–49.
12. Adami G, Fassio A, Rossini M, et al. Machine learning to characterize bone biomarkers profile in rheumatoid arthritis. *Front Immunol* 2023; 14: 1291727.
13. Pilotto Heming C, Niemeyer Filho P, Moura-Neto V, Aran V. Recent advances in the use of liquid biopsy to fight central nervous system tumors. *Cancer Treat Res Commun* 2023; 35: 100709.
14. Aili Y, Maimaitiming N, Mahemuti Y, et al. Liquid biopsy in central nervous system tumors: The potential roles of circulating miRNA and exosomes. *Am J Cancer Res* 2020; 10(12): 4134.
15. Müller C, Holtschmidt J, Auer M, et al. Hematogenous dissemination of glioblastoma multiforme. *Sci Transl Med* 2014; 6(247): 247ra101.
16. Orzan F, De Bacco F, Lazzarini E, et al. Liquid biopsy of cerebrospinal fluid enables selective profiling of glioma molecular subtypes at first clinical presentation. *Clin Cancer Res* 2023; 29(7): 1252–66.
17. Teplyuk NM, Mollenhauer B, Gabriely G, et al. MicroRNAs in cerebrospinal fluid identify glioblastoma and metastatic brain cancers and reflect disease activity. *Neuro Oncol* 2012; 14(6): 689–700.
18. Akers JC, Hua W, Li H, et al. A cerebrospinal fluid microRNA signature as biomarker for glioblastoma. *Oncotarget* 2017; 8(40): 68769–79.
19. Wang ZQ, Zhang MY, Deng ML, et al. Low serum level of miR-485–3p predicts poor survival in patients with glioblastoma. *PloS one* 2017; 12(9): e0184969.
20. Northcott PA, Buchhalter I, Morrissy AS, et al. The whole-genome landscape of medulloblastoma subtypes. *Nature* 2017; 547(7663): 311–17.
21. Zhang L, Zhang S, Yao J, et al. Microenvironment-induced PTEN loss by exosomal microRNA primes brain metastasis outgrowth. *Nature* 2015; 527(7576): 100–4.
22. Bonner ER, Bornhorst M, Packer RJ, et al. Liquid biopsy for pediatric central nervous system tumors. *NPJ Precis Oncol* 2018; 2: 29.

23. Escudero L, Llort A, Arias A, et al. Circulating tumour DNA from the cerebrospinal fluid allows the characterisation and monitoring of medulloblastoma. *Nat Commun* 2020; 11(1): 5376.
24. Herrgott GA, Snyder JM, She R, et al. Detection of diagnostic and prognostic methylation-based signatures in liquid biopsy specimens from patients with meningiomas. *Nat Commun* 2023; 14(1): 5669.
25. Herrgott GA, Asmaro KP, Wells M, et al. Detection of tumor-specific DNA methylation markers in the blood of patients with pituitary neuroendocrine tumors. *Neuro Oncol* 2022; 24(7): 1126–39.
26. Donati S, Aurilia C, Palmini G, et al. MicroRNAs as potential biomarkers in pituitary adenomas. *Noncoding RNA* 2021; 7(3): 55.
27. Pan C, Diplas BH, Chen X, et al. Molecular profiling of tumors of the brainstem by sequencing of CSF-derived circulating tumor DNA. *Acta Neuropathol* 2019; 137(2): 297–306.
28. Stallard S, Savelieff MG, Wierzbicki K, et al. CSF H3F3A K27M circulating tumor DNA copy number quantifies tumor growth and in vitro treatment response. *Acta Neuropathol Commun* 2018; 6(1): 80.
29. Zhang L, Ridgway LD, Wetzel MD, et al. The identification and characterization of breast cancer CTCs competent for brain metastasis. *Sci Transl Med* 2013; 5(180): 180ra48.
30. Li M, Chen J, Zhang B, et al. Dynamic monitoring of cerebrospinal fluid circulating tumor DNA to identify unique genetic profiles of brain metastatic tumors and better predict intracranial tumor responses in non-small cell lung cancer patients with brain metastases: A prospective cohort study (GASTO 1028). *BMC Med* 2022; 20(1): 398.
31. Kubelt C, Brändl B, van Bömmel A, et al. PATH–45. Intrapigliom rapid sequencing diagnosis of brain tumors. *Neuro Oncol* 2022; 24(7): vii160–1.
32. Menna G, Piaser Guerrato G, Bilgin L, et al. Is there a role for machine learning in liquid biopsy for brain tumors? A systematic review. *Int J Mol Sci* 2023; 24(11): 9723.
33. Mouliere F, Smith CG, Heider K, et al. Fragmentation patterns and personalized sequencing of cell-free DNA in urine and plasma of glioma patients. *EMBO Mol Med* 2021; 13(8): e12881.
34. Theakstone AG, Brennan PM, Jenkinson MD, et al. Rapid spectroscopic liquid biopsy for the universal detection of brain tumours. *Cancers* 2021; 13(15): 3851.
35. Sol N, In 't Veld SGJG, Vancura A, et al. Tumor-educated platelet RNA for the detection and (pseudo)progression monitoring of glioblastoma. *Cell Rep Med* 2020; 1(7): 100101.
36. Mattox AK, Yang B, Douville C, et al. The mutational landscape of spinal chordomas and their sensitive detection using circulating tumor DNA. *Neuro Oncol Adv* 2020; 3(1): vdaa173.
37. Cheng L, Duan W, Guan J, et al. Detection of glioma-related hotspot mutations through sequencing of cerebrospinal fluid (CSF)-derived circulating tumor DNA: A pilot study on CSF-based liquid biopsy for primary spinal cord astrocytoma. *Neurospine* 2023; 20(2): 701–8.
38. Szymanski JJ, Sundby RT, Jones PA, et al. Cell-free DNA ultra-low-pass whole genome sequencing to distinguish malignant peripheral nerve sheath tumor (MPNST) from its benign precursor lesion: A cross-sectional study. *PLoS Med* 2021; 18(8): e1003734.
39. Mattox AK, Douville C, Silliman N, et al. Detection of malignant peripheral nerve sheath tumors in patients with neurofibromatosis using aneuploidy and mutation identification in plasma. *eLife* 2022; 11: e74238.
40. Wright DW, Kellermann A, McGuire LC, et al. CDC grand rounds: Reducing severe traumatic brain injury in the United States. *MMWR Morb Mortal Wkly Rep* 2013; 62(27): 549–52.
41. Wang KK, Yang Z, Zhu T, et al. An update on diagnostic and prognostic biomarkers for traumatic brain injury. *Expert Rev Mol Diagn* 2018; 18(2): 165–80.
42. Papa L, Brophy GM, Welch RD, et al. Time course and diagnostic accuracy of glial and neuronal blood biomarkers GFAP and UCH-L1 in a large cohort of trauma patients with and without mild traumatic brain injury. *JAMA Neurol* 2016; 73(5): 551–60.
43. Bazarian JJ, Welch RD, Caudle K, et al. Accuracy of a rapid glial fibrillary acidic

protein/ubiquitin carboxyl-terminal hydrolase L1 test for the prediction of intracranial injuries on head computed tomography after mild traumatic brain injury. *Acad Emerg Med* 2021; 28(11): 1308–17.
44. National Spinal Cord Injury Statistical Center. Available from: https://sites.uab.edu/nscisc/ (Accessed April 2026).
45. Griffin JF, Davis MC, Ji JX, et al. Quantitative magnetic resonance imaging in a naturally occurring canine model of spinal cord injury. *Spinal Cord* 2015; 53(4): 278–84.
46. Mathew M, Mezue WC, Chikani MC, et al. Correlation of quantitative MRI parameters with neurological outcome in acute cervical spinal cord injury. *J West Afr Coll Surg* 2021; 11(1): 5–10.
47. Azad TD, Ran KR, Liu J, et al. A future blood test for acute traumatic spinal cord injury. *Biomarkers* 2023; 28(8): 703–13.
48. Yang Z, Bramlett HM, Moghieb A, et al. Temporal profile and severity correlation of a panel of rat spinal cord injury protein biomarkers. *Mol Neurobiol* 2018; 55(3): 2174–84.
49. Light M, Minor KH, DeWitt P, et al. Multiplex array proteomics detects increased MMP-8 in CSF after spinal cord injury. *J Neuroinflammation* 2012; 9: 122.
50. Kuhle J, Gaiottino J, Leppert D, et al. Serum neurofilament light chain is a biomarker of human spinal cord injury severity and outcome. *J Neurol Neurosurg Psychiatry* 2015; 86(3): 273–9.
51. Kwon BK, Streijger F, Fallah N, et al. Cerebrospinal fluid biomarkers to stratify injury severity and predict outcome in human traumatic spinal cord injury. *J Neurotrauma* 2017; 34(3): 567–80.
52. Kyritsis N, Torres-Espín A, Schupp PG, et al. Diagnostic blood RNA profiles for human acute spinal cord injury. *J Exp Med* 2021; 218(3): e20201795.
53. Wang L, Wang B, Liu J, Quan Z. Construction and analysis of a spinal cord injury competitive endogenous RNA network based on the expression data of long noncoding, micro- and messenger RNAs. *Mol Med Rep* 2019; 19(4): 3021–34.
54. Cheng X, Xu J, Yu Z, et al. LncRNA Xist contributes to endogenous neurological repair after chronic compressive spinal cord injury by promoting angiogenesis through the miR-32–5p/notch-1 axis. *Front Cell Dev Biol* 2020; 8: 744.
55. Tigchelaar S, Streijger F, Sinha S, et al. Serum MicroRNAs reflect injury severity in a large animal model of thoracic spinal cord injury. *Sci Rep* 2017; 7(1): 1376.
56. Ma X, Ma T, Chang L, et al. Correlation between miRNA-124, miRNA-544a, and TNF-α levels in acute spinal cord injury. *Spinal Cord* 2022; 60(9): 779–83.
57. Tigchelaar S, Gupta R, Shannon CP, et al. MicroRNA biomarkers in cerebrospinal fluid and serum reflect injury severity in human acute traumatic spinal cord injury. *J Neurotrauma* 2019; 36(15): 2358–71.
58. Tarhini AA, Stuckert J, Lee S, et al. Prognostic significance of serum S100B protein in high-risk surgically resected melanoma patients participating in Intergroup Trial ECOG 1694. *J Clin Oncol* 2009; 27(1): 38–44.
59. Chatterjee P, Pedrini S, Stoops E, et al. Plasma glial fibrillary acidic protein is elevated in cognitively normal older adults at risk of Alzheimer's disease. *Transl Psychiatry* 2021; 11(1): 27.
60. Adeoye O, Hornung R, Khatri P, Kleindorfer D. Recombinant tissue-type plasminogen activator use for ischemic stroke in the United States: A doubling of treatment rates over the course of 5 years. *Stroke* 2011; 42(7): 1952–5.
61. Wijerathne H, Witek MA, Baird AE, Soper SA. Liquid biopsy markers for stroke diagnosis. *Expert Rev Mol Diagn* 2020; 20(8): 771–88.
62. Undén J, Strandberg K, Malm J, et al. Explorative investigation of biomarkers of brain damage and coagulation system activation in clinical stroke differentiation. *J Neurol* 2009; 256(1): 72–7.
63. Hjalmarsson C, Bjerke M, Andersson B, et al. Neuronal and glia-related biomarkers in cerebrospinal fluid of patients with acute ischemic stroke. *J Cent Nerv Syst Dis* 2014; 6: 51–8.
64. Dambinova SA, Betterman K, Glynn T, et al. Diagnostic potential of the NMDA receptor peptide assay for acute ischemic stroke. *PloS one* 2012; 7(7): e42362.

65. Singh HV, Pandey A, Shrivastava AK, et al. Prognostic value of neuron specific enolase and IL-10 in ischemic stroke and its correlation with degree of neurological deficit. *Clin Chim Acta* 2013; 419: 136–8.
66. Bustamante A, López-Cancio E, Pich S, et al. Blood biomarkers for the early diagnosis of stroke: The stroke-chip study. *Stroke* 2017; 48(9): 2419–25.
67. Bustamante A, Mancha F, Macher HC, et al. Circulating cell-free DNA is a predictor of short-term neurological outcome in stroke patients treated with intravenous thrombolysis. *J Circ Biomark* 2016; 5: 1849454416668791.
68. Vajpeyee A, Wijatmiko T, Vajpeyee M, Taywade O. Cell free DNA: A novel predictor of neurological outcome after intravenous thrombolysis and/or mechanical thrombectomy in acute ischemic stroke patients. *Neurointervention* 2018; 13(1): 13–19.

6

Diagnostic Applications of Artificial Intelligence in Neuro-Oncology

UMMEY HANI, DAVID J. PARK AND STEVEN D. CHANG

INTRODUCTION

Central nervous system (CNS) tumors represent a major global health burden, with more than 250,000 new cases reported annually worldwide.[1] These tumors embody some of the most challenging pathologies in medicine, requiring a multimodal and multidisciplinary approach to optimize patient outcomes. The diagnostic pathway typically begins with a neurological examination, followed by advanced neuroimaging, biopsy, histopathological evaluation and molecular profiling. Definitive treatment planning often involves consensus discussions within a specialized tumor board, bringing together neurosurgeons, neuroradiologists, neuropathologists and neuro-oncologists.[2]

Despite these collective efforts and significant advances in recent decades, malignant CNS tumors, particularly gliomas, continue to carry poor prognoses. Gliomas account for over 80% of malignant intracranial tumors, with glioblastoma alone responsible for at least 10000 deaths annually in the United States.[3] These sobering statistics underscore the urgency of continued progress in surgical neuro-oncology, diagnostics and adjunctive therapies.

The evolution of neuro-oncology: A historical perspective

The roots of neuro-oncology lie in the earliest explorations of brain anatomy, yet the field's modern foundation was established in the early twentieth century. Harvey Cushing, widely regarded as the father of modern neurosurgery, pioneered refined surgical techniques and, together with Percival Bailey in 1926, introduced the first histogenetic classification of gliomas. Around the same time, Walter Dandy revolutionized intracranial imaging with ventriculography (1918) and pneumoencephalography (1919), while Egas Moniz's introduction of cerebral angiography (1927) and the mid-twentieth-century adoption of planar tomography advanced neurodiagnostic imaging further.

The 1970s brought transformative developments with the advent of computed tomography (CT) and, soon after, magnetic resonance imaging (MRI), which fundamentally reshaped brain tumor diagnosis, surgical navigation and postoperative monitoring.[4] Surgical precision likewise advanced in the 1960s and 1970s with the introduction of the operating microscope and microsurgical techniques by Gazi Yasargil. Together, these innovations marked a shift toward safer, more effective tumor resections.

Functional preservation gradually became central to neuro-oncological surgery. Wilder Penfield's cortical stimulation mapping in 1937, leading to the creation of the iconic "homunculus," was later refined by Ojemann in 1977 and extended by Berger in 1992 to protect eloquent cortical regions during tumor resections. More recently, Duffau and others have integrated connectome-based surgery and white matter tractography, embedding principles of network neuroscience into operative planning.[5,6]

DOI: 10.1201/9781003471165-6

Parallel to these surgical and imaging milestones, the molecular era of neuro-oncology began to unfold. The WHO's first formal classification of CNS tumors in 1979 has since evolved to incorporate immunohistochemistry (IHC) and key molecular markers, such as IDH mutations and 1p/19q codeletion, fundamentally reshaping both diagnostic criteria and treatment strategies. Today, neuro-oncology stands as a multidisciplinary specialty at the intersection of microsurgery, molecular biology, and advanced imaging, driven by the shared goal of maximizing tumor control while preserving neurological function.[5,7]

Current diagnostic challenges in neuro-oncology

The management of CNS tumors remains fraught with challenges that limit diagnostic precision and timely treatment. Tumor heterogeneity, variable treatment responses, disparities in access to advanced care and the scarcity of reliable biomarkers all contribute to diagnostic uncertainty and suboptimal outcomes.[8,9]

MRI remains the cornerstone of neuro-oncological imaging, but it is not without limitations. Standard non-contrast sequences are often insufficient for visualizing tumor margins, while gadolinium-based contrast agents, though indispensable, carry risks of neurotoxicity, nephrogenic systemic fibrosis and long-term tissue deposition. Moreover, gadolinium enhancement relies on disruption of the blood–brain barrier (BBB), meaning that infiltrative tumors such as glioblastomas may remain partially invisible on imaging, complicating assessments of true tumor extent.[10–12]

Another persistent diagnostic dilemma is distinguishing between tumor recurrence, treatment-related pseudoprogression and radiation necrosis. Advanced MRI techniques such as magnetic resonance spectroscopy (MRS), diffusion tensor imaging (DTI), functional MRI (fMRI), diffusion-weighted imaging (DWI), susceptibility-weighted imaging (SWI), chemical exchange saturation transfer (CEST) and perfusion-weighted imaging are increasingly used to address these limitations.[13,14] Nevertheless, interobserver variability, machine-to-machine inconsistency, and uneven distribution of expertise across centers continue to restrict the reliability of these tools.

In this context, artificial intelligence (AI) has emerged as a transformative force in CNS tumor diagnostics. By leveraging machine learning (ML) and deep learning (DL) algorithms, AI systems are able to process vast imaging and molecular datasets, automate complex segmentation tasks and detect subtle imaging patterns beyond human perception.[15] Convolutional neural networks (CNNs), in particular, have shown remarkable utility in analyzing MRI and histopathological images, facilitating tumor grading, treatment response monitoring and prognostic predictions.[12] **Table 6.1** summarizes all the different ways AI can enhance diagnostic accuracy in neuro-oncology. **Figure 6.1** demonstrates a visual AI workflow in Neuro-Oncology Diagnostics.

Table 6.1 Summary of AI applications in neuroimaging and tumor analysis, highlighting methods, outputs and clinical impacts

Application area	AI methods	Key outputs	Clinical impact / Utility
Neuroimaging (MRI, CT, PET)	Convolutional Neural Networks (CNNs), Deep Learning Reconstruction (DLR), Vision Transformers (ViTs), Capsule Networks (CapsNet)	Tumor detection, classification (e.g. glioblastoma vs metastases), segmentation, improved image quality	Faster and more accurate identification of tumors, improved pre-surgical planning, differentiation of true progression versus pseudoprogression
Segmentation	CNNs, U-Net, Multi-encoder single-decoder CNNs, CapsNet, Vision Transformers	Tumor boundaries, whole-tumor maps, sensitivity/precision metrics, Dice coefficient	Accurate tumor delineation for surgery, radiation planning, volumetric monitoring; reduces manual annotation burden

Table 6.1 (*Continued*)

Application area	AI methods	Key outputs	Clinical impact / Utility
Radiomics	Feature extraction (wavelet, Laplacian, Gabor transforms), ML models	Quantitative tumor features: Shape, texture, heterogeneity, vascular patterns	Personalized predictive models, prognosis prediction, treatment planning, integration with genomic / histopathology data
Radiogenomics / Virtual biopsy	DL–based radiomics, CNNs, Transformer models, AI-integrated optical histology (e.g. DeepGlioma)	Molecular alterations (IDH, 1p/19q, ATRX, MGMT, EGFR), predicted histology, gene mutation status	Non-invasive molecular profiling, risk stratification, guides chemotherapy / surgical strategy, supports tumor board decisions
Transformer-based architectures	Swin Transformer, SPP-U-Net, RMTF-Net	Tumor segmentation, molecular prediction	Improved precision in heterogeneous tumor regions, scalable performance, combines imaging and molecular profiling
Workflow / Clinical decision support	AI outputs integrated into tumor boards, virtual biopsy dashboards	Objective risk scores, rapid molecular insights, treatment guidance	Reduces diagnostic timelines, informs multidisciplinary decision-making, safer management of high-risk/pediatric tumors

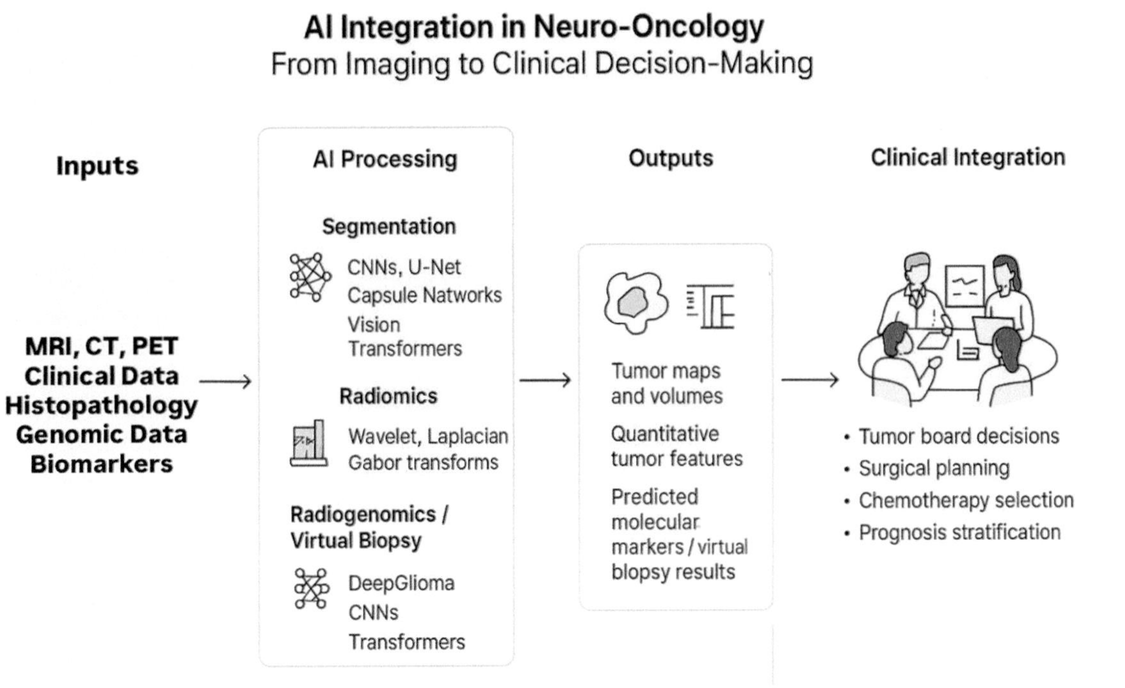

Figure 6.1 A visual AI workflow in neuro-oncology diagnostics showing how multimodal imaging and molecular data integrated with AI provide clinicians with rapid, reproducible and actionable insights, supporting decision-making in tumor boards, surgical planning and personalized treatment strategies.

Yet, despite these advances, the integration of AI into clinical workflows faces significant obstacles. Data heterogeneity, lack of standardization across imaging protocols, limited multi-institutional validation and ethical concerns surrounding bias and transparency remain barriers to adoption.[16,17] Concerns over generalizability across populations further highlight the need for robust validation and equitable implementation.[18] Until such challenges are addressed, the promise of AI in neuro-oncology will remain partially unrealized, and many patients risk suboptimal treatment stratification and outcomes.

Artificial intelligence in neuroimaging for diagnosis

AI applications in MRI, CT and PET have significantly advanced the ability to detect, classify and segment brain tumors, as well as differentiate between true tumor progression and treatment-related changes such as pseudoprogression. In many tasks, DL models now outperform conventional imaging analysis techniques.[19,20]

Image pre-processing and enhancement

AI has improved pre-processing pipelines by correcting motion artifacts, normalizing image intensity, reducing noise and resampling scans for consistency. These steps ensure that downstream analyses, such as radiomics or segmentation, are more reliable.[20,21] In addition, AI supports multimodal image registration that aligns MRI, CT and PET scans, allowing for better tumor mapping and surgical planning.[20] Emerging DL reconstruction (DLR) techniques enhance resolution and edge sharpness, improving detection of subtle lesions such as pituitary microadenomas and metastases.[15]

Tumor classification and detection

AI-based classification models have shown high-diagnostic performance across multiple tumor types. For example, spatial convolutional attention inception (SCAT) networks, a type of convolutional neural network (CNN), can distinguish glioblastoma (GBM) from solitary brain metastases with an accuracy of over 92%.[22] Similarly, CNN-based methods have been applied to predict glioma grade, identify pediatric posterior fossa tumors, and classify lesions on dynamic PET imaging, often matching or even exceeding radiologist performance.[12,23] Other ML approaches, such as random forest (RF) classifiers, which are ensemble models that combine multiple decision trees, have been used to predict the primary source of brain metastases using MRI-based texture features.[24]

Segmentation techniques

Accurate tumor segmentation, which refers to outlining the tumor boundary and separating it from normal brain tissue, is essential for treatment planning. Segmentation approaches range from manual (very accurate but labor-intensive), to semi-automatic (AI-assisted with human oversight), and now fully automated DL methods, which include CNNs, Capsule Networks (CapsNets), and vision transformers (ViTs).[15,20,25] CapsNets are an evolution of neural networks designed to capture spatial hierarchies between parts of an object, requiring relatively less data. This is an advantage given the limited size of brain tumor imaging datasets. ViTs, on the other hand, leverage self-attention mechanisms to model long-range dependencies across an image, enabling robust segmentation performance and scalability when trained on large datasets.

Modern DL–based segmentation achieves very high agreement with expert tumor annotations. For example, models often report Sørensen–Dice coefficients above 0.9 for whole-tumor regions.[26] This metric quantifies the overlap between AI predictions and the actual tumor outlines, where 1.0 indicates a perfect match. These models combine information from multiple MRI sequences to produce a single, clearer tumor map, improving the accuracy of tumor delineation, as demonstrated in studies such as the BraTS 2020 challenge.[27] Architectures such as U-Net, a CNN designed for biomedical image segmentation, and its variants, have become standard. U-Net–based methods applied to black-blood MRI achieved a sensitivity of 93% and precision of 85% in detecting brain metastases.[28] In pediatric posterior fossa tumors, modified DL models such as ResNeXt have achieved an area under the receiver operating characteristic curve (AUROC) of 0.99 for tumor detection and 0.92 for subtype classification.[29]

Radiomics for neuro-oncology

Radiomics refers to converting medical images into quantitative features that capture tumor shape, texture, intensity patterns and heterogeneity. These features can then be linked to clinical outcomes, prognosis or molecular alterations.[30,31] For instance, wavelet transforms decompose MRI scans into multiple frequency bands, highlighting both fine and coarse textural patterns within a tumor. Laplacian operators accentuate edges, improving detection of sharp tumor boundaries and Gabor transforms enhance vascular patterns and tissue microarchitecture, aiding in characterizing angiogenic activity within tumors.[12,32,33]

When integrated with demographic, histopathological and genomic data, these radiomic features can be used to generate highly personalized predictive models for patient care.

ARTIFICIAL INTELLIGENCE IN MOLECULAR PROFILING AND VIRTUAL BIOPSY OF CNS TUMORS

From histopathology to virtual biopsy

Traditionally, the diagnosis and classification of CNS tumors have relied on invasive histopathology and molecular sequencing. While tissue sampling remains the gold standard, it carries risks of morbidity, sampling bias and logistical delays. The advent of radiogenomics has opened the possibility of a "virtual biopsy," where imaging enhanced by AI predicts key molecular markers and genomic profiles. This approach not only aids diagnosis but also has the potential to guide treatment decisions, stratify prognosis and reduce the need for repeat biopsies, particularly in surgically inaccessible lesions.

Radiogenomics extends radiomics by linking imaging features to molecular and genetic tumor profiles. DL-based radiomics, which automatically learns discriminative features without manual engineering, has achieved high accuracy in tumor classification and prognostication.[20] Multiparametric MRI radiomics has also been shown to predict gene mutations, epigenetic modifications and signaling pathway alterations, supporting precision medicine approaches in gliomas and other CNS tumors.[30]

In addition to radiogenomic approaches, AI systems are being developed to accelerate and complement traditional molecular diagnostics. Molecular classification is critical for prognostication and personalized therapy, yet timely testing can be delayed, affecting surgical and adjuvant decisions. One such example is DeepGlioma, an AI-based platform that integrates optical histology with genomic data to predict molecular alterations, including IDH mutation, 1p/19q co-deletion and ATRX mutation, used in adult-type diffuse glioma classification. In preliminary multicenter studies, it achieved high accuracy in molecular prediction, demonstrating how AI can serve as a potential adjunct to conventional laboratory testing.[8]

Key molecular biomarkers and imaging correlates

The 2016 WHO classification integrated molecular alterations with histology, establishing markers such as IDH mutation, 1p/19q codeletion, MGMT promoter methylation and epidermal growth factor receptor (EGFR) alterations as critical determinants of prognosis and therapy. Mutant IDH gliomas are associated with longer survival and distinct imaging phenotypes such as hypoenhancement, higher apparent diffusion coefficient (ADC) values and T2-FLAIR mismatch.[34] CNN-based models have achieved accuracies up to 99% AUC in predicting IDH mutation status using multiparametric MRI.[35] Emerging transformer-based architectures, such as the Swin Transformer, have further improved accuracy (AUC 0.965 internally), even without refined tumor segmentation.[36] MGMT promoter methylation is found in ~33–57% of gliomas; this marker predicts sensitivity to alkylating agents like temozolomide. Radiomic studies combining perfusion and conventional MRI have achieved prediction accuracies of 61–83%, while DL models have reported even higher accuracies (up to 95%) using only T2-weighted inputs.[34] EGFR alterations, especially the EGFRvIII splice variant, are detected in ~40% of glioblastomas. EGFR mutations are linked to aggressive phenotypes and deep peritumoral infiltration.[30,37,38] Radiomic classifiers using perfusion MRI and multiparametric features achieve 80–85% accuracy. 1p/19q codeletion is present in ~30% of lower-grade gliomas and defines oligodendroglioma when combined with IDH mutation. Imaging correlates include poorly circumscribed borders, left frontal predominance and heterogeneous signals. CNN approaches have predicted codeletion with accuracies up to 93%.[34]

Beyond these, AI has also been applied to rarer glioma subtypes and pediatric entities. For example, *BRAF* V600E and BRAF fusions in pediatric low-grade gliomas have been predicted from FLAIR-based radiomics with external validation AUCs up to 0.85, while H3 K27M mutations in diffuse midline gliomas have been identified with AUCs above 0.90.[39–41] These findings highlight the broadening scope of AI-enabled radiogenomics beyond common adult gliomas.

Emerging transformer-based architectures

Building on the success of CNNs and CapsNets, transformer-based architectures have recently emerged as a powerful approach for brain tumor segmentation. Leveraging self-attention mechanisms, these models can capture long-range dependencies within imaging data, enabling more precise delineation of complex tumor boundaries and heterogeneous regions. Transformer models such as SPP-U-Net, RMTF-Net and Swin Transformer have demonstrated superior performance compared to conventional CNN-based methods, not only in segmentation accuracy but also in predicting molecular characteristics like IDH mutation status.[36,42,43]

These models benefit from transfer learning and data augmentation strategies, which enhance robustness and efficiency even with limited training datasets. Additionally, unsupervised anomaly detection capabilities allow transformers to identify both pixel- and image-level outliers, potentially flagging atypical tumor regions without requiring labeled data. Collectively, these advancements position transformers as a versatile and high-performing tool, complementing existing CNN and CapsNet frameworks, and bridging the gap between image segmentation and molecular profiling in neuro-oncology.

Clinical implications of virtual biopsy

AI-enabled molecular profiling has the potential to transform neuro-oncology workflows by shortening diagnostic timelines, guiding risk stratification and informing treatment decisions even before invasive procedures. For example, non-invasive identification of MGMT promoter methylation can directly influence chemotherapy planning, while predicting IDH mutation status may inform prognosis and surgical strategy. In practice, AI outputs could be integrated into tumor board discussions, supporting multidisciplinary decision-making by providing rapid, objective and reproducible molecular insights. Virtual biopsy approaches are especially valuable in pediatric tumors and diffuse midline gliomas, where surgical sampling carries high risk, enabling timely and safer treatment planning without delaying clinical care.

ETHICAL DILEMMAS, CHALLENGES AND FUTURE OF AI IN NEURO-ONCOLOGY DIAGNOSTICS

The rapid integration of AI into neuro-oncology has raised profound ethical, technical and regulatory challenges. While the potential to improve diagnostic accuracy, streamline workflows and enable virtual biopsies is undeniable, the use of AI in such a high-stakes clinical domain brings new dilemmas that require scrutiny.

ETHICAL DILEMMAS IN AI-ASSISTED NEURO-ONCOLOGY

One of the most widely discussed ethical concerns is the opacity of DL systems, often described as the "black box problem." CNNs underpinning many AI tools make it difficult for clinicians to fully interpret or explain outputs to patients. This lack of transparency risks undermining the principles of informed consent, limiting opportunities for error detection, and raising liability questions when AI-assisted decisions lead to adverse outcomes.[44,45] Equally concerning is the potential erosion of clinician autonomy, as reliance on AI could weaken professional judgment and shift responsibility away from the physician.[45]

The prognostic applications of AI carry particularly heavy moral weight. Machine-generated survival predictions and treatment forecasts influence life-defining decisions, including end-of-life care planning. Errors in these outputs could lead to premature withdrawal of treatment or undue prolongation of suffering, especially when uncertainty is not adequately communicated to patients and families. These issues are compounded in neuro-oncology, where cognitive impairment is common, complicating consent and shared decision-making.[46]

Privacy is another pressing concern. AI systems in neuro-oncology often integrate multimodal datasets, including imaging, genomic and clinical information, all of which heightens the risk of re-identification. Balancing the need for large, diverse datasets against patient confidentiality requires robust governance frameworks that can ensure data security, regulate secondary use and protect vulnerable patient groups.[44]

Finally, questions of justice and equity arise when algorithms are trained on non-representative datasets. Underrepresentation of minority populations risks perpetuating existing disparities in CNS tumor outcomes, while unequal access to AI-enhanced care could deepen socioeconomic and geographic divides. Ensuring fairness requires deliberate bias mitigation strategies, systematic auditing and diverse dataset curation.[44]

Implementation challenges

Technical and logistical barriers also hinder clinical adoption. A major challenge lies in data heterogeneity; differences in imaging acquisition, annotation practices and pre-processing pipelines between institutions limit model generalizability. Similarly, most existing models perform well retrospectively but lack prospective validation or multi-institutional trials, creating uncertainty about real-world reliability.[47]

Clinical adoption further depends on workflow integration. Surveys of neuro-oncologists reveal concerns about overreliance, deskilling and disruptions to established practices. Without proper education and transparent communication of limitations, AI risks becoming a burden rather than a support in clinical workflows.[48]

Regulatory and governance considerations

Traditional regulatory pathways are poorly suited for adaptive AI systems that evolve after deployment. Current frameworks lack clear guidance on issues such as post-market surveillance, liability and continuous model updating. There is a growing consensus on the need for comprehensive governance frameworks, including institutional AI oversight committees, standardized documentation and accountability mechanisms.[45]

Patient autonomy and trust

AI adoption must respect and reinforce patient autonomy. This is especially challenging in neuro-oncology, where cognitive impairments often complicate consent. Tailored consent frameworks, surrogate decision-making protocols and transparent communication are essential. Above all, the physician–patient relationship must remain central, with AI positioned as a decision-support tool rather than a replacement for clinical judgment.[45]

BIAS, FAIRNESS AND ALGORITHMIC JUSTICE

Bias in AI reflects and amplifies existing disparities in healthcare. Historical inequities, underrepresentation in datasets and socioeconomic barriers to advanced imaging all contribute to biased outputs. Addressing these concerns requires diverse data collection, fairness-aware algorithm design, and mandatory subgroup performance reporting. Continuous monitoring after deployment is equally critical to ensure equitable care across populations.[44,49]

Future directions

Looking forward, several priorities emerge. First, explainable AI is crucial for fostering trust and accountability, allowing clinicians and patients to understand the reasoning behind outputs.[44,45] Second, data standardization and interoperability are needed to enable robust cross-institutional validation.[47] Third, rigorous prospective trials comparing AI-assisted with conventional decision-making will be essential to establish clinical utility.[45]

From an ethical standpoint, specialized consent frameworks for cognitively impaired patients, multidisciplinary ethics committees, and adaptive regulatory pathways will help balance innovation with patient protection. Education will also play a central role: clinicians require training to interpret AI responsibly, while patients and families need accessible resources to understand its role in their care.[50,51]

Research gaps

Despite rapid progress, significant gaps remain. Few studies address long-term outcomes of AI adoption, including its impact on clinical skills and healthcare systems. Implementation science approaches are underutilized, and patient perspectives, particularly among underrepresented groups, remain largely absent from current research. Addressing these gaps will be vital for safe and equitable deployment.

CONCLUSION

Integrating AI into neuro-oncology is both a game-changer and a serious ethical challenge. The tools are already delivering real clinical value: better tumor detection, classification and segmentation from MRI/CT/PET; improved image quality that speeds and sharpens pre-surgical planning; and AI-driven radiomics and radiogenomics that enable "virtual biopsy" for non-invasive molecular insights. When coupled with clinical decision support and tumor board integration, these systems reduce diagnostic timelines, provide objective risk signals and help tailor therapy to the individual patient.

To make these gains safe and durable, the path forward must be disciplined and patient-centered. That means multidisciplinary collaboration, prospective and multisite validation, continuous monitoring for bias and model drift, clear reporting and governance of data use and workflows that augment, and not replace, clinical judgment. If we keep equity, transparency and patient welfare at the core, AI can responsibly accelerate precision care in neuro-oncology.

REFERENCES

1. Al-Rahbi A, Al-Mahrouqi O, Al-Saadi T. Uses of artificial intelligence in glioma: A systematic review. *Med Int (Lond)* 2024; 4(4): 40.
2. Khalafallah AM. Quantifying the utility of a multidisciplinary neuro-oncology tumor board. *J Neurosurg* 2020; 135(1): 87–92.
3. Ibrahim M, Muhammad Q, Zamarud A, et al. Navigating glioblastoma diagnosis and care: Transformative pathway of artificial intelligence in integrative oncology. *Cureus* 2023; 15(8): e44214.
4. De Jesus O. Neurosurgical breakthroughs of the last 50 years: A historical journey through the past and present. *World Neurosurg* 2025; 196: 123816.
5. de la Garza-Salazar JG, Juarez-Sánchez P, Arrieta-Rodríguez O, et al. History of neuro-oncology: Towards a new frontier. In: Monroy-Sosa A, Chakravarthi SS, de la Garza-Salzar JG, et al. (eds). *Principles of Neuro-Oncology*. Cham: Springer; 2020, pp. 1–14.
6. Castillo M. History and evolution of brain tumor imaging: Insights through radiology. *Radiology* 2014; 273(2 Suppl): S111–25.
7. Miller J, Filipe L, McBrayer SK, et al. Isocitrate dehydrogenase (IDH) mutant gliomas: A Society for Neuro-Oncology (SNO) consensus review on diagnosis, management, and future directions. *Neuro Oncol* 2022; 25(1): 4–25.
8. Hollon T, Jiang C, Chowdury A, et al. Artificial-intelligence-based molecular classification of diffuse gliomas using rapid, label-free optical imaging. *Nat Med* 2023; 29(4): 828–32.
9. Moassefi M, Shahriar Faghani, Erickson B. Artificial intelligence in neuro-oncology: Predicting molecular markers and response to therapy. *Med Res Arch* 2024; 12(6).
10. Domingo JL, Semelka RC. Gadolinium toxicity: Mechanisms, clinical manifestations, and nanoparticle role. *Arch Toxicol* 2025; 99(10): 3897–916.
11. Semelka RC, Ramalho M. Gadolinium deposition disease: Current state of knowledge and expert opinion. *Investig Radiol* 2023; 58(8): 523–9.
12. Rafanan J, Ghani N, Kazemeini S, et al. Modernizing neuro-oncology: The impact of imaging, liquid biopsies, and AI on diagnosis and treatment. *Int J Mol Sci* 2025; 26(3): 917.
13. Villanueva-Meyer JE, Mabray MC, Cha S. Current clinical brain tumor imaging. *Neurosurgery* 2017; 81(3): 397–415.
14. García-Figueiras R, Baleato-González S, Padhani AR, et al. Advanced imaging of colorectal cancer: From anatomy to molecular imaging. *Insights Imaging* 2016; 7(3): 285–309.
15. Park JE. Artificial intelligence in neuro-oncologic imaging: A brief review for clinical use cases and future perspectives. *Brain Tumor Res Treat* 2022; 10(2): 69–75.
16. Rahimi S. Going beyond the brick: Assessing and supporting creativity using AI-powered digital games. *Creat Res J* 2023; 37: 275–83.
17. Chong PL, Vaigeshwari V, Mohammed Reyasudin BK, et al. Integrating artificial intelligence in healthcare: Applications, challenges, and future directions. *Future Sci OA* 2025; 11(1): 2527505.

18. Urooj F, Tameezuddin A, Khalid Z, et al. Use of artificial intelligence and radio genomics in neuroradiology and the future of brain tumour imaging and surgical planning in low- and middle-income countries. *J Pak Med Assoc* 2024; 74(3 (Supple 3): S51–S63.
19. Chukwujindu E, Faiz H, Al-Douri S, et al. Role of artificial intelligence in brain tumour imaging. *Eur J Radiol* 2024; 176: 111509.
20. Al-Kadi OS, Al-Emaryeen R, Al-Nahhas S, et al. Empowering brain cancer diagnosis: Harnessing artificial intelligence for advanced imaging insights. *Rev Neurosci* 2024; 35(4): 399–419.
21. Abdel Razek AAK, Alksas A, Shehata M, et al. Clinical applications of artificial intelligence and radiomics in neuro-oncology imaging. *Insights Imaging* 2021; 12(1): 152.
22. Lv C, Shu X-J, Chang H, et al. Classification of high-grade glioblastoma and single brain metastases using a new SCAT-inception model trained with MRI images. *Front Neurosci* 2024; 18: 1349781.
23. Blanc-Durand P, Van Der Gucht A, Schaefer N, et al. Automatic lesion detection and segmentation of 18F-FET PET in gliomas: A full 3D U-Net convolutional neural network study. *PLoS One* 2018; 13(4): e0195798.
24. Ortiz-Ramón R, Andrés Larroza, Ruiz-España S, et al. Classifying brain metastases by their primary site of origin using a radiomics approach based on texture analysis: A feasibility study. *Eur Radiol* 2018; 28(11): 4514–23.
25. Sabour S, Frosst N, Hinton GE. Dynamic routing between capsules. arXiv:1710.09829v2, 2017.
26. Wu S, Li H, Quang D, Guan Y. Three-plane-assembled deep learning segmentation of gliomas. *Radiol Artif Intell* 2020; 2(2): e190011.
27. Center for Biomedical Image Computing & Analytics. Brain Tumor Segmentation (BraTS) Challenge. Available from: https://www.med.upenn.edu/cbica/brats/ (Accessed April 2026).
28. Yae Won Park, Ji Eun Park, Sung Soo Ahn, et al. Deep learning-based metastasis detection in patients with lung cancer to enhance reproducibility and reduce workload in brain metastasis screening with MRI: A multi-center study. *Cancer Imaging* 2024; 24(1): 32.
29. Quon JL, Bala W, Chen LC, et al. Deep learning for pediatric posterior fossa tumor detection and classification: A multi-institutional study. *Am J Neuroradiol* 2020; 41(9): 1718–25.
30. Kickingereder P, Bonekamp D, Nowosielski M, et al. Radiogenomics of glioblastoma: Machine learning–based classification of molecular characteristics by using multiparametric and multiregional MR imaging features. *Radiology* 2016; 281: 907–18.
31. Shofty B, Artzi M, Ben Bashat D, et al. MRI radiomics analysis of molecular alterations in low-grade gliomas. *Int J Comput Assist Radiol Surg* 2018; 13(4): 563–71.
32. Ahmad M, Hassan M, Shafi I, Osman A. Classification of tumors in human brain MRI using wavelet and support vector machine. *IOSR J Comput Eng* 2012; 8: 25–31.
33. Kumar V, Gu Y, Basu S, et al. Radiomics: The process and the challenges. *Magn Reson Imaging* 2012; 30: 1234–48.
34. Rudie JD, Rauschecker AM, Bryan RN, et al. Emerging applications of artificial intelligence in neuro-oncology. *Radiology* 2019; 290(3): 607–18.
35. Patel SH, Poisson LM, Brat DJ, et al. T2-FLAIR mismatch, an imaging biomarker for IDH and 1p/19q status in lower-grade gliomas: A TCGA/ TCIA project. *Clin Cancer Res* 2017; 23(20): 6078–85.
36. Lan Y, Zou S, Qin B, Zhu X. Potential roles of transformers in brain tumor diagnosis and treatment. *Brain X* 2023; 1(2).
37. Heimberger AB, Hlatky R, Suki D, et al. Prognostic effect of epidermal growth factor receptor and EGFRvIII in glioblastoma multiforme patients. *Clin Cancer Res* 2005; 11(4): 1462–6.
38. Tykocinski ES, Grant RA, Kapoor GS, et al. Use of magnetic perfusion-weighted imaging to determine epidermal growth factor receptor variant III expression in glioblastoma. *Neuro Oncol* 2012; 14(5): 613–23.
39. Ahmed S, Elsayed I. Availability and affordability of PET tracers, the challenges and opportunities in developing countries. *Egypt J Nucl Med* 2022; 25: 1–7.

40. Weinberg BD, Kuruva M, Shim H, Mullins ME. Clinical applications of magnetic resonance spectroscopy (MRS) in of brain tumors: From diagnosis to treatment. *Radiol Clin N Am* 2021; 59: 349–62.
41. Douglas DB, Iv M, Douglas PK, et al. Diffusion tensor imaging of TBI: Potentials and challenges. *Top Magn Reson Imaging* 2015; 24: 241–51.
42. Pinaya WHL, Tudosiu PD, Gray R, et al. Unsupervised brain imaging 3D anomaly detection and segmentation with transformers. *Med Image Anal* 2022; 79: 102475.
43. Anaya-Isaza A, Mera-Jiménez L, Verdugo-Alejo L, Sarasti L. Optimizing MRI-based brain tumor classification and detection using AI: A comparative analysis of neural networks, transfer learning, data augmentation, and the cross-transformer network. *Eur J Radiol Open* 2023; 10: 100484.
44. Khalighi S, Reddy K, Midya A, et al. Artificial intelligence in neuro-oncology: Advances and challenges in brain tumor diagnosis, prognosis, and precision treatment. *NPJ Precis Oncol* 2024; 8(1): 80.
45. Khan AA, Ibad H, Ahmed KS, et al. Deep learning applications in neuro-oncology. *Surg Neurol Int* 2021; 12: 435.
46. Lissak IA, Edlow BL, Rosenthal E, Young MJ. Ethical considerations in neuroprognostication following acute brain injury. *Semin Neurol* 2023; 43(5): 758–67.
47. Li XT, Huang RY. Standardization of imaging methods for machine learning in neuro-oncology. *Neurooncol Adv* 2021; 2(Suppl 4): iv49–55.
48. Li M, Xiong X, Xu B, Dickson C. Chinese oncologists' perspectives on integrating AI into clinical practice: Cross-sectional survey study. *JMIR Form Res* 2024; 8: e53918.
49. Ienca M, Ignatiadis K. Artificial intelligence in clinical neuroscience: Methodological and ethical challenges. *AJOB Neurosci* 2020; 11(2): 77–87.
50. Singh R, Kassis G, Sbaih O, et al. Big data in neurosurgery: A guideline on data structures, machine learning models, and ethical considerations. *Oper Neurosurg* 2025; Online ahead of print.
51. Quinn TP, Coghlan S. Readying medical students for medical AI: The need to embed AI ethics education. arXiv:2109.02866v1, 2021.

7

Detection and Diagnosis of Cerebrovascular Lesions Using Artificial Intelligence

SIMON LEVINSON, HENK VAN VOORST AND JEREMY J. HEIT

INTRODUCTION

Cerebrovascular diseases pose a significant challenge to global health, contributing to high rates of morbidity and mortality. This chapter provides an overview of the ways in which Artificial Intelligence (AI) is transforming cerebrovascular diseases' diagnosis and reviews the relevant AI techniques most commonly employed in patients with cerebrovascular disease.

Objectives

The primary goal of this chapter is to establish a foundation for understanding the intersection of AI and cerebrovascular disease diagnostics.

- *Educational Foundation*: Provide readers with essential knowledge about cerebrovascular diseases and the significance of AI in modern medicine.
- *Contextual Framework*: Explore how AI technologies are applied in diagnosing and managing cerebrovascular conditions.

OVERVIEW OF CEREBROVASCULAR DISEASES

Cerebrovascular diseases encompass a range of medical conditions that affect the blood vessels and blood supply to the brain. Disruptions in cerebral blood flow can lead to serious neurological deficits and are a leading cause of long-term disability and death worldwide.

Definition and types

STROKE

A stroke occurs when the blood supply to part of the brain is interrupted or reduced, preventing brain tissue from getting oxygen and nutrients. Strokes are classified into two main types:

- *Ischemic*: Caused by narrowing or blockage in an artery that supplies blood to the brain. This form of stroke comprises approximately 85% of all types of strokes.
- *Hemorrhagic*: Occurs when a weakened blood vessel ruptures and bleeds into the brain or surrounding tissues. There are several common non-traumatic causes of hemorrhagic stroke.
  - *Hypertensive hemorrhage*: Caused by the rupture of a small artery due to acute or chronic hypertension.
  - *Aneurysms*: An aneurysm is a bulge or ballooning in a blood vessel wall, often occurring in arteries at the base of the brain. If an aneurysm ruptures, it can lead to a hemorrhagic stroke with the majority of the hemorrhage in the subarachnoid space that overlies the brain surface.

DOI: 10.1201/9781003471165-7

- *Arteriovenous malformations*: Arteriovenous malformations (AVMs) are abnormal tangles of blood vessels connecting arteries and veins, which disrupt normal blood flow and oxygen circulation. They can occur in the brain and increase the risk of bleeding or seizures.
- *Fistulae*: Fistulae of the dural or pial vessels can occur in the brain or spine and involve abnormal connections between arteries and veins and can result in bleeding.

EPIDEMIOLOGY AND CLINICAL SIGNIFICANCE

Cerebrovascular diseases are among the leading causes of death and disability globally. According to the World Health Organization (WHO), stroke is the second leading cause of death and the third leading cause of disability worldwide (as measured by disability adjusted life years, [DALY]) with a global annual cost of over $721 billion.[1–3] In the period 1990–2022, incidence has increased by 70% and there has been a 143% incidence in DALYs.[3] The high prevalence and increasing global health and economic burden of these conditions underscores the need for effective diagnostic tools and treatment strategies.[4]

THE ROLE OF AI IN CEREBROVASCULAR DIAGNOSTICS

AI is revolutionizing medicine. AI's ability to process large datasets and recognize complex patterns makes it an invaluable tool in modern practice. Particularly in cerebrovascular disease, with its high prevenance and morbidity, AI is already changing the way conditions are diagnosed and treated.

BOX 7.1 Ischemic stroke overview impact and risk factors

- *Global impact*: Millions of people suffer from strokes annually, with significant socioeconomic implications due to long-term care needs.
- *Risk factors*: Hypertension, diabetes, smoking and high cholesterol are common risk factors that contribute to the development of cerebrovascular diseases.[4]
- *Clinical challenges*: Early detection and accurate diagnosis are critical for improving patient outcomes, but traditional diagnostic methods can be time-consuming and may miss subtle abnormalities.[5]

BOX 7.2 Specific relevance to neurosurgery and cerebrovascular diagnostics

- *Enhanced imaging analysis*: AI algorithms can analyze medical images more quickly and accurately than traditional methods, detecting anomalies that may be overlooked by the human eye.[6–8]
- *Predictive modeling*: Machine learning (ML) models can predict patient outcomes, such as the likelihood of aneurysm rupture or stroke recurrence, facilitating proactive clinical decisions.[7]
- *Surgical planning*: AI assists neurosurgeons in planning complex procedures by simulating surgical approaches and predicting potential complications.[6,8,9]

FUNDAMENTALS OF AI IN DIAGNOSTICS OF CEREBROVASCULAR DISEASE

Key types of AI technologies revolutionizing disease diagnosis include ML, deep learning (DL), natural language processing (NLP), and computer vision. ML is a framework that can be optimized to execute a specific task without being explicitly programed to do so. (**Figure 7.1**). It works by generalizing from examples, making it effective where manual programming isn't feasible. The key to ML is combining three main components: representation (defining possible solutions), evaluation (measuring solution quality) and optimization (selecting the best solution). The approach allows for generalizations to be made from a training dataset.[10] DL refers to a subset of ML that is often based on neural networks with multiple layers that excels in interpreting complex medical imaging data, enhances diagnostic accuracy for conditions like cerebrovascular diseases by highlighting anomalies in MRI or CT scans. NLP allows AI systems to understand and interpret unstructured clinical notes and medical

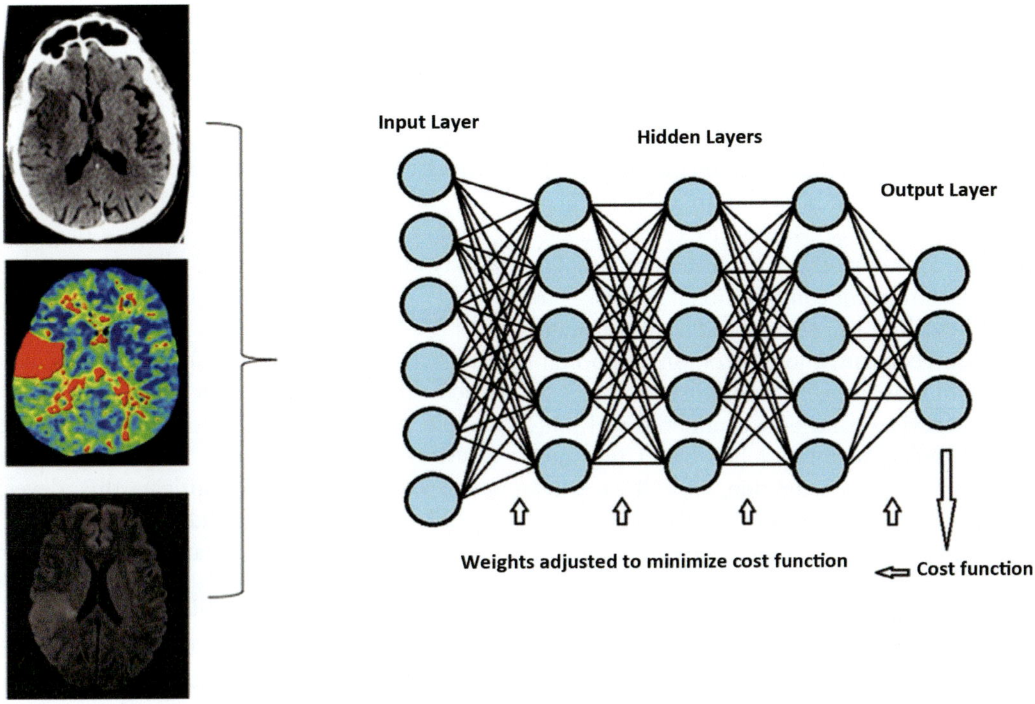

Figure 7.1 An illustration of artificial neural networks, a branch of machine learning. The input layer is the first layer, followed by a configurable number of hidden layers and an output layer. Each layer is made up of nodes or neurons. (Reproduced under Creative Commons License 4.0 from Pacchiano et. al., 2023.[27])

literature and extracts valuable information that can inform diagnosis and treatment plans. Computer vision enables the automated analysis of medical images and detects abnormalities with high precision and consistency. Together, these AI technologies enhance clinical decision-making, reduce diagnostic errors and contribute to more personalized and effective patient care.

Data sources for training AI models

Training AI models to diagnose cerebrovascular diseases relies heavily on the choice and quality of data sources, which profoundly affect model performance and generalizability. Potential data sources include medical imaging datasets, electronic health records (EHRs), clinical registries, genomic data and wearable device outputs. Each of these sources, while valuable, present specific challenges that must be managed to develop effective and ethical AI systems.

Medical imaging data—such as Magnetic Resonance imaging (MRI), computed tomography (CT), positron emission tomography (PET) and digital subtraction angiography (DSA)—are crucial for visualizing cerebrovascular structures and pathologies. These images can be obtained from public repositories such as the ISLES and MICCAI datasets or from hospital archives.[11] However, inconsistency in imaging protocols, machine settings and operator techniques can introduce variabilities. Annotation errors and incomplete data further compromise quality, which potentially misleads AI models if not addressed properly.

EHRs offer a wealth of information, including unstructured clinical notes, structured lab results, medication records, vital signs and demographic data. Despite their richness, EHRs often suffer from inconsistencies, missing values, erroneous data entry and potential biases due to overrepresentation of certain populations. Privacy regulations such as the Health Insurance Portability and Accountability Act (HIPAA) and General Data Protection Regulation (GDPR) also limit access to patient data, making it challenging to compile large, diverse datasets necessary for robust AI training.

Clinical registries and cohort studies, such as stroke registries and longitudinal research studies, like the Framingham Heart Study, provide standardized and often high-quality data over extended periods. While valuable for predictive modeling, these sources may not fully represent the general population and can be subject to the same access limitations as EHRs.

Genomic and biomarker data, including genetic profiles and proteomic information, offer insights into individual predispositions to cerebrovascular diseases. However, these datasets are complex and require significant computational resources to process. They also raise ethical and legal considerations around consent, anonymization and potential misuse of sensitive genetic information.

Wearable devices contribute continuous real-time data on physiological metrics like blood pressure, heart rate and oxygen saturation, as well as activity levels relevant to stroke recovery and prevention. Integrating this data with traditional medical sources poses technical challenges due to differences in data formats and scales. Additionally, standardization issues can complicate data aggregation and analysis.

Bias and lack of representativeness are significant pitfalls across all data sources. Overrepresentation of specific demographic groups—such as adults over children, males over females, or certain ethnicities—can result in AI models that do not generalize well to broader populations.[12–14] Data from tertiary care centers might not reflect cases seen in primary care or rural settings. Imbalanced datasets, particularly concerning rare conditions like AVMs, can lead models to become biased toward more prevalent diseases, reducing sensitivity to less common but clinically significant conditions.[15]

AI model development is complicated by technical challenges such as high-computational resource demands from large datasets and the risk of overfitting when trained on limited or non-representative data, which can undermine clinical utility. Ethical concerns like patient privacy and issues of model generalizability and bias also need to be addressed. To mitigate these issues, data augmentation and synthesis techniques can balance datasets by increasing training examples for underrepresented classes. Cross-institutional collaborations enhance data diversity and share the burden of data annotation. Federated learning enables models to be trained across multiple sites without sharing raw data, reducing privacy concerns. Adhering to standardized data collection and annotation protocols decreases variability and facilitates multimodal data integration.

AI model development

Developing and validating AI models that accurately diagnose cerebrovascular diseases involves complex challenges that must be carefully addressed to ensure their effectiveness, reliability and ethical deployment in clinical settings. Three primary issues are overfitting, lack of generalizability and transparency.

OVERFITTING

This occurs when a model is over optimized for a specific training dataset that results in excellent in-sample performance but poor generalizability in external datasets, resulting in poor performance on new, unseen data. To mitigate this, developers should employ robust validation techniques like cross-validation and use separate testing datasets.[6,16]

LACK OF GENERALIZABILITY

Lack of generalizability arises when AI models trained on data from specific demographics or single institutions fail to perform adequately across diverse patient populations due to variations in genetic backgrounds, lifestyle factors, imaging protocols and disease prevalence. Ensuring diversity in training data and using fairness-aware ML techniques can promote equity and improve model performance across different groups.

TRANSPARENCY AND INTERPRETABILITY

Transparency and interpretability are also critical; many AI models function as "black boxes," that hinder trust by physicians and other medical providers. Incorporating interpretable algorithms or explainability techniques, such as attention maps in imaging analysis, can enhance transparency and allow physicians to understand and verify AI-generated conclusions.[17,18]

Integrating AI models into existing clinical workflows has practical hurdles. The AI system must be compatible with hospital information systems and imaging equipment, and requires collaboration between software developers, IT professionals and clinical staff (*see* "Applications of AI"). Training physicians to effectively use AI tools and interpret their outputs is essential to ensure these technologies augment clinical decision-making without adding complexity or significant time burdens. Additionally, AI models intended for clinical use must undergo rigorous evaluation by regulatory bodies like the US Food and Drug Administration (FDA) or the European Medicines Agency (EMA), and demonstrate safety, efficacy and reliability through clinical trials and extensive testing.

Evaluating the performance of AI models necessitates careful selection of metrics that reflect both accuracy and clinical utility. While traditional metrics such as accuracy, sensitivity and specificity provide a foundational understanding, metrics such as positive predictive value (PPV) and negative predictive value (NPV) offer direct insight into the model's practical implications in patient care. Balancing sensitivity with PPV ensures the AI model delivers reliable and actionable results. In cases of class imbalance, common in medical datasets, the area under the precision-recall curve (AUC-PR) becomes more informative than the area under the receiver operating curve (AUROC).[19,20] By thoroughly addressing these challenges, researchers and physicians can develop robust, trustworthy AI tools that enhance the diagnosis and management of cerebrovascular diseases and ultimately improve patient outcomes while aligning with ethical and clinical standards.

APPLICATIONS OF AI IN CEREBROVASCULAR DIAGNOSTICS

Advancements in **computer vision models** have profoundly impacted neuroradiology by enhancing the analysis and interpretation of complex brain imaging data. **Classification models** such as Visual Geometry Group (VGG), Residual Network (ResNet) and DenseNet have been pivotal in identifying patterns associated with cerebrovascular diseases. For example, ResNet's deep residual learning framework allows for the training of very deep neural networks by mitigating the vanishing gradient problem and enabling detection of subtle anomalies in imaging data that might be overlooked by the human eye. DenseNet further improves feature propagation and reduces redundancy by connecting each layer to every other layer in a feed-forward fashion, enhancing diagnostic precision.

Segmentation models like U-Net and its successor nnU-Net have revolutionized image segmentation tasks in medical imaging. U-Net's encoder-decoder architecture is specifically designed for biomedical image segmentation, which allows for precise delineation of anatomic structures and pathologic regions such as ischemic lesions or aneurysms. nnU-Net extends this by automatically configuring itself to adapt to any given dataset without manual intervention, streamlining the segmentation process and reducing the need for extensive parameter tuning.[11,21] This automation accelerates workflow efficiency and consistency in image analysis.

The introduction of **transformer-based models** like the vision transformer (ViT) has opened new horizons in medical image analysis. Originally developed for NLP, transformers have been adapted to capture long-range dependencies in image data, providing a global context that enhances pattern recognition. For neuroradiologists, transformer models facilitate more comprehensive image assessments by effectively integrating information across the entire image, which is particularly beneficial in detecting diffuse or complex cerebrovascular pathologies.[22,23]

Collectively, these advanced computer vision models have significantly augmented the capabilities of neuroradiologists. They enhance diagnostic accuracy by providing quantitative analyses and highlighting regions of interest, reduce interpretation time through automation and enable the handling of large volumes of imaging data with consistency and precision, ultimately improving patient outcomes in the diagnosis and management of cerebrovascular diseases.

Clinical and technical limitations

Studies have underscored several challenges in translating AI into effective clinical practice.[30,31] False positives and negatives remain a concern, particularly when detecting subtle ischemic changes. In Wardlaw's review, the sensitivity for ischemia detection across various AI platforms ranged from 44% to 83%, with specificity from 57% to 93%. For large vessel occlusion (LVO) detection, sensitivities varied from 80% to 96%, and specificities from 90% to 98%, depending on imaging quality and patient factors.[30] AI's sensitivity to variables such as scan quality and head movement may limit its reliability, suggesting the need for rigorous testing standards and validation in diverse clinical settings.

DIAGNOSIS OF OTHER CEREBROVASCULAR LESIONS

Recent advancements in AI have demonstrated significant potential for enhancing the detection of intracranial aneurysms, particularly with DL on

CASE STUDY 7.1: STROKE DIAGNOSIS

A 72-year old woman is found by her husband at 8 AM with difficulty speaking and right-sided weakness. Emergency services suspect a stroke on arrival and the patient is brought to the CT scanner on arrival to the Emergency Department. Her National Institutes of Health Stroke Score (NIHSS) is 21 and she is noted to have no movement of her right leg or arm, slurred speech and drooping of the right face. The CT scan demonstrates a left-sided stroke in the middle cerebral artery. The reviewing neuroradiologist uses perfusion metrics that are automatically processed and analyzed by RapidAI™ to determine the ischemic core and penumbra sizes. The patient is deemed to have a favorable score to penumbra ratio (**Figure 7.2**), which allows her to be immediately taken to the neurointerventional radiology suite where a neurointerventional surgeon removes the clot and the arteries are noted to be patent at the end of the procedure. Over the next several days, she regains near complete function of her right side and her speech continues to improve. She is discharged to a rehab facility where she is expected to make an excellent recovery.

AI has become an integral part of stroke diagnosis and management, offering tools that enhance speed, accuracy and efficiency in clinical decision-making. Stroke, being a time-sensitive medical emergency with a complex decision-making algorithm, benefits from AI technologies that expedite the diagnostic process, help minimize missed cases and facilitate prompt treatment. Multiple companies have developed AI solutions that assist healthcare professionals in identifying stroke types, assessing severity and determining the most appropriate interventions.

RapidAI[24,25] is one of the leading platforms in this domain. Utilizing advanced algorithms, RapidAI analyzes imaging data from CT scans and MRIs to quickly detect signs of ischemic stroke

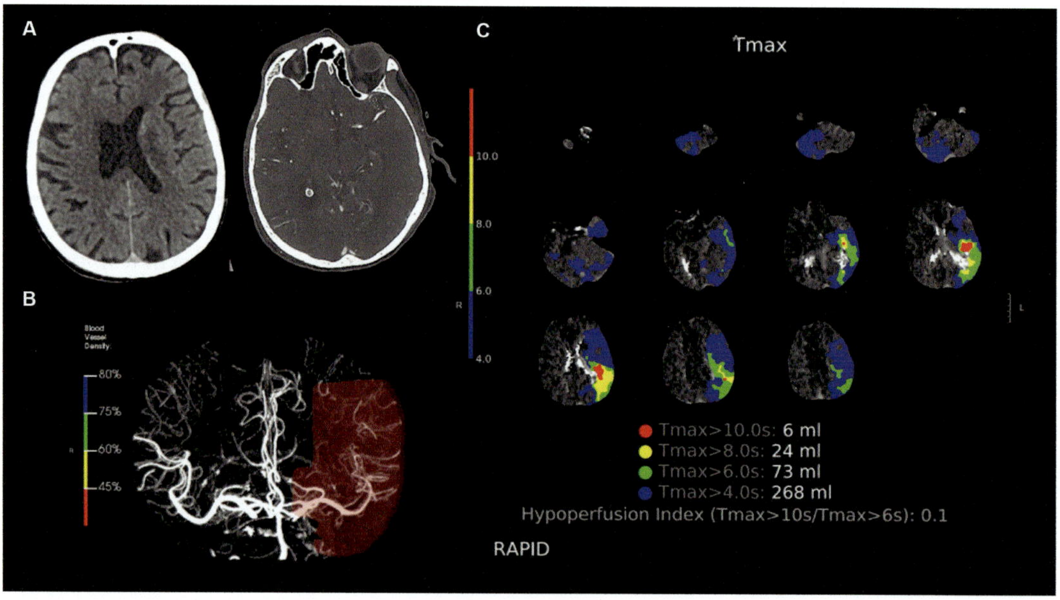

Figure 7.2 Representative case. Panel A demonstrates a non-contrast CT scan on the left and a CT angiography examination on the right demonstrating a clot on the distal left M1 segment of the middle cerebral artery. Panel B is a analysis performed by the automated software RapidAI™ highlighting an area of relative vessel hypodensity, indicating decreased blood flow. Panel C demonstrates aggregate time-to-maximum (T max) perfusion measurements indicating slow flow in the MCA territory. Together, these findings are consistent with an infarct in the distal left M1 vessel and the patient was treated with mechanical thrombectomy.

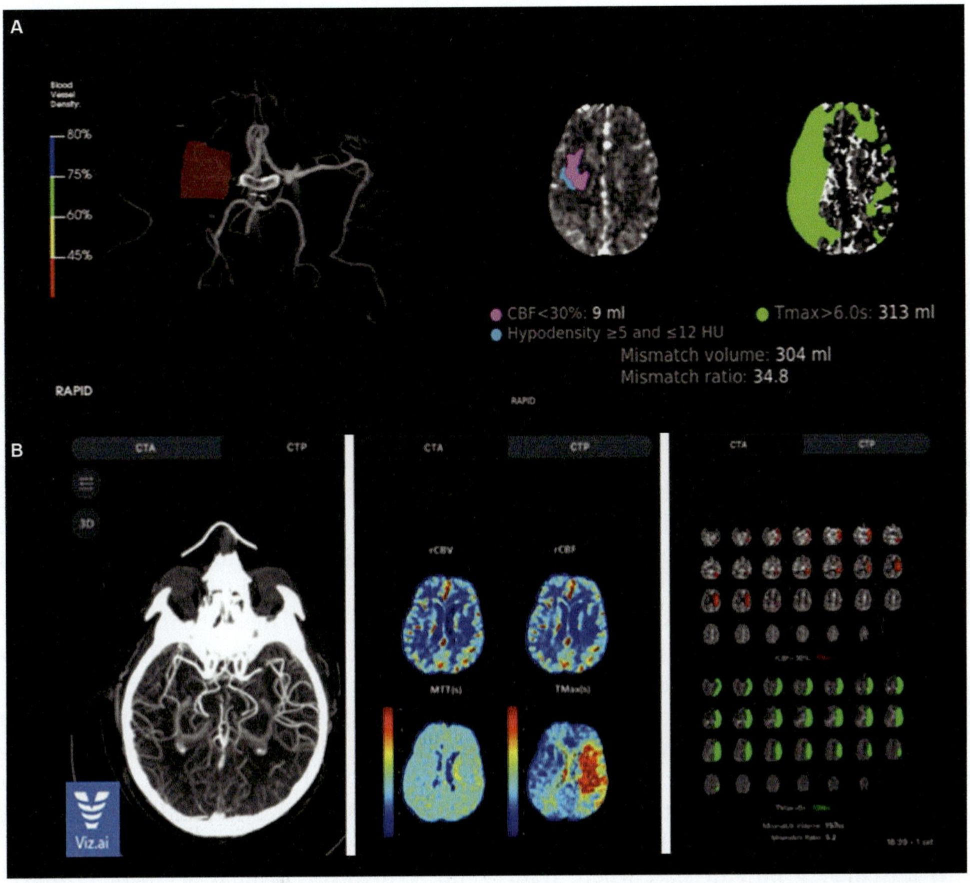

Figure 7.3 Example of ischemic stroke rendered in two AI software packages. In Panel A, processing performed by RAPID-LVO software showing flow reduction (vessel density < 45% in right M1); RAPID software also calculates CBF and T max for volume and mismatch ratio, crucial for endovascular treatment planning. Panel B shows an example of Viz.ai data processing; in this case, LVO is detected and software automatically alerts the stroke team. (Reproduced under Creative Commons licenses 4.0 from Pacchiano et. al., 2023.[27])

and hemorrhage. The software provides automated assessments of brain perfusion and tissue viability, highlighting areas with reduced blood flow that may still be salvageable. By delivering rapid and precise imaging analyses, RapidAI enables clinicians to make timely decisions regarding reperfusion therapies such as thrombectomy or thrombolysis and provides a communication platform for the team (**Case Study 7.1**, **Figures 7.2** and **7.3**). Other products, such as Rapid ASPECTS seeks to identify an Alberta Stroke Program Early CT Score (ASPECTS) score through an ML algorithm to help with treatment eligibility decisions. Last, RAPID ICH (intracerebral hemorrhage) can analyze non-contrast CT scans to identify possible intracranial hemorrhage using a validated AI algorithm.

Another example is Viz.ai,[26,27] which offers an AI-powered platform designed to synchronize stroke care. Viz.ai's software employs deep learning algorithms to analyze CT angiography images and automatically detect large vessel occlusions (LVOs). Similarly, the system alerts the stroke team, reducing the time between imaging and treatment initiation (**Figure 7.3**). This rapid notification system is crucial in time-sensitive scenarios where every minute counts. Viz.ai's platform also includes communication tools that allow team members to share images and consult in real time, enhancing collaborative decision-making (*see* **Figure 7.2**).

Aidoc[28] and Avicenna.AI[29] are two other companies focusing on detecting intracranial hemorrhages and occlusions, prioritizing cases needing urgent attention using pattern recognition and ML.

In addition to these companies, ongoing research and development in AI models—such as convolutional neural networks (CNNs) and transformer architectures—continue to enhance the field. For example, advanced computer vision models like **U-Net** for image segmentation and ResNet for image classification have been instrumental in improving the accuracy of stroke detection algorithms. These models enable precise delineation of stroke lesions and facilitate the differentiation between types of stroke, which is essential for effective treatment planning.

CT angiography (CTA) images. A study involving a large multicenter dataset from China introduced a CTA-based AI model, developed to assist clinicians in accurately identifying aneurysms.[32,33] The AI model exhibited a sensitivity of 95.7%, surpassing the diagnostic performance of clinicians alone, whose sensitivity reached only 65.8% on average. Additionally, the AI model demonstrated high patient-level and lesion-level accuracy, with clinicians showing improved diagnostic performance when assisted by AI (AUC 0.878 vs 0.795 without AI). By acting as a "second reader," the model effectively reduced missed cases, particularly for smaller aneurysms less than 5 mm in size, where traditional CTA interpretation often falls short.[33,34] This AI assistance not only boosted diagnostic sensitivity but also decreased reading times and facilitated adoption among clinicians, with a 92.6% acceptance rate in real-world applications. Implementing AI as a supplemental diagnostic tool thus offers substantial promise for both improving detection rates of intracranial aneurysms and minimizing the risk of life-threatening complications like subarachnoid hemorrhage.

AI applications in cerebrovascular imaging extend beyond aneurysm detection, offering innovative solutions across detection, prediction and treatment planning for other cerebrovascular diseases. For instance, AI models support early detection and segmentation of AVMs, leveraging methods such as skeletonization and fuzzy clustering to enhance visualization of complex vascular structures.[35] In predicting rupture risks and other outcomes, ML algorithms incorporate hemodynamic, morphological and clinical data, aiding in identifying high-risk patients and informing personalized treatment plans.[36] Additionally, AI techniques have been developed to assist in real-time procedural guidance, like catheter tracking during endovascular treatments, significantly reducing procedural time and complexity for physicians.[37] Few of these techniques have yet made a significant impact on clinical practice when compared to stroke given the lower prevalence of these diseases and more complex AI processing needed.

AI technologies have also attempted to be applied to intracranial hemorrhage (ICH) diagnosis, to enable earlier detection and more accurate assessment of hematoma volume.[24] Traditional ICH diagnosis involves manual segmentation techniques, which are time-consuming and can delay intervention. AI models, particularly CNNs, address this by automating detection and quantification of hematomas directly from non-contrast CT (NCCT) scans, allowing for rapid volume calculations that align closely with manual estimates.[38]

These models can detect various ICH subtypes—including subarachnoid, intraventricular and subdural hemorrhages—as well as associated features like hematoma expansion (HE), a critical prognostic indicator that typically increases morbidity risk. However, in a recent study assessing the effectiveness of a system designed to detect ICH to support a tele radiology practice, over 50,000 CT scans were reviewed. It was found there was actually an *increase* in radiologist time to review scans overall due to increased length of time to review falsely positive scans (4465/56745 CT scans were false positives), underscoring that not all systems will be effective during their initial implementation and may, in fact, cause more work or delays than a non-AI-enhanced system.[39]

Overall, many efforts are being made to aid in the diagnosis of cerebrovascular lesion with AI. Care and careful study need to be undertaken though to ensure these systems are providing a direct benefit to providers, patients and the healthcare system.

AI for cerebrovascular surgery

While ML techniques hold great potential for cerebrovascular diagnosis as discussed, there are also potential use for cases in the operating room (OR).

Microvascular anastomosis, a complex and skill-intensive surgical procedure, poses a considerable clinical challenge, requiring extensive practice, commitment and resilience to master. To better understand this technique, Gonzalez-Romo et al. analyzed hand motion during microvascular anastomosis using a CNN to track 21 hand positions. This study involved six participants—two experts, two intermediates and two novices—who performed the procedure without any restrictions on their hand movements and it was aimed at improving trainee education but could, one day, be used to train more advanced models to assist surgeons intraoperatively.[8,40]

Robotic-assisted procedures are not common in open cerebrovascular surgery but are widely used in other surgical subspecialities. Future AI systems could learn from surgical videos and other inputs to train robotic surgical tools or provide real-time feedback to surgeons while operating.

FUTURE DIRECTIONS IN AI FOR CEREBROVASCULAR DIAGNOSIS

Advancements in AI continue to reshape the landscape of cerebrovascular diagnostics. This section explores future directions in AI technologies, the expansion of data sources, collaborative efforts, standardization and potential innovations that may further enhance diagnosis and treatment in cerebrovascular diseases.

Trends and advancement in AI technologies

EXPLAINABLE AI AND INTERPRETABILITY

As AI models grow more complex, the need for explainable AI (XAI) becomes crucial, especially in medicine where understanding a model's predictions is vital for clinical trust. XAI aims to make AI decisions transparent to clinicians using techniques like saliency maps, attention mechanisms and model-agnostic methods such as local interpretable model-agnostic explanations (LIME) and SHapley Additive exPlanations (SHAPs). By revealing features influencing diagnoses, XAI might enhance collaboration between AI systems and healthcare professionals, ensuring AI supports rather than obscures clinical decision-making. Explainability in medical AI may also result in faster clinical uptake, as physicians will be more likely to use an AI model that can clearly explain how it comes to its conclusions. From a medicolegal liability standpoint, XAI might have benefits if incorrect judgments are made. Clear regulatory frameworks are required that specify who is responsible and what are acceptable and unacceptable errors.

TRANSFER LEARNING

Transfer learning entails the fine-tuning of pre-trained models to new tasks with limited additional training. By leveraging models trained on large datasets such as ImageNet or large medical imaging databases, AI systems can apply learned features to cerebrovascular diagnostics, especially when domain-specific data are scarce. By building on established models' rich features, fewer labeled training data are required to achieve high performance. Transfer learning has been successful in medical imaging and will continue to play a significant role in AI advancements for cerebrovascular disease diagnosis. However, it remains challenging to find the optimal (supervised) training task and dataset to develop the most appropriate model to use for transfer learning.

ALTERNATIVE SUPERVISION TECHNIQUES AND FOUNDATION MODELS

Scarcity of labeled medical data challenges AI training. Unsupervised and self-supervised learning allow models to learn from unlabeled data by capturing underlying patterns from simulated transformations and can, therefore, use much more data during training which can lead to better representation of image features in models. Initial self-supervised techniques for computer vision models (contrastive learning) relied on the ability of DL models to correct transformation of images such as rotation and cropping. Nowadays, large language models (LLMs) are often used to extract complex text embeddings from radiological reports. These text embeddings are subsequently deployed to train models using the corresponding images. The considerable scalability of these image-to-text models and performance gain for various tasks has resulted in the frequent use of the term "foundation model." Foundation models, in turn, can be used in a transfer learning setting where additional supervised fine-tuning is used, or in a setting where few or zero-shot learning techniques are used to directly make predictions. Although several 2D medical imaging foundation models exist, 3D models representing the entire brain have yet to be developed or be made available to the public. In cerebrovascular diagnostics, such techniques can produce robust models that detect rare conditions or adapt to new imaging modalities with limited supervision; they are also able to perform tasks such as image segmentation and quantitively analyzing images.

CHALLENGES IN DOMAIN AND TASK ADAPTATION

Common issues of AI models in medicine are the overemphasis on easy to predict cases and therefore an underrepresentation and poorer performance for rare and more challenging cases. As a result, many AI models are good at predicting the obvious but have, besides automation of certain tasks, only a limited added value to evaluation by a clinician. Whereas a first improvement would be to fine-tune models using transfer learning, this might lead to "catastrophic forgetting"; after fine-tuning, the performance for the initial easier cases might drop considerably and could therefore underperform for the initial task. Alternative weighted data sampling techniques during training have been proposed to negate these issues. Active learning and hard example mining optimize model performance while reducing annotation efforts. In active learning, models request expert annotations on uncertain cases, making labeling more efficient by focusing on informative samples. Hard example mining adapts the training to focus on uncertain cases, enhancing its ability to handle challenging diagnostics. These techniques can produce more accurate, generalizable AI models in cerebrovascular diagnostics, even with limited annotated data.

MACHINE LEARNING OPERATIONS

Machine learning operations (MLOps) is becoming increasingly important in healthcare, though not yet widely adopted. MLOps involves practices and tools for deploying, monitoring and maintaining ML models in production. Implementing MLOps ensures AI models in cerebrovascular diagnostics are up to date, reliable and perform optimally, including automating workflows and managing data pipelines. As AI integrates into clinical settings, adopting MLOps will be essential to sustain AI benefits over time.

Expansion of data sources

INCORPORATION OF REAL-TIME DATA AND WEARABLE DEVICES

Integrating real-time data from wearable devices enhances cerebrovascular diagnostics by providing continuous monitoring of physiological parameters like blood pressure, heart rate and oxygen saturation. These data streams feed into AI models, enabling reinforcement learning where models adapt based on ongoing inputs and outcomes. This approach allows for early detection of cerebrovascular events, personalized risk assessments and timely interventions. However, challenges such as data quality, patient privacy and integrating wearable data into existing healthcare systems must be addressed.

LARGER AND MORE DIVERSE DATASETS

Access to larger and more diverse datasets is crucial for developing AI models that generalize well across different populations. Compiling extensive imaging databases and clinical repositories enhances model robustness and reduces biases. Techniques like data augmentation and synthetic data generation can further expand training datasets, allowing models to learn from a wider variety of cases. Nonetheless, assembling and sharing large datasets involve navigating complex legal and ethical considerations, especially regarding patient privacy and data protection regulations.

In addition, many pathologies that physicians are interested in have a low incidence, but potentially severe implications if not correctly identified. Therefore, training models on highly homogenous datasets may make these rare or challenging cases more difficult to diagnosis. One way to address this is to underweigh routine high-incidence cases and overweigh the lower-incidence, more complex cases in model training, thus emphasizing the variability in the dataset.[41] Furthermore, extensive validation can warrant safe and reliable use of AI in cerebrovascular care.

EXPANDING COLLABORATION

Advancing AI in cerebrovascular diagnostics necessitates collaboration across institutions to pool resources, expertise and data, overcoming the limitations of single-center studies and producing more generalizable models. Legal and regulatory barriers like patient privacy laws pose challenges to data sharing. However, secure cloud solutions from providers such as Amazon Web Services (AWS), Google and Microsoft offer compliant environments for collaboration. For example, Microsoft Azure has clearance in Europe to handle high-risk Protected Health Information in ML applications. Despite their availability, these platforms are often underutilized in the medical community. Increasing awareness of these secure tools can facilitate broader collaborations while ensuring compliance with data protection regulations.

Developing standardized protocols and benchmarks is crucial for the consistent development and evaluation of AI models. Standardization streamlines data collection, annotation and reporting processes, enabling accurate comparisons between different models and studies. Yet, variability in clinical practices, equipment and patient populations makes achieving standardization challenging. An alternative approach is to develop adaptable AI techniques that can be validated across diverse settings. By focusing on the robustness and flexibility of models rather than rigid standards, the medical community can advance AI applications that accommodate real-world complexities.

Future innovations in cerebrovascular diagnostics

Predictive modeling using AI holds promise for shifting from reactive diagnostics to proactive prevention of cerebrovascular diseases. By analyzing comprehensive datasets—including genetic information, lifestyle factors and environmental exposures—AI models can identify individuals at high risk for conditions like stroke or aneurysm formation, potentially improving public health.

AI can also inform and optimize therapeutic interventions for cerebrovascular diseases. For instance, AI can help determine whether an aneurysm patient would benefit more from an endovascular procedure or medical management. Additionally, AI-driven simulations and virtual reality (VR) tools can enhance surgical planning and training, improving precision and reducing the risk of complications.

Techniques such as supervised learning have been used as the first step to developing useful AI applications and newer models are now often trained with unsupervised methods. When combined with more robust datasets, these may support models that can be adaptable to specific tasks while also still able to generalize across a wide range of cases.

It is essential to have methods to accurately assess an AI model's real-world impact. Reader studies as well as retrospective and prospective clinical evaluation of AI models can help determine when AI models are effectively performing their intended function. While AI has shown impressive capabilities in controlled settings and in its initial wide deployment to aid in the detection of ischemic stroke, it remains uncertain if AI applications can enhance medical decision-making, the diagnostic process or improve patient outcomes. Reader studies can give a first insight into when an AI application might provide added value to the diagnostic process or when it fails. Retrospective cohorts or clinical trials might be considered to evaluate if AI applications can be used to accurately estimate imaging markers associated with certain outcomes or with the benefit of a specific treatment. Insights from such reader studies and retrospective clinical studies can be used to design prospective studies. Prospective studies and clinical trials are necessary to validate AI tools, identify their strengths and limitations and ensure they contribute positively to clinical outcomes. Integrating AI into treatment decisions requires careful consideration to complement, not replace, clinicians' expertise. Designing AI systems with user-centric interfaces and providing training programs can promote effective collaboration between humans and machines, preventing overreliance on AI outputs and unintended consequences in patient care.

CONCLUSION

In summary, the future of AI in cerebrovascular diagnosis is poised to bring significant advancements that enhance patient care. Embracing XAI, leveraging new learning paradigms, integrating multimodal data and fostering collaborative efforts are essential steps toward realizing this potential. Addressing challenges related to data availability, standardization and ethical considerations will be critical in ensuring that AI technologies are developed responsibly and effectively. Ultimately, through careful innovation and evaluation, AI can play a transformative role in the prevention, diagnosis and treatment of cerebrovascular diseases, leading to improved outcomes for patients worldwide.

REFERENCES

1. World Health Organization. *Neurological Disorders: Public Health Challenges.* Geneva: World Health Organization; 2006.
2. Thomas H, Diamond J, Vieco A, et al. Global atlas of cardiovascular disease 2000–2016: The path to prevention and control. *Glob Heart* 2018; 13: 143–63.
3. Feigin VL, Brainin M, Norrving B, et al. World Stroke Organization (WSO): Global stroke fact sheet 2022. *Int J Stroke* 2022; 17: 18–29.
4. Cowen L (ed). *Stroke: Pathophysiology, Diagnosis, and Management.* Philadelphia: Elsevier; 2022.
5. Hankey GJ, Macleod M, Chen C, et al. (eds). *Warlow's Stroke: Practical Management.* Hoboken: Wiley-Blackwell; 2019.
6. Awuah WA, Adebusoye FT, Wellington J, et al. Recent outcomes and challenges of artificial intelligence, machine learning, and deep learning in neurosurgery. *World Neurosurg X* 2024; 23: 100301.
7. Fiani B, Pasko KBD, Sarhadi K, Covarrubias C. Current uses, emerging applications, and clinical integration of artificial intelligence in neuroradiology. *Rev Neurosci* 2022; 33: 383–95.
8. Tangsrivimol JA, Schonfeld E, Zhang M, et al. Artificial intelligence in neurosurgery: A state-of-the-art review from past to future. *Diagnostics (Basel)* 2023; 13: 2429.
9. Bravo J, Wali AR, Hirshman BR, et al. Robotics and artificial intelligence in endovascular neurosurgery. *Cureus* 2022; 14: e23662.
10. Ghaffar Nia N, Kaplanoglu E, Nasab A. Evaluation of artificial intelligence techniques in disease diagnosis and prediction. *Discov Artif Intell* 2023; 3: 5.
11. Hernandez Petzsche MR, de la Rosa E, Hanning U, et al. ISLES 2022: A multi-center magnetic resonance imaging stroke lesion segmentation dataset. *Sci Data* 2022; 9: 762.
12. Noseworthy PA, Attia ZI, Brewer LPC, et al. Assessing and mitigating bias in medical artificial intelligence. *Circ Arrhythm Electrophysiol* 2020; 13(3): e007988.
13. Straw, I. The automation of bias in medical Artificial Intelligence (AI): Decoding the past to create a better future. *Artif Intell Med* 2020; 110: 101965.
14. Mittermaier M, Raza MM, Kvedar JC. Bias in AI-based models for medical applications: challenges and mitigation strategies. *NPJ Digit Med* 2023; 6(1): 113.
15. Tejani AS, Ng YS, Xi Y, Rayan JC. Understanding and mitigating bias in imaging artificial intelligence. *Radiographics* 2024; 44: e230067.
16. Charilaou P, Battat, R. Machine learning models and over-fitting considerations. *World J Gastroenterol* 2022; 28: 605–7.
17. Changhez J, James S, Jamala F, et al. Evaluating the efficacy and accuracy of AI-assisted diagnostic techniques in endometrial carcinoma: A systematic review. *Cureus* 2024; 16: e60973.
18. Kaczmarczyk R, Wilhelm TI, Martin R, Roos J. Evaluating multimodal AI in medical diagnostics. *NPJ Digit Med* 2024; 7: 1–5.
19. Park SH, Han K. Methodologic guide for evaluating clinical performance and effect of artificial intelligence technology for medical diagnosis and prediction. *Radiology* 2018; 286: 800–9.
20. Varoquaux G, Cheplygina V. Machine learning for medical imaging: Methodological failures and recommendations for the future. *NPJ Digit Med* 2022; 5: 1–8.
21. Abbasi H, Orouskhani M, Asgari S, Zadeh SS. Automatic brain ischemic stroke segmentation with deep learning: A review. *Neurosci Inform* 2023; 3: 100145.
22. Al-hammuri K, Gebali F, Kanan A, Chelvan IT. Vision transformer architecture and applications in digital health: A tutorial and survey. *Vis Comput Ind Biomed Art* 2023; 6(1): 14.
23. Shamshad F, Khan S, Zamir SW, et al. Transformers in medical imaging: A survey. *Med Image Anal* 2023; 88: 102802.

24. Heit JJ, Honce JM, Yedavalli VS, et al. RAPID aneurysm: Artificial intelligence for unruptured cerebral aneurysm detection on CT angiography. *Radiology* 2022; 31(10): 106690.
25. Rapid AI. Aneurysm, pulmonary embolism and stroke software platform powered by AI. Available from: https://www.rapidai.com (Accessed April 2026).
26. Viz.ai. AI-Powered Care Coordination. Viz.ai, the Proven AI-Powered Care Coordination Platform. Available from: https://www.viz.ai/ (Accessed April 2026).
27. Pacchiano F, Tortora M, Criscuolo S, et al. Artificial intelligence applied in acute ischemic stroke: From child to elderly. *Radiol Med* 2023; 129: 83–92.
28. Aidoc. Clinical AI Company. Rapid Responses, Smarter Care. Available from: https://www.aidoc.com/ (Accessed April 2026).
29. Avicenna. Empowering Radiology With AI-based Tools. Available from: https://avicenna.ai/ (Accessed April 2026).
30. Wardlaw JM, Mair G, von Kummer R, et al. Accuracy of automated computer-aided diagnosis for stroke imaging: A critical evaluation of current evidence. *Stroke* 2022; 53: 2393–403.
31. Murray NM, Unberath M, Hager GD, Hui FK. Artificial intelligence to diagnose ischemic stroke and identify large vessel occlusions: A systematic review. *J Neurointerv Surg* 2020; 12: 156–64.
32. Joo B, Choi HS, Ahn SS, et al. A deep learning model with high standalone performance for diagnosis of unruptured intracranial aneurysm. *Yonsei Med J* 2021; 62: 1052–61.
33. Hu B, Shi Z, Lu L, et al. A deep-learning model for intracranial aneurysm detection on CT angiography images in China: A stepwise, multicentre, early-stage clinical validation study. *Lancet Digit Health* 2024; 6: e261–71.
34. Kuwabara M, Ikawa F, Sakamoto S, et al. Effectiveness of tuning an artificial intelligence algorithm for cerebral aneurysm diagnosis: A study of 10,000 consecutive cases. *Sci Rep* 2023; 13: 16202.
35. You WC, W YT, Hong JS, et al. Detection and segmentation of arteriovenous malformation lesions using a two-stage deep learning strategy. *Int J Radiat Oncol Biol Phys* 2022; 114: e108.
36. Mallma MJR, Vilca-Aguilar M, Zuloaga-Rotta L, et al. Machine learning approach for analyzing 3-year outcomes of patients with brain arteriovenous malformation (AVM) after stereotactic radiosurgery (SRS). *Diagnostics (Basel)* 2023; 14: 22.
37. Robertshaw H, Karstensen L, Jackson B, et al. Artificial intelligence in the autonomous navigation of endovascular interventions: A systematic review. *Front Hum Neurosci* 2023; 17: 1239374.
38. Schmitt N, Mokli Y, Weyland CS, et al. Automated detection and segmentation of intracranial hemorrhage suspect hyperdensities in non-contrast-enhanced CT scans of acute stroke patients. *Eur Radiol* 2021; 32: 2246–54.
39. Del Gaizo AJ, Osborne TF, Shahoumian T, Sherrier R. Deep learning to detect intracranial hemorrhage in a national teleradiology program and the impact on interpretation time. *Radiol Artif Intell* 2024; 6: e240067.
40. Gonzalez-Romo NI, Hanalioglu S, Mignucci-Jiménez G, et al. Quantification of motion during microvascular anastomosis simulation using machine learning hand detection. *Neurosurg Focus* 2023; 54: E2.
41. Jogan M, Kurada S, Vasisht S, et al. Quality over quantity? The role of data quality and uncertainty for AI in surgery. *Global Surg Educ* 2024; 3: 79.

8

Artificial Intelligence Usage by Robotics in Neurosurgery

MICHAEL D. MONTEREY, YASSINE GUENNOUN AND MICHAEL Y. WANG

INTRODUCTION

Neurosurgical procedures require intimate spatial, anatomic and physiological knowledge as well as precise and delicate manipulation of neural tissue. The adoption of technology has been vital in improving patient outcomes, reducing morbidity and lowering healthcare costs. Furthermore, the trend of adopting minimally invasive surgical techniques is the driving force behind technological advancements in surgical care to improve patient outcomes.[1] This is reflected economically by the estimated global minimally invasive surgery revenue in 2024 to be $79.3 billion and projected to reach $173.9 billion by 2029.[2]

Progression in the field of neurosurgery is one that has largely been intertwined with technological advancements. Moreover, neurosurgery is well suited for the adoption of new technologies, specifically robotics.[3] The implementation of surgical robots is becoming more commonplace for neurosurgical procedures such as intracranial biopsies, placement of intracranial leads, spinal instrumentation and many more.[4] Neurosurgical adoption of robotic surgery is fundamental due to the enhanced surgical technique of procedures, the push toward minimally invasive techniques and ultimately, to improve the patient experience.

Similarly, artificial intelligence (AI) has rapidly been implemented in the field of medicine. There has been a prominent impact of AI in neurosurgery specifically in diagnosis, preoperative planning, diagnostics/imaging and postoperative outcomes (Patel et al. 2025).[5] This is demonstrated by the growing number of publications pertaining to AI and usage within neurosurgery.[6]

Therefore, it seems only natural that a symbiotic relationship would develop between surgical robots and AI. The convergence of AI and robotics in neurosurgery represents one of the most profound technological advancements in the field of medicine. Together, AI and robotics promise to elevate the standards of neurosurgical procedures, enhancing outcomes, minimizing risks and expanding the horizons of what is surgically feasible. This chapter will examine the synergy of robotics and AI in neurosurgery and future directions.

Evolution of robotics

Historically, neurosurgery relied heavily on the exceptional skill and steady hand of the surgeon. However, even the most skilled practitioners are subject to the limitations of human dexterity and endurance. The introduction of robotic systems has mitigated these limitations by providing tremor-free, consistent and highly precise control. In 1985, neurosurgery was the first field to implement a surgical robot with a successful stereotactic biopsy with the assistance of Unimation PUMA (Programable Universal Machine for Assembly) 560.[7] This was then followed with the first Food and Drug Administration (FDA)- approved neurosurgical

DOI: 10.1201/9781003471165-8

robotic device in 2014, the NeuroMate robot (Integrated Surgical Systems, Sacramento, CA, USA). This slow development of neurosurgical robots is not due to lack of creativity or desire but more likely attributable to the delicate nature of neurosurgical procedures and the requirement of technology to accommodate to these tasks.[8]

Globally, there is a growing number of neurosurgeons implementing surgical robots with an estimated 85% of neurosurgeons within the United States expressing interest in embracing robotics.[9,10] FDA has approved 49 surgical robots as of 2023, and this number is expected to increase substantially over the coming years.[11] Financial incentives for development of robotics are evident as the market is valued at over $3 billion.[10] Consequently, a competitive landscape has developed with Johnson & Johnson Medtech, Medtronic, Globus Medical, Stryker and Zimmer Biomet competing in the robotic market. Economical resistance exists due to the high costs of surgical robots but new pay models such as Robotic-as-a-Service (RaaS), which is a lease for products, will help to expand the market beyond academic institutions and into more rural areas. Furthermore, patients are more commonly seeking robotic surgery and minimally invasive techniques due to improved results in shorter hospital stays, smaller incisions, fewer infections and less pain.[12,13] Although only a small percentage of surgeries are completed with robotics, aggressive adoption is to be expected due to increasing affordability and improved patient outcomes.

From a surgical technical standpoint, there is known and expected variability regarding surgical techniques, capabilities and patient outcomes.[14] This inconsistency among surgeons is largely due to experience. Surgical robots have the transformative power to improve the precision of surgery and help standardize procedures. This has been repeatedly demonstrated by the high degree of accuracy of pedicle screw placement during spine surgery.[15] Furthermore, no surgeon is immune to the human attributes of errors of fatigue. Robotics eliminates this technical fault due to indefatigability with the hopes of preserving or extending a surgeon's career.

Surgical robots are classified based on the level of autonomy performed, ranging from Level 0, robot assistance or no robotic autonomy, to Level 5, full autonomy.[16] Of the current FDA approved surgical robots 86% were deemed Level 1 and there are no existing fully autonomous robots.[11] Thus, most available robotic systems function as "closed-loop" systems, in which the robot only executes an action after surgeon input. Perhaps a more appropriate vernacular for this technology would be "cobot."

Therefore, today robotic systems integrate artificial intelligence primarily at the level of image-based planning, navigation and guided execution. Clinically deployed platforms use preoperative imaging to define trajectories that are registered intraoperatively and executed by robots, with AI-adjacent components supporting image fusion, segmentation, fiber tracking and workflow consistency. Systems from Medtronic, Globus Medical, Brainlab and Zimmer Biomet exemplify this paradigm, in which software-generated surgical plans are physically realized through robotic alignment and guidance. While these platforms are widely validated and globally deployed, their core contribution lies in improving accuracy, reproducibility and workflow integration rather than enabling adaptive or autonomous intraoperative decision-making.

Notable exceptions exist within highly specialized clinical contexts. For example, the CyberKnife robot displays advanced autonomous functions in performing brain and spine radiosurgery under human supervision as it can adjust to real-time imaging and patient posture to provide precise radiation treatment.[17] However, advancements across lower-level robots indicates a promising future as we strive to develop more sophisticated and autonomous robotic surgical systems.[18]

This shift is reflected in current research efforts aimed at integrating perception, planning and control within unified frameworks, thereby pushing robotics toward higher functional autonomy. Frontier platforms such as Robeauté are developing intracerebral microrobots designed to navigate within brain tissue, a setting that demands robust onboard perception, localization and autonomous control and is now advancing toward first-in-human evaluation. Therapeutic systems such as AI-driven robotic laser ablation, including collaborations between Monteris and Symphony Robotics, use image-based planning and computer vision to target complex or irregular lesions, illustrating a direct commercialization pathway for AI-guided intervention. Supporting these advances, newer planning software and regulatory approvals are increasingly defining how imaging, surgical plans and robotic execution are linked within a single workflow. FDA documentation for systems such as those from Zeta Surgical and Brain Navi now explicitly describes how software, navigation and robotic guidance are intended to work together in the operating room, creating a clear and standardized framework.

In summary, although neurosurgery has been slower to adopt surgical robotics relative to other specialties, technological advancements have provided a pathway to navigate the complex neuroanatomy and for the implantation of robotics to be a mainstay in the neurosurgical operating room.

Technical aspects of artificial intelligence

Artificial intelligence has become commonplace in almost all aspects of everyday life. Thus, its adoption into a variety of medical fields was inexorable, including neurosurgery. These algorithms analyze patient data to offer predictive insights that inform surgical decision-making. The systems can assess risk factors, simulate outcomes based on different intervention strategies, and optimize treatment plans. By correlating historical data with intraoperative feedback, AI-driven decision support systems help neurosurgeons adjust their approaches dynamically, ensuring the highest levels of patient safety and efficacy.

Several recent examples illustrate how these capabilities are now being incorporated directly into surgical systems. Vision-guided robotic suturing, in which deep learning supports real-time instrument control and soft tissue interaction, has demonstrated promising results.[19] In microsurgical contexts, AI methods that combine anatomical segmentation with instrument tracking provide structured input that can inform semi-autonomous robotic actions.[20] Computer vision and deep learning are also being applied to improve real-time navigation and trajectory planning.[21] Collectively, these developments reflect a shift from clinician-in-the-loop assistive perception toward robotic systems that can meaningfully guide or execute well-defined surgical tasks, while maintaining human oversight.

Image-guided AI-driven robotics in neurosurgery

One of the most significant applications of AI in neurosurgery is image guidance. The desire to move toward more minimally invasive surgeries, the collaboration of AI and robotics is well suited. As AI is significantly well adapted in imaging processing. Neuronavigation stands to garner significant benefit. By accounting for anatomical variations among patients, the image processing prowess of AI allows exact reconstruction of relevant neuroanatomy during surgical planning to avoid iatrogenic injury to critical structures. This is exemplified as previously stated in spine surgery with more accurate pedicle screw placement. Perhaps this is best embodied in complex tumor resections. Multiple studies have shown the utility of AI in assisting with safe tumor resection, which ultimately resulted in more complete tumor resection.[22–24] Furthermore, automated segmentation algorithms have the invaluable ability to demarcate tumors, blood vessels and neural pathways all resulting in better surgical planning and resulting in improved surgical outcomes.[22] Similarly, in Lateral Lumbar interbody fusion, AI-enhanced ultrasound imaging had a greater than 95% accuracy of lumbar plexus nerve detection.[25]

While image-based AI improves anatomical accuracy, a parallel line of research focuses on understanding the temporal structure of surgery itself. Recent advances allow these systems to model entire surgical workflows over long procedures, enabling reliable identification of procedural steps across complex robotic cases.[26,27] Methods that require only limited or coarse labeling have further improved scalability, reducing the need for extensive manual annotation.[28] Early studies also show that surgical phases can be reliably identified even in complex and variable procedures, allowing this information to be used alongside navigation and instrument tracking to assist the surgeon during higher-risk steps.[29]

Computer vision can also be used to tailor surgical strategy. Models trained on patient-specific data are increasingly used to support personalized neurosurgical planning, including prediction of postoperative seizure outcomes from interictal intracranial EEG in epilepsy surgery[30] and estimation of achievable extent of resection from imaging and anatomical features in glioblastoma surgery.[31] When integrated into robotic planning and navigation platforms, such patient-specific outcome predictions can guide the surgical strategy and intraoperative decision-making.

Moreover, the integration of real-time intraoperative imaging into robotic platforms enables continuous self-updating control loops. Modern robotic systems increasingly use ML to combine robot motion data, navigation information and real-time imaging to adapt surgical trajectories during a procedure. Conceptually, this can be understood through reinforcement learning, where a system learns how to act by observing its environment, taking actions and updating its behavior based on feedback toward a defined surgical goal, an approach that has been widely explored in robotic surgery research.[32] This framework allows robotic systems to adjust motion in response to anatomical deformation, uncertainty, or new imaging information rather than relying solely on fixed preoperative plans.

Recent work demonstrates how models can fuse different modalities to enable adaptive navigation and trajectory adjustment during surgery, including simulation-based training of robotic systems that integrate ultrasound feedback for navigation in complex anatomy.[33] Complementary approaches show that patient-specific, real-time segmentation of brain ultrasound can provide continuously updated anatomical information to support navigation.[34]

However, intraoperative imaging introduces additional challenges, as modalities such as ultrasound are noisy, operator-dependent and difficult to interpret consistently, limiting their use for robust real-time learning despite demonstrated feasibility of real-time tumor detection and workflow integration.[35,36]

Finally, although haptic feedback is widely recognized as critical for safe navigation and automation, especially in endovascular neurosurgery, its limited availability, sensing constraints and latency have led most current systems to rely predominantly on visual and kinematic cues.[37,38] Collectively, these factors explain why vision-centric learning dominates current neurosurgical robotic systems, while data availability, annotation burden and reliable multimodal sensing remain the primary barriers to more autonomous capabilities.

Future directions

As image navigation is a vital aspect of AI-robotic surgery, further advances in imaging have been explored via augmented reality and virtual reality (AR/VR). When AR/VR are implemented for surgical navigation with robotics it has been proven produces comparable levels of accuracy to conventional methods (such fluoroscopic imaging) with improvements in procedural efficiency and radiation reduction.[39] Additionally, it is postulated that AR with instrument tracking may aid the surgeon in detecting alignment issues while conducting manual manipulations such as drilling, but the accuracy of these operations can be increased further through the inclusion of robotics.[38] Regardless, the implementation of AR/VR is likely to be gradual as it would require further safety regulations and adaptation of its own technology (i.e. AR headsets).

Another frontier is integration with telemedicine. Spinal surgery has been completed via a remote 5G wireless network displaying proof of concept.[39] Similarly, endovascular telerobotic interventions for peripheral vascular disease and coronary arteries provide an outline for potential remote stroke care.[40] The prospect of telerobotic surgery is a continuing emerging field and has the potential to bring specialized care to more rural populations.

Despite these expanding capabilities, several core components of current neurosurgical workflows remain largely non–machine-learning–driven, limiting adaptability during surgery. Navigation and robotic guidance systems typically rely on preoperative registration and do not continuously update the patient model after dural opening, or brain shift, leading to progressive inaccuracy midcase. Learning-based image updating and linking preoperative MRI with intraoperative ultrasound or video offer a direct path to maintaining accurate targets in real time, with fully automated brain-shift compensation already demonstrated in neurosurgical settings.[41] Similarly, trajectory planning in robotics is often open-loop, with plans generated preoperatively and executed with limited intraoperative replanning; machine learning-based safe planning methods could enable continuous trajectory adjustment under uncertainty.[42]

Beyond geometry and planning, several perception- and context-related gaps remain. Most robotic systems do not perform real-time anatomical recognition from operative views, leaving the surgeon responsible for mentally tracking critical structures while the robot provides positioning or holding assistance. ML-based intraoperative anatomy recognition can introduce context-aware constraints.[43] In addition, robotic platforms lack awareness of surgical workflow or phase; phase recognition models validated in neurosurgical procedures demonstrate how procedural context could be used to trigger navigation overlays or constraints at the appropriate time.[44]

CHALLENGES AND LIMITATIONS

As with any implementation of new technology AI usage by robotics raises several ethical questions. AI algorithms are intimately involved in medical diagnosis and treatment planning. It is currently ambiguous who will assume responsibility if a patient experiences a negative outcome. It is suggested accountability would be distributed among the physician, the software provider, algorithm creator and the entity supplying the data.[45] Thus, clear guidelines will need to be defined to ensure patient safety and address medicolegal issues.

AI also is contingent upon large datasets and the question of patient privacy is of concern.

Machine learning development for neurosurgical robotics depends primarily on high-quality visual data, which can result in biased decision-making. This could result in worsening of already present healthcare disparities.[45] Operative video, endoscopic, microscopic and increasingly intraoperative ultrasound, is currently the most critical modality, supporting tasks such as instrument recognition, workflow understanding, event detection and real-time guidance.[46] However, progress is constrained by major bottlenecks, including the scarcity of large, well-annotated surgical video datasets, significant heterogeneity in viewpoints, lighting, anatomy, and instrumentation, and persistent domain shift across institutions and platforms.[47] Recent open-source dataset efforts represent an important field response to these limitations by enabling more scalable training and benchmarking, even when not neurosurgery-specific.[48]

To mitigate this data bottleneck, AI is increasingly integrated into robotic systems to enable objective skill evaluation as a means of generating large-scale, standardized and high-quality surgical data. By analyzing robot kinematics, instrument motion, and operative video, these systems can consistently quantify technical performance and procedural variability across surgeons and institutions.[49,50] Importantly, weakly supervised and self-supervised learning approaches allow surgical steps and behaviors to be learned directly from unannotated or heterogeneously labeled video, substantially reducing annotation burden while improving dataset scalability and consistency.[51] When embedded within robotic platforms, these capabilities transform routine surgical activity into training-ready datasets that support model development, quality improvement and future adaptive robotic assistance.

The relationship of AI and robotic surgery and the push toward autonomous surgical robots requires regulatory bodies tasked with establishing standards to ensure rigorous safety standards are met and continuous post-market analysis.

Finally, there are significant financial limitations to implementation of both AI algorithms and surgical robots. High upfront purchase cost, ongoing maintenance and infrastructure upgrades are all potential financial burdens to deter hospital systems in adopting the new technology.[53] However, it could be argued that robotic surgery resulting in shorter hospital stays, shorter surgery and decreased complications could offset these costs.

Conclusion

Artificial intelligence and robotics synergistically are exceptionally powerful tools that have transformed the landscape of neurosurgery. AI's capacity for rapid data analysis in collaboration with the precision of robotic systems, mean that neurosurgical procedures have become more accurate, less invasive and significantly safer. While challenges remain, including high costs, regulatory hurdles and ethical considerations, the benefits of this technological integration are clear. The continued evolution of machine learning, combined with advances in AR/VR, will lead to a future in which neurosurgery will be more standardized, predictable, efficient and tailored to individual patient needs.

As AI and robotics systems continue to advance, they will not only expand the range of treatable neurosurgical conditions but also provide the ability to reach and treat more rural populations. Ongoing research, coupled with rigorous clinical validation, will be critical in ensuring that these technologies are adopted safely and ethically into everyday surgical practice. Ultimately, the responsibility of the integration and use of this new technology largely falls on the surgeon, and it is wise that we educate ourselves appropriately as we adopt this technology. The future of neurosurgical practice is now a symbiotic relationship of surgeon expertise and advanced technology creating new standards for surgical care.

REFERENCES

1. Khan NR, Clark AJ, Lee SL, et al. Surgical outcomes for minimally invasive vs open transforaminal lumbar interbody fusion: An updated systematic review and meta-analysis. *Neurosurgery* 2015; 77(6): 847–74; discussion 874.
2. MarketsandMarkets. Minimally invasive medical robotics, imaging & visualization systems market [Internet]. MarketsandMarkets; [cited 2025 Mar 14]. Available from: https://www.marketsandmarkets.com/Market-Reports/minimally-invasive-medical-robotics-imaging-visualization-systems-market-787.html (Accessed July 2026).
3. Attenello FJ, Lee B, Yu C, et al. Supplementing the neurosurgical virtuoso: Evolution of automation from mythology to operating room adjunct. *World Neurosurg* 2014; 81(5–6): 719–29.
4. Khanna O, Beasley R, Franco D, DiMaio S. The path to surgical robotics in neurosurgery. *Oper Neurosurg (Hagerstown)* 2021; 20(6): 514–20.
5. Patel T, Ibrahim HY, Henna F, et al. A narrative review on artificial intelligence in neurosurgery: Ethical challenges and implementation considerations. *Ann Med Surg (Lond)* 2025; 87(12): 8654–63.
6. El-Hajj VG, Gharios M, Edström E, Elmi-Terander A. Artificial intelligence in neurosurgery: A bibliometric analysis. *World Neurosurg* 2023; 171: 152–158.e4.
7. Bagga V, Bhattacharyya D. Robotics in neurosurgery. *Ann R Coll Surg Engl* 2018; 100(6 Suppl): 22–6.
8. Wang MY, Goto T, Tessitore E, Veeravagu A. Introduction: Robotics in neurosurgery. *Neurosurg Focus* 2017; 42(5): E1.
9. Stumpo V, Staartjes VE, Klukowska AM, et al. Global adoption of robotic technology into neurosurgical practice and research. *Neurosurg Rev* 2021; 44(5): 2675–87.
10. Bain & Company. Navigating the next wave of surgical robotics [Internet]. 2023 Feb 9. Available from: https://www.bain.com/insights/navigating-the-next-wave-of-surgical-robotics/ (Accessed July2026).
11. Lee A, Baker TS, Bederson JB, et al. Levels of autonomy in FDA-cleared surgical robots: A systematic review. *NPJ Digit Med* 2024; 7: 103.
12. Chuchulo A, Ali A. Is robotic-assisted surgery better? *AMA J Ethics* 2023; 25(8): E598–604.
13. Menger RP, Savardekar AR, Farokhi F, Sin A. A cost-effectiveness analysis of the integration of robotic spine technology in spine surgery. *Neurospine* 2018; 15(3): 216–24.
14. Satkunasivam R, Klaassen Z, Ravi B, et al. Relation between surgeon age and postoperative outcomes: A population-based cohort study. *CMAJ* 2020; 192(15): E385–92.
15. Rasouli JJ, Shao J, Neifert S, et al. Artificial intelligence and robotics in spine surgery. *Global Spine J* 2021; 11(4): 556–64.
16. Yang GZ, Cambias J, Cleary K, et al. Medical robotics—regulatory, ethical, and legal considerations for increasing levels of autonomy. *Sci Robot* 2017; 2:eaam8638.
17. Kilby W, Dooley JR, Kuduvalli G, et al. The CyberKnife robotic radiosurgery system in 2010. *Technol Cancer Res Treat* 2010; 9(5): 433–52.
18. Attanasio A, Scaglioni B, De Momi E, Valdastri P. Autonomy in surgical robotics. 2021; 4: 651–79.
19. Vargas HF, Vivas A, Bastidas S, et al. Advances towards autonomous robotic suturing: Integration of finite element force analysis and instantaneous wound detection through deep learning. *Biomed Signal Process Control* 2025; 101: 107181.

20. Sugiyama T, Tang M, Sugimori H, et al. Artificial intelligence-integrated video analysis of vessel area changes and instrument motion for microsurgical skill assessment. *Sci Rep* 2025; 15(1): 27898.
21. Gan Z, Xu X, Li F, et al. Deep learning-based clinical decision support system for intracerebral hemorrhage: An imaging-based AI-driven framework for automated hematoma segmentation and trajectory planning. *Neurosurg Focus* 2025; 59(1): E5.
22. Tangsrivimol JA, Schonfeld E, Zhang M, et al. Artificial intelligence in neurosurgery: A state-of-the-art review from past to future. *Diagnostics (Basel)* 2023; 13(13): 2429.
23. Williams S, Layard Horsfall H, Funnell JP, et al. Artificial intelligence in brain tumour surgery—an emerging paradigm. *Cancers (Basel)* 2021; 13(19): 5010.
24. Xu J, Meng Y, Qiu K, et al. Applications of artificial intelligence based on medical imaging in glioma: current state and future challenges. *Front Oncol* 2022; 12: 892056.
25. Carson T, Ghoshal G, Cornwall GB, et al. Artificial intelligence-enabled, real-time intraoperative ultrasound imaging of neural structures within the psoas: Validation in a porcine spine model. *Spine (Phila Pa 1976)* 2021; 46(3): E146–E152.
26. Liu Y, Boels M, Garcia-Peraza-Herrera LC, et al. LoViT: Long video transformer for surgical phase recognition. *Med Image Anal* 2025; 99: 103366.
27. Pérez A, Rodríguez S, Ayobi N, et al. MuST: Multi-scale transformers for surgical phase recognition. arXiv [Preprint]. 2024; arXiv:2407.17361v1.
28. Ding X, Yan X, Wang Z, et al. Less is more: surgical phase recognition from timestamp supervision. *IEEE Trans Med Imaging* 2023; 42(6): 1897–910. 46. Collins JW, Marcus HJ, Ghazi A, et al. Ethical implications of AI in robotic surgical training: a Delphi consensus statement. Eur Urol Focus. 2021. doi:10.1016/j.euf.2021.04.006.
29. Fareed J, Raju B, Nagaraj A, et al. Uncharted waters of machine and deep learning for surgical phase recognition in neurosurgery. *World Neurosurg* 2022; 160:4–12.
30. Partamian H, Jahromi S, Corona L, et al. Machine learning on interictal intracranial EEG predicts surgical outcome in drug resistant epilepsy. *NPJ Digit Med* 2025; 8(1): 138.
31. Kernbach JM, Schroeder U, Hakvoort K, et al. Enhancing decision-making in glioblastoma surgery through an explainable human-AI collaboration: An international multicenter model development and external validation study. *NPJ Precis Oncol* 2025; 9(1): 387.
32. Guanglin J, Gao Q, Zhang T, et al. A heuristically accelerated reinforcement learning-based neurosurgical path planner. *Cyborg Bionic Syst* 2023; 4: 0026.
33. Ao Y, Moghani M, Mittal M, et al. SonoGym: high performance simulation for challenging surgical tasks with robotic ultrasound. arXiv [Preprint]. 2025; arXiv:2507.01152v1.
34. Dorent R, Torio E, Haouchine N, et al. Patient-specific real-time segmentation in trackerless brain ultrasound. arXiv [Preprint]. 2024; arXiv:2405.09959v1.
35. Cepeda S, Esteban-Sinovas O, Romero R, et al. Real-time brain tumor detection in intraoperative ultrasound: From model training to deployment in the operating room. *Comput Biol Med* 2025 ;193: 110481.
36. Šteňo A, Buvala J, Babková V, et al. Current limitations of intraoperative ultrasound in brain tumor surgery. *Front Oncol* 2021; 11: 659048.
37. Wagner CR, Phillips T, Roux S, Corrigan JP. Future directions in robotic neurosurgery. *Oper Neurosurg (Hagerstown)* 2021; 21(4): 173–80.
38. Burström G, Nachabe R, Persson O, Edström E. Augmented and virtual reality instrument tracking for minimally invasive spine surgery. *Spine (Phila Pa 1976)* 2019; 44(15): 1097–104.
39. Tian W, Fan M, Zeng C, et al. Telerobotic spinal surgery based on 5G network: The first 12 cases. *Neurospine* 2020; 17(1): 114–20.
40. Berczeli M, Britz GW, Loh T, Lumsden AB. Telerobotic endovascular interventions and their potential for cerebrovascular treatment. *Tex Heart Inst J* 2022; 49(2): e217608.

41. Li C, Evans LT, Hong J, et al. Fully automated image updating for brain shift compensation after dural opening. *J Neurosurg* 2026; 144(1): 206–16.
42. Ao Y, Esfandiari H, et al. SafeRPlan: Safe deep reinforcement learning for intraoperative planning of pedicle screw placement. *Med Image Anal* 2025; 99: 103345.
43. Khan DZ, Valetopoulou A, Das A, et al. Artificial intelligence assisted operative anatomy recognition in endoscopic pituitary surgery. *NPJ Digit Med* 2024; 7(1): 314.
44. González-Cebrián Á, Bordonaba S, Pascau J, et al. Attention in surgical phase recognition for endoscopic pituitary surgery: Insights from real-world data. *Comput Biol Med* 2025; 191: 110222.
45. Collins JW, Marcus HJ, Ghazi A, et al. Ethical implications of AI in robotic surgical training: a Delphi consensus statement. *Eur Urol Focus* 2021. doi:10.1016/j.euf.2021.04.006.
46. Buyck F, Vandemeulebroucke J, Ceranka J, et al. Computer-vision based analysis of the neurosurgical scene: a systematic review. *Brain Spine* 2023; 3: 102706.
47. Rueckert T, Rueckert D, Palm C. Methods and datasets for segmentation of minimally invasive surgical instruments in endoscopic images and videos: A review of the state of the art. *Comput Biol Med* 2024; 169: 107929.
48. Xu Z, Wang H, Huang Y, et al. Spine endoscopic atlas: An open-source dataset for surgical instrument segmentation. *Sci Data* 2025; 12(1): 1611.
49. Cui Z, Ma R, Yang CH, et al. Capturing relationships between suturing sub-skills to improve automatic suturing assessment. *NPJ Digit Med* 2024; 7(1): 152.
50. Lam K, Chen J, Wang Z, et al. Machine learning for technical skill assessment in surgery: A systematic review. *NPJ Digit Med* 2022; 5(1): 24.
51. Sreeram K, Chen K, Bhattacharyya K. Weakly supervised pre-training for surgical step recognition using unannotated and heterogeneously labeled videos. *Int J Comput Assist Radiol Surg* 2025; 21: 267–77.
52. Peng Y, Liu Y, Lai S, et al. Global trends and prospects in health economics of robotic surgery: a bibliometric analysis. *Int J Surg.* 2023;109:3896-904.

9

The Compass of the Future: Machine Learning-Guided Navigation in Spine Surgery

RISHI JAIN, DILLAN PRASAD, MEHUL MITTAL, NIKHIL SRIRAM, JOSHUA M. TENNYSON, NOAH B. DREWES, SACHIN GOVIND, CHRISTOPHER S. AHUJA, NADER S. DAHDALEH AND NAJIB EL TECLE

INTRODUCTION

Artificial intelligence (AI) and machine learning (ML) techniques have increasingly gained traction in spine surgery as tools to characterize disease and support clinical decision-making. As these technologies move from analytical applications to the operating room (OR), they promise to reshape the capabilities of surgical navigation. Standard navigation systems enable the surgeon to visualize patient anatomy and plan implant trajectories; ML-based platforms extend this by improving image segmentation, reconstruction and registration, while supporting continuous intraoperative adaptation. In practice, these advances have translated to higher pedicle screw placement accuracy, decreased radiation exposure and reduced surgeon fatigue.[1–3] This chapter introduces ML architectures foundational to these developments and describes how they support current spine navigation and robotic systems. Finally, we discuss novel multimodal approaches that aim to progress toward greater intraoperative intelligence, where navigation evolves from static image guidance to context-aware, real-time surgical support. By bridging computational principles with clinical relevance, we aim to highlight the current state and demonstrated potential of intelligent navigation systems in spine surgery.

HISTORY OF NEURONAVIGATION

Neuronavigation has its roots in cranial surgery, where frameless stereotactic platforms enabled image-guided localization with improved precision and safety relative to predecessors. Bucholz and colleagues' 2002 patent formally introduced systems capable of correlating preoperative imaging with patient anatomy without the need for rigid frames, allowing surgeons to target intracranial lesions with greater accuracy and reduced operative morbidity.[4] The technology's success in cranial procedures catalyzed rapid adaptation to the spine, a particularly valuable domain as exposure and visualization can be limited. Early translation to spine surgery relied on anatomic landmarks and dynamic reference arrays (DRAs), and Foley and Smith demonstrated that registering dorsal spinal elements to a DRA could stabilize tracking accuracy in the presence of physiologic movement, paving the way for the first navigated pedicle screw insertions.[5] Over the next decade, the introduction of intraoperative 3D imaging (O-arm, intraoperative CT) improved registration accuracy across multilevel constructs and minimally invasive corridors, reducing cumulative drift.

The primary clinical objective of early-generation surgical navigation systems was error reduction.

DOI: 10.1201/9781003471165-9

High-quality meta-analyses of randomized controlled trials have since confirmed achievement of this endpoint, reporting superior accuracy and lower complication rates with navigated pedicle screw placement compared to fluoroscopy-guided approaches.[3,6] However, radiation exposure now represents an additional major driver of innovation; fluoroscopy-based navigation, though effective, also subjects patients and OR staff to greater intraoperative radiation doses.[7] Machine vision-based navigation systems provide a workaround, introducing structured light surface mapping and computer vision (CV) algorithms to execute registration without repeat fluoroscopy. A randomized prospective study evaluating 429 pedicle screw insertions found that FLASH Navigation (7D Surgical, Toronto) reduced total intraoperative radiation time by 94.3% and total intraoperative radiation dose by 97.8% relative to standard 3D fluoroscopy approaches.[8] Although preoperative CT remains necessary, FLASH patients benefited from 34.4% and 41.0% reductions in preoperative CT dose and postoperative total dose length product, respectively, with equivalent accuracy of screw placement.[8]

These developments lay the foundation for the current generation of ML-based navigation, in which the goal is no longer simply enhanced visualization but to continuously maintain an accurate—and sometimes interactive—representation of patient anatomy as it changes intraoperatively.

EMERGING APPLICATIONS OF ML IN NEURONAVIGATION FOR THE SPINE

Surgical navigation is a data-fusion problem; ML models take multimodal preoperative data and render patient-specific anatomy that can be used for planning and updated intraoperatively as necessary. From these images, the system generates surface and bony landmarks, labels vertebrae and soft tissue features and extracts safe boundaries.[9] As computing power expands, these models may soon integrate multidimensional video data (low-dose fluoroscopy or optical video streams) to refine registration in real time as tissue is manipulated or hardware placed. For surgeons, this translates to reliable targeting with fewer rescans and steadier execution during reduction and rod contouring. An overview of each phase, and the ML architectures that support them (**Table 9.1**) follows.

Image segmentation, registration and processing

After multimodal imaging has been obtained, data is segmented to distinguish critical anatomic and operative features including vertebrae, intervertebral discs, soft tissue and cord. As a foundational step, accurate segmentation allows surgeons and software to know exactly where each spinal element is.

Traditional segmentation approaches have relied on anatomic atlases, strict statistical shape models and active contouring.[10,11] However, they often require manual fine-tuning and struggle with variability in anatomy or image quality.[10] Deep learning (DL) architectures, such as residual- or convolutional-based architectures (including U-Nets), have become popular for their ability to learn features and produce precise pixel/voxel-level labels.[12] For example, U-Net-based models can take a CT or MRI of the spine and output a segmented volume highlighting each vertebra, enabling greater automation and flexibility with preserved spatial resolution.[10] Transformer-based methods extend this further by incorporating self-attention mechanisms to better capture global spatial relationships across the spine; they can also integrate time series input, including depth-sensing data or surgical footage.[13,14] Models such as Spine-Transformers and LumVertCancNet enable precise vertebral labeling and cancellous-bone segmentation on CT, while even Meta's Segment Anything Model has shown generalizability to pathologic anatomy.[13–15] Today's state-of-the-art spine segmentation algorithms are highly accurate on standardized benchmarks. Models trained and tested on large datasets, such as the VerSe (Vertebral Segmentation) spine CT challenge and xVertSeg data, routinely achieve Dice similarity coefficient scores greater than 0.90 for vertebral segmentation and greater than 95% correct vertebral level identification, particularly when anatomic priors are incorporated into the network or post-processing pipeline.[16–19]

Once structures are segmented, the system must establish registration, or the spatial alignment between the patient's actual anatomy and the preoperative imaging. These steps determine where the patient is in space relative to the navigation system, allowing instrument tip locations to be displayed accurately on the segmented "map."

Traditional approaches rely on rigid matching of bony landmarks or surface contours, but this assumes that anatomy remains fixed throughout the case. However, in deformity correction and with complex instrumentation, osteotomies, rod reduction and soft tissue tensioning can alter segmental alignment, producing registration drift that diminishes navigational accuracy and increases the risk of pedicle breach or injury.[20] ML-augmented registration can maintain fidelity by coupling biomechanical priors with adaptive segmentation. Once a segmentation scaffold is established, hybrid registration frameworks combine rigid alignment of vertebral bodies with elastic modeling of surrounding soft tissues to account for expected deformation patterns.[21] This allows the navigation system to maintain a stable reference frame even as individual segments rotate, translate, or deform during osteotomy and rod engagement. Low-dose optical or fluoroscopic inputs processed by CNNs can refine registration without repeat CT scans, as shown in trials with FLASH machine-vision guidance.[8]

Image reconstruction

Traditionally, 3D convolutional neural networks (CNNs), recurrent neural networks (RNNs) and variational autoencoders (AEs) have been favored architectures for image reconstruction.[22] In current spine neuronavigation, the most clinically pertinent reconstruction tasks include generating 3D volumes from CT or MRI input to enable perioperative trajectory planning and improving intraoperative image quality or real-time mapping.[23,24] DL plays a critical role in denoising and processing segmentation masks, as well as "stacking" meshes to create a tangible volume that retains anatomically accurate positioning of spinal elements in 3D space.[25] These methods are also valuable in facilitating metal-artifact reduction to improve bone-implant conspicuity and measurement fidelity at lower radiation dose (which directly benefits registration stability and screw accuracy around hardware), as well as mitigating the need for excessive, radiation-necessitating imaging modalities by means of intelligent interpolation.[26,27] Although the need for loss function optimization often limits results observed empirically, 3D reconstructions have been noted as similar—if not superior—to existing preoperative planning methods. Abel et al. noted equivalent virtual pedicle screw placement, as measured by screw angulation and lateral distances to defined planes, on standard CT and CNN-3D-reconstructed MRI.[24]

Generative adversarial networks (GANs) have also recently emerged as a powerful framework for reconstruction in spinal neuronavigation applications, particularly in the context of inter- and intramodality conversion (e.g. low-dose CT to high-quality CT, CT to MRI, etc.). In GAN architecture, a generator is trained to create synthetic images that a discriminator attempts to distinguish from real imaging, subsequently generating high-volume, high-fidelity synthetic data.[28] Using this approach, Saravi et al. demonstrated that GAN-based synthesis can fuse features across modalities (X-ray and CT) to reduce radiation exposure while preserving bony detail necessary for planning and generation of 3D volumes.[29] Yang and colleagues took this a step further, using CT-derived simulated bi-planar X-ray images to train a modified 2D to 3D-GAN that automatically reconstructed 3D spine structures.[30] While direct extensions to navigation have not been thoroughly explored with GAN-derived output, they have demonstrated near equivalent performance to more traditional DL methods. Pure GAN, GAN-CNN, or GAN-attention-based methods therefore stand to significantly improve such approaches while paving the path for enhanced intraoperative navigation in practice, including the planning of bony cuts, optimization of mixed rigid and elastic structure registration, and improved accuracy of alignment in complex pathologies.[21]

INTRAOPERATIVE DYNAMIC TRACKING AND VISUALIZATION

Intraoperative tracking and visualization represent the final stage of ML-based processing for spinal neuronavigation. While conventional navigation has historically employed fudicial markers or, more recently, standalone cameras with limited feedback abilities, marrying CV with visualization tools has demonstrated notable value in adapting to the unpredictable nature of the operating room. Continuous AI-assisted tracking transforms navigation from a static reference into a real-time safety system. During deforming correction or rod placement, even millimeter-scale vertebral motion can shift planned screw trajectories beyond safe margins and disrupt the initial registration. Optical and motion adaptive frameworks in early clinical and simulation studies demonstrate that live tracking (calibrated and tracked probes, etc.) can maintain registration fidelity as anatomy shifts, reducing dependence on repeat fluoroscopy.[8,31–33] In one study, Liebmann et al. demonstrated that the exposed posterior elements can be automatically segmented and tracked in real time without fiducials or repeated fluoroscopy, allowing the navigation model to update continuously as spinal position shifts.[31] In cadaveric validation, this marker-less dynamic registration maintained sub-2–3 mm target accuracy during simulated pedicle screw placement.[31] For surgeons, these systems translate into fewer confirmatory scans, steadier screw trajectories and reduced cumulative operative time. When surface changes are large (as in osteotomies or general deformity correction), intelligent intraoperative navigation systems can also use radiographs or long-film/tomosynthesis and use learned 2D-to-3D registration/synthesis to "re-anchor" the model.[34,35] Han et al. highlighted how architectures such as long short-term memory (LSTM) networks can additionally be used to fine-tune tracking of time-series tasks, such as the respiratory motion of vertebrae, intraoperatively.[33] As models become capable of integrating and processing a greater number of features in real time, their ability to detect positioning of instrumentation, adhere to planned trajectory and assist in avoiding unintentional breaches will also improve.[36]

Augmented reality (AR) surgical navigation systems provide an intuitive interface for intraoperative navigation, overlaying anatomy and trajectories directly onto the operative field. These platforms do not require the same multi-phase set-up as DRAs and instead often use optical cameras, standard imaging data and CV frameworks for landmark detection and intraoperative tracking. Feature detection and CV algorithms such as speeded-up robust features (SURF) and oriented FAST and rotated BRIEF (ORB) operate by extracting stable surface key points and aligning them with preoperative imaging, allowing the AR system to lock the virtual spine model to exposed anatomy in real time.[32] Technologies such as Medivis's SurgicalAR and Novarad's VisAR platforms have rapidly gained popularity for offering high-resolution, auto-segmented 3D visualizations with high-accuracy object recognition and tracking abilities.[37] Of note, SurgicalAR's positional accuracy was found to exceed that of in-market surgical navigation tracking systems and the FDA's ASTM-F2554–18 consensus standard.[38] In practice, this reduces reliance on repeated attention shifts to external monitors and promotes intuitive spatial understanding, particularly in minimally invasive corridors. However, challenges remain with AR systems, including the limited ability to annotate and model complex presentations—such as deformities and vasculature—lack of extensive training datasets, and subpar rendering latencies.[39] The growing popularity of consumer AR/VR technologies, such as the Apple VisionPro, supports open-access innovation and may offer a potentially unique, "crowd-sourced" solution to overcome these barriers (**Figure 9.1**).

Hybrid approaches that combine segmentation, reconstruction and real-time feedback are increasingly being explored to execute context-aware navigation. The aim is not necessarily full automation, but rather to enable systems that can suggest or maintain safe instrument paths as anatomy shifts or as exposure evolves. Zhang and colleagues demonstrated the potential of a composite workflow, integrating multitask segmentation and 3D reconstruction with model-free reinforcement learning for anterior spine surgery path planning.[40] Within its foundational Markov Decision Process (MDP) framework, the model evaluated many possible approach trajectories and selected the one that minimized risk while maximizing target exposure.[40] Qi et al. also shared promising results, using a 3D U-Net architecture to segment vertebrae, identify key landmarks and propose trajectories for pedicle screw placement.[41] As the first of its kind, the model obtained an impressive

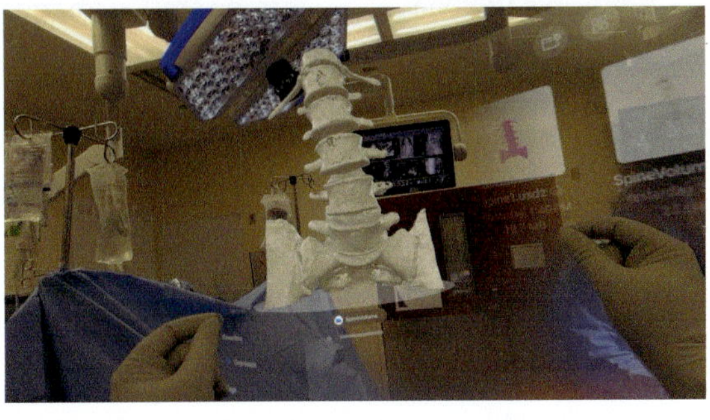

Figure 9.1 An interactive, patient-specific 3D spine volume as viewed on the Apple Vision Pro for intraoperative visualization (Northwestern Memorial Hospital).

93% rate of "good" and "excellent" path determination (i.e. screw trajectory, depth, etc.) ratings by a panel of expert surgeons.[41] Another group highlighted the performance of a 3D-U-Net algorithm in selecting pedicle screw placement based on preoperative computed tomography (CT) data. When compared to freehand surgical screw placements, the model had a significantly higher proportion of cases classified as Gertzbein Grade A (ideal placement) and frequently identified more biomechanically appropriate screw length and diameter compared to manual planning.[42] Clinically, these systems demonstrate the potential to standardize planning, reduce cognitive load during multilevel fixation and provide decision support in complex surgeries.

ROBOTIC SYSTEMS AND NAVIGATION

While rapid advances in robotics and CV promise to evolve robotic neurosurgical technologies, current approaches rely largely on navigational assistance during human-controlled operations. Since 2015, the FDA has replaced the term "surgical robots" with "robotically assisted surgical devices" (RAS) to emphasize that no FDA-approved systems fully possess autonomous decision-making capacity, reiterate the surgeon's sole responsibility

Table 9.1 Overview of key ML terms and model architectures

Method	Role in spine neuronavigation	Clinical relevance
Convolutional neural networks (CNNs)	Extract anatomic boundaries and identify bony structures on CT/MRI; used for vertebra segmentation and screw trajectory mapping	Provides consistent vertebral labeling and pedicle boundary identification, reducing reliance on manual segmentation and visual estimation
3D U-Net and related volumetric CNNs	Perform full spine segmentation in three dimensions with preserved anatomic detail	Enables accurate preoperative planning and ensures that navigation overlays rest on correct anatomy
Autoencoders (AEs)/ Variational AEs	Generate cleaned or enhanced reconstructions from noisy, low-dose or incomplete scans.	Allows usable imaging with less radiation or incomplete data
Transformer-based models	Capture global spatial relationships across multiple vertebrae and regions	Improves segmentation stability in deformity, anatomic variants and long constructs
Recurrent neural networks (RNNs)	Model sequential changes in intraoperative images	Tracks ongoing anatomic change rather than assuming the spine is static (i.e. mitigates registration drift)
LSTM networks (a type of RNN)	Predict small, periodic movements (e.g. respiration) and maintain overlay alignment	Prevents navigation drift during respiration or table adjustments
Generative adversarial networks (GANs)	Produce synthetic imaging and execute inter- or intramodality imaging conversions	Allows CT-equivalent planning while reducing radiation exposure
Reinforcement learning (RL)	Optimize surgical tasks and tool guidance pathways through a reward–punishment learning model	Potential future applications include robotic screw path optimization and automated deformity correction planning, but not yet standard in the OR

for the case, and perhaps quell speculative concern about robots wholly replacing physicians and care providers.[43]

Yang and colleagues proposed a 2017 framework detailing six stages of surgical automation, including:

1. No autonomy
2. Robot assistance
3. Task autonomy
4. Conditional autonomy
5. High autonomy
6. Full autonomy[44]

Progressing through the stages implies increased robotic decision-making while decreasing human involvement. An example of a Yang level 2 robotic system could filter tremor and enforce trajectory constraints, reducing fatigue and enhancing precision. At level 3, robots can execute pre-planned steps such as drilling or screw placement. A recent review by Lee et al. identified 49 FDA-approved robotic surgery devices from 2015 to 2023 and classified them according to the Yang framework.[43] Of these 49 systems, eight have indications for spine surgery, with common procedures including pedicle screw insertion all but one and spacer placement. And of these eight systems, all were classified as Yang autonomy Level 2 (robot assistance; requiring continuous surgeon control), though the FDA has approved four Yang Level 3 (task autonomy; execute pre-planned actions without continuous surgeon control) and three Yang Level 4 (conditional autonomy; generate patient-specific strategies for a procedure) systems for specialties outside of spine and neurosurgery. Among spine platforms, Cirq (Brainlab, Munich) is notable in that its integrated planning ecosystem incorporates AI/ML-based imaging and anatomic recognition tools, but the robotic arm itself remains a Level 2 system requiring surgeon-driven decision-making and execution.[43] Our own analysis concurs with Lee and colleagues in that no FDA-approved or non-FDA-approved experimental spine surgical technologies merit Yang Level 5 or 6 classification, supporting that limited commercial systems use true ML for navigated or robotically assisted surgery (RAS).[45]

LOOKING AHEAD

As AI/ML-enabled navigation technologies advance in spine surgery, their integration into robotic platforms and intraoperative navigation workflows continues to expand. One particularly promising domain is intraoperative safety monitoring, where algorithms can predict or detect adverse events. In a recent cadaveric study, Massalimova et al. trained a CNN on vibroacoustic sensor data collected during pedicle drilling and correctly identified 98% of cortical breach events demonstrating the feasibility of AI-based failsafe frameworks for intraoperative navigation.[46] Such approaches could also be applied to detecting dural tears, vascular injury or cerebrospinal fluid (CSF) leak, by synthesizing immediate feedback from torque, pressure and impedance sensors. Defining clinically validated intraoperative "checkpoints" will be imperative as these systems evolve toward higher degrees of autonomy.

Beyond intraoperative safety, ML integration is expanding the continuum of spinal care. For instance, the use of wearable sensors within standard spinal care paradigms can inform patient-specific treatment plans, capturing biomechanical recovery data for predictive modeling of outcomes and informed personalization of postoperative management.[47] As semi-autonomous systems mature, these data streams may also guide adaptive robotic planning and optimization of intervention in a manner that best fits a given clinical phenotype. Such iterative feedback could be of value for patients undergoing repeat or sequential surgeries. While wearables data represent one additional dimension that can be incorporated in intelligent surgical planning or navigation systems, it captures the broader transition toward multimodal data integration. In the future, navigation platforms are expected to synthesize information from radiomic signatures, pertinent video footage and patients' longitudinal medical histories to both create dynamic surgical maps and suggest novel approaches.

It is important to note that these advances introduce several ethical and regulatory considerations. As commonly cited, AI models require large quantities of sensitive patient data for training. Ensuring robust data security, appropriate data ownership and utilization and informed patient consent is essential. As a result of these privacy concerns, establishing diverse, voluminous datasets within spine surgery has proved challenging, and institutions' hesitancy to share data continues to grow.[48] Synthetic learning is a developing, AI-enabled method to mitigate privacy risks, and GANs are increasingly being leveraged to generate volumes of data that do not put patient information at risk; such an approach provides a private medium for reliable classification and large-scale implementation of ML tools.[48,49] The FDA has also taken preemptive measures to lay definitive bounds; in 2021, they launched the Artificial Intelligence and Machine Learning Software as a Medical Device (AI/ML SaMD) Action Plan to guide the oversight and lifecycle management of AI-driven technologies in healthcare.[50] Establishing rigorous validation, transparency and auditability standards will be essential before higher levels of surgical automation can be safely adopted.

CONCLUSION

The progressive integration of ML-driven navigation, decision support and robotics has the potential to expand access to high-quality spine care. Rather than replacing spine surgeon judgment, these technologies may help standardize critical steps and mitigate unwanted variability that stems from differences in training environment, surgeon experience and institutional resources. Such systems could also support remote collaboration and mentoring, broadening access to advanced techniques in regions that most require it.

As spine surgery enters a new era, the value of intelligent navigation systems lies in their careful and intentional integration into existing care frameworks. An understanding of which ML architectures are best suited for certain tasks, how intraoperative feedback should be interpreted and where surgeon judgment remains critical will determine whether these systems meaningfully improve care. At its best, the future of spine surgery will represent a thoughtful convergence of evidence-based operative principles, data-driven augmentation and traditional clinical intuition.

REFERENCES

1. Bcharah G, Gupta N, Panico N, et al. Innovations in spine surgery: A narrative review of current integrative technologies. *World Neurosurg* 2024; 184: 127–36.
2. Overley SC, Cho SK, Mehta AI, Arnold PM. Navigation and robotics in spinal surgery: Where are we now? *Neurosurgery* 2017; 80(3 Suppl): S86–99.
3. Shuman WH, Valliani AA, Chapman EK, et al. Intraoperative navigation in spine surgery: Effects on complications and reoperations. *World Neurosurg* 2022; 160: e404–11.
4. Bucholz RD. System for indicating the position of a surgical probe within a head on an image of the head. USA, 2002.
5. Foley KT, Smith MM. Image-guided spine surgery. *Neurosurg Clin N Am* 1996; 7(2): 171–86.
6. Yang Z, Sun Y, Deng C, et al. Comparative efficacy of robotic-assisted and freehand techniques for pedicle screw placement in spinal disorders: A meta-analysis and systematic review. *J Robot Surg* 2024; 18(1): 121.
7. Bratschitsch G, Leitner L, Stücklschweiger G, et al. Radiation exposure of patient and operating room personnel by fluoroscopy and navigation during spinal surgery. *Sci Rep* 2019; 9(1): 17652.
8. Malham GM, Munday NR. Comparison of novel machine vision spinal image guidance system with existing 3D fluoroscopy-based navigation system: A randomized prospective study. *Spine J* 2022; 22(4): 561–9.
9. Qadri SF, Shen L, Ahmad M, et al. CT-based automatic spine segmentation using patch-based deep learning. *Int J Intell Syst* 2023; 2023: 1–14.
10. Saeed MU, Dikaios N, Dastgir A, et al. An automated deep learning approach for spine segmentation and vertebrae recognition using computed tomography images. *Diagnostics (Basel)* 2023; 13(16): 2658.
11. Qian X, Wang J, Guo S, Li Q. An active contour model for medical image segmentation with application to brain CT image. *Med Phys* 2013; 40(2): 021911.
12. Lessmann N, van Ginneken B, de Jong PA, Išgum I. Iterative fully convolutional neural networks for automatic vertebra segmentation and identification. *Med Image Anal* 2019; 53: 142–55.
13. Zhang Y, Shi Z, Wang H, et al. LumVertCancNet: A novel 3D lumbar vertebral body cancellous bone location and segmentation method based on hybrid Swin-transformer. *Comput Biol Med* 2024; 171: 108237.

14. Tao R, Liu W, Zheng G. Spine-transformers: Vertebra labeling and segmentation in arbitrary field-of-view spine CTs via 3D transformers. *Med Image Anal* 2022; 75: 102258.
15. Khazanchi R, Govind S, Jain R, et al. Zero-shot segmentation of spinal vertebrae with metastatic lesions: an analysis of Meta's Segment Anything Model 2 and factors affecting learning free segmentation. *Neurosurg Focus* 2025; 59(1): E18.
16. Sekuboyina A, Husseini ME, Bayat A, et al. VerSe: A Vertebrae labelling and segmentation benchmark for multi-detector CT images. *Med Image Anal* 2021; 73: 102166.
17. Meng D, Boyer E, Pujades S. Vertebrae localization, segmentation and identification using a graph optimization and an anatomic consistency cycle. *Comput Med Imaging Graph* 2023; 107: 102235.
18. Xiong X, Graves SA, Gross BA, et al. Lumbar and thoracic vertebrae segmentation in CT scans using a 3D multi-object localization and segmentation CNN. *Tomography* 2024; 10(5): 738–60.
19. Cheng P, Yang Y, Yu H, He Y. Automatic vertebrae localization and segmentation in CT with a two-stage Dense-U-Net. *Sci Rep* 2021; 11(1): 22156.
20. Shin JH, Yanamadala V, Cha TD. Computer-assisted navigation for real time planning of pedicle subtraction osteotomy in cervico-thoracic deformity correction. *Oper Neurosurg* 2019; 16(4): 445–50.
21. Huesman R, Klein G, Kimdon JA, et al. Deformable registration of multi-modal data including rigid structures. *IEEE Trans Nucl Sci* 2002; 50(3): 389–92.
22. Rahman H, Khan AR, Sadiq T, et al. A systematic literature review of 3D deep learning techniques in computed tomography reconstruction. *Tomography* 2023; 9(6): 2158–89.
23. Jecklin S, Jancik C, Farshad M, et al. X23D-intraoperative 3D lumbar spine shape reconstruction based on sparse multi-view x-ray data. *J Imaging* 2022; 8(10): 271.
24. Abel F, Lebl DR, Gorgy G, et al. Deep-learning reconstructed lumbar spine 3D MRI for surgical planning: Pedicle screw placement and geometric measurements compared to CT. *Eur Spine J* 2024; 33(11): 4144–54.
25. Chen Y, Gao Y, Fu X, et al. Automatic 3D reconstruction of vertebrae from orthogonal bi-planar radiographs. *Sci Rep* 2024; 14(1): 16165.
26. Sun J, Li H, Yu T, et al. Application of metal artifact reduction algorithm in reducing metal artifacts in post-surgery pediatric low radiation dose spine computed tomography (CT) images. *Quant Imaging Med Surg* 2024; 14(7): 4648–58.
27. Luchmann D, Jecklin S, Cavalcanti NA, et al. Spinal navigation with AI-driven 3D-reconstruction of fluoroscopy images: An ex-vivo feasibility study. *BMC Musculoskelet Disord* 2024; 25(1): 925.
28. Jeong JJ, Tariq A, Adejumo T, et al. Systematic review of generative adversarial networks (GANs) for medical image classification and segmentation. *J Digit Imaging* 2022; 35(2): 137–52.
29. Saravi B, Guzel HE, Zink A, et al. Synthetic 3D spinal vertebrae reconstruction from biplanar x-rays utilizing generative adversarial networks. *J Pers Med* 2023; 13(12): 1642.
30. Yang CJ, Lin CL, Wang CK, et al. Generative adversarial network (GAN) for automatic reconstruction of the 3D spine structure by using simulated bi-planar x-ray images. *Diagnostics (Basel)* 2022; 12(5): 1121.
31. Liebmann F, von Atzigen M, Stütz D, et al. Automatic registration with continuous pose updates for marker-less surgical navigation in spine surgery. *Med Image Anal* 2024; 91: 103027.
32. Manni F, Elmi-Terander A, Burström G, et al. Towards optical imaging for spine tracking without markers in navigated spine surgery. *Sensors (Basel)* 2020; 20(13): 3641.
33. Han Z, Tian H, Han X, et al. A respiratory motion prediction method based on LSTM-AE with attention mechanism for spine surgery. *Cyborg Bionic Syst* 2024; 5: 0063.
34. Frisk H, Burström G, Persson O, et al. Automatic image registration on intraoperative CBCT compared to surface matching registration on preoperative CT for spinal navigation: Accuracy and workflow. *Int J Comput Assist Radiol Surg* 2024; 19(4): 665–75.

35. Zhang X, Uneri A, Huang Y, et al. Deformable 3D–2D image registration and analysis of global spinal alignment in long-length intraoperative spine imaging. *Med Phys* 2022; 49(9): 5715–27.
36. Kim KH, Koo HW, Lee BJ. Deep learning-based localization and orientation estimation of pedicle screws in spinal fusion surgery. *Korean J Neurotrauma* 2024; 20(2): 90–100.
37. Felix B, Kalatar SB, Moatz B, et al. Augmented reality spine surgery navigation: Increasing pedicle screw insertion accuracy for both open and minimally invasive spine surgeries. *Spine (Phila Pa 1976)* 2022; 47(12): 865–72.
38. Morley CT, Arreola DM, Qian L, et al. Mixed reality surgical navigation system; Positional accuracy based on food and drug administration standard. *Surg Innov* 2024; 31(1): 48–57.
39. Park JJ, Tiefenbach J, Demetriades AK. The role of artificial intelligence in surgical simulation. *Front Med Technol* 2022; 4: 1076755.
40. Zhang Q, Li M, Qi X, et al. 3D path planning for anterior spinal surgery based on CT images and reinforcement learning. *2018 IEEE International Conference on Cyborg and Bionic Systems (CBS)*, 2018: 317–21.
41. Qi X, Meng J, Li M, et al. An automatic path planning method of pedicle screw placement based on preoperative CT images. *IEEE Trans Med Robot Bionics* 2022; 4: 403–13.
42. Jia S, Weng Y, Wang K, et al. Performance evaluation of an AI-based preoperative planning software application for automatic selection of pedicle screws based on computed tomography images. *Front Surg* 2023; 10: 1247527.
43. Lee A, Baker TS, Bederson JB, Rapoport BI. Levels of autonomy in FDA-cleared surgical robots: A systematic review. *NPJ Digit Med* 2024; 7(1): 103.
44. Yang GZ, Cambias J, Cleary K, et al. Medical robotics-Regulatory, ethical, and legal considerations for increasing levels of autonomy. *Sci Robot* 2017; 2(4): eaam8638.
45. Sadagopan NS, Prasad D, Jain R, et al. Beyond AI and robotics: The dawn of surgical automation in spine surgery. *Artif Intell Surg* 2024; 4(4): 387–400.
46. Massalimova A, Timmermans M, Cavalcanti N, et al. Automatic breach detection during spine pedicle drilling based on vibroacoustic sensing. *Artif Intell Med* 2023; 144: 102641.
47. Haddas R, Lawlor M, Moghadam E, et al. Spine patient care with wearable medical technology: State-of-the-art, opportunities, and challenges: A systematic review. *Spine J* 2023; 23(7): 929–44.
48. Schonfeld E, Veeravagu A. Demonstrating the successful application of synthetic learning in spine surgery for training multi-center models with increased patient privacy. *Sci Rep* 2023; 13: 12481.
49. Giuffrè M, Shung DL. Harnessing the power of synthetic data in healthcare: Innovation, application, and privacy. *NPJ Digit Med* 2023; 6(1): 186.
50. Singh V, Cheng S, Kwan AC, Ebinger J. United States Food and Drug Administration regulation of clinical software in the era of artificial intelligence and machine learning. *Mayo Clin Proc Digit Health* 2025; 3(3): 100231.

10

Artificial Intelligence for Surgical Workflow Analysis

DANYAL Z. KHAN AND HANI J. MARCUS

What is surgical workflow analysis?

Surgical workflow analysis is the systematic codification of a surgical procedure into its constituent components.[1,2] It seeks to break down a complex intervention into its fundamental building blocks, to gain a more in-depth understanding of the intervention and to allow structured comparative analysis between interventions.[1,2] Its inception is intertwined with the advent of surgical data science—a rapidly advancing field which seeks to digitise, codify and analyse surgical patient pathways to enable in-depth service evaluation, more robust comparative surgical research and advancements in technological tools (e.g. artificial intelligence [AI]) to enable more personalized surgical care and improve surgical outcomes.[3] Surgical workflow analysis shares these goals and is the focused operative phase of the surgical patient pathway.

The components that make up surgical workflow are complex, frequently debated and are rapidly developing as our understanding of the field grows.[1,4] This evolution is largely driven by the advancements in technological instruments we use to perform surgery (e.g. microscopes/endoscopes, navigation and robotics) and our ability to analyse data (e.g. computer vision [CV] technology).

One conceptual approach is to consider the *5 Ws and H* of a surgery—what, why, when, where, who and how? Analysing **purposeful events** encompasses "What is being performed?" "Why is it being performed?" and "When is this being performed?" **Anatomy** localizes this movement and the "Where?" whilst the **instrument**, as an extension of the surgeon, represents the "Who?" The "How is the performance?" is related to characteristics such as **surgical skill** and **errors**, both heavily influenced by operative difficulty.

Each of these components is first organised into taxonomies, and then intertwined into ontologies.[4,5] Taxonomies classify and organise items into a hierarchy. For relatively discrete and defined objects such as anatomy and instruments, this is often straightforward (e.g. scissors). However, this is more difficult to define for purposeful events and the analysis of the character of events (e.g. surgical skill, surgical errors) or objects (e.g. anatomic variants). The taxonomy of purposeful events has been the recent focus of the surgical workflow community and is best showcased by the SAGES Annotation Framework guidelines and related works (**Table 10.1**), which deconstructs surgeries into phases, steps, tasks, actions and gestures.[1,4,6–9] However, there is considerable heterogeneity in the use of these terms in the literature.

Workflow ontologies are then formed by relating these taxonomies to each other in a clinically relevant and machine-readable fashion (**Figure 10.1**). It is easiest to ground workflow ontologies in an event taxonomy first (**Table 10.1**) as this sets the level of granularity desired, and drives the complexity and specificity of the linkages with the objects and characteristic taxonomies. Furthermore, these

DOI: 10.1201/9781003471165-10

Table 10.1 Surgical event hierarchical taxonomy

Domain	Definition	Example
Phase	Highest level temporal component of an operation for segmentation purposes; phases are divided into Access, Execution of Surgical Objectives and Closure	Nasal phase (endonasal pituitary surgery)—encompassing the beginning of surgery until entry into the sphenoid sinus
Step	Procedure-specific segment to accomplish a clinically meaningful goal, without which the procedure cannot be completed. Steps need not be performed in a specific order. Steps can be interrupted. Steps do not have to be unique to that operation alone (i.e. a step can be present across similar procedures)	Identification and dissection of the hepatocystic triangle (cholecystectomy surgery)
Task	Sub-component of a step. Composed of a series of actions to accomplish a goal. More than one task must be completed to carry out a step	Exposing and skeletonizing the cystic duct and artery (cholecystectomy surgery)
Action	A primitive component of a task. A series of actions are required to complete a task. Most often represented by a verb. Triplets: Verb x Anatomy x Instrument	Coagulating named artery using bipolar
Gestures	Poorly defined. Atomic surgical gestures largely derived from kinematic data from robotic surgery. In theory, describes the smallest definable interactions between surgeon, instrument tip and tissue. Defined as a discrete movement occurring as a continuous motion preceded and followed by a period without motion—often with spatial, temporal and force components	Left-to-right blunt dissection from X-Y-Z to X-Y-Z, at X m/s, with X N force.

Derived from Meireles et al.[4]

purposeful events contextualise the other components of workflow, and are therefore the core of any workflow ontology. At the highest level, i.e. "phase" level events, general anatomic regions can be vaguely linked with high-level purposeful goals—for example, an Access phase where superficial anatomic structures are traversed to access a surgical target. At more granular levels, specific events can be linked with specific objects or characteristics—for example, "action" events are composed of a verb (e.g. suturing) performed using a specific instrument (e.g. needle holder) on specific anatomic structures (e.g. dura).

By applying these workflow ontologies to operations, we can compare two surgeries in a quantitative manner. A more in-depth understanding of variations in surgical procedures is crucial for comparative research in surgery, which has historically been hampered by our inability to standardize interventions and account for differences in interventions during randomized controlled trials (RCTS), for example. Further, variations in surgical performance are almost universally linked with varying surgical outcomes, and thus understanding these variations can improve surgical audit, help surgeons drive improvements in surgical performances and may also assist with decision support (e.g. predicting surgical outcomes).[3,10] Practically speaking, the cornerstone of surgical workflow analysis is through analysis of surgical video, which may be supplemented by other data sources (e.g. kinematic or haptic data from robots).

Neurosurgery is an ideal candidate for surgical workflow analysis and a surgical data science approach to evidence synthesis.[11,12] Operations are among the most complex and variable of any

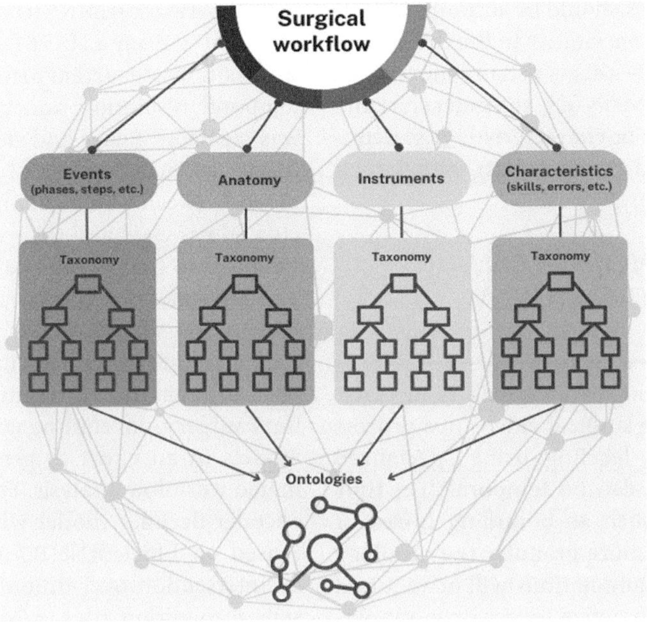

Figure 10.1 Overview of surgical workflow analysis, which conceptually involves linking taxonomies for events, objects (anatomy and instruments) and characteristics into ontologies. (Image made using CanvaPro, with taxonomy icon from Puspito at the NounProject.)

surgical speciality, and there is a relative paucity of traditional high-level evidence (e.g. RCTs) to guide practice. Further, neurosurgery is inherently ripe for digitization by virtue of the technology used to perform the majority of cranial and spinal operations—the operating microscope or endoscope, for example.

CREATING NEUROSURGICAL WORKFLOW ANALYSIS ONTOLOGIES

Prior to recording and applying workflow analysis surgical video, it is crucial to develop, standardize and validate an ontology framework, tailored to the procedure in question, set at an appropriate level of granularity.[13] Currently, creating this framework is most frequently done using a modified Delphi consensus approach.[13] This is composed of multiple phases, starting with a literature review and preliminary framework generation, which is then iterated through multiple rounds of surveys and/or meetings with key stakeholders. Ideally, stakeholders would involve an international panel of surgical experts and would include scientists with expertise in surgical data science. There are numerous examples of such processes in neurosurgery—heralded by an ontology of surgical steps for endoscopic pituitary surgery, and more recently, microscopic vestibular schwannoma resection and lumbar decompression.[13–15] To encompass the wide variation of surgical techniques used across centres, parts of the ontologic framework can be labeled as "core" (required to complete the operation) and "optional" (varies case-to-case or surgeon-to-surgeon).[13–15] Developing these standardized, clinically applicable and machine-readable frameworks is crucial for consistent workflow analysis within centres and across multiple centres.[4]

Crucially, such frameworks should consider carefully the level of granularity desired, as this not only influences ontology creation (as per above) but also the practical analysis of surgical videos (more granular frameworks, generate more frequent and shorter duration workflow events). The desirable characteristics of ontology frameworks are best summarized by the SAGES Annotation Framework Guidance and include having a clear hierarchy with temporal (events such as steps) and spatial features (e.g. anatomy); defined and non-redundant categories; and flexibility for edge cases (e.g. free text entry options).[4]

Ideally, each framework should be accompanied by a user guide to reduce variability in the interpretation of the framework—this is usually more of an issue for recognizing events (e.g. the exact start and end of a surgical step) or characteristic (e.g. defining skill domains and rating scales), rather than instruments or anatomy.[4,16]

PERFORMING WORKFLOW ANALYSIS USING SURGICAL VIDEO AND AI

Once an agreed ontology framework is in place, this can be used to tag surgical videos in a process called annotation or labeling using specialized software. Annotation can be temporal (i.e. time stamps) or spatial (such as bounding boxes or polygon masks). The more granular the ontology framework, the more annotations will be required per video. It is good practice to perform annotations in duplicate to calculate inter-annotator variability (suggesting ontology improvements or further annotator training is needed) and to resolve annotation errors or discrepancies.[4,16] As annotating software advances, many of them have developed time-saving features such as interpolation and object tracking. If done manually, this annotation is still extremely labor-intensive posing limitations to its upscaling and analysis.

However, recent advances in AI, more specifically CV, have allowed this operative workflow analysis to be generated automatically and accurately.[17,18] In the surgical AI community, this has largely been driven through community competitions such as the EndoVis challenge, which adapted artificial neural networks (ANNs) such as AlexNet (from the preceding ImageNet challenge) to endoscopic gastrointestinal surgery videos (creating EndoNet).[19,20] The first example of such AI models for surgical workflow analysis in neurosurgery was based on these models and applied to endoscopic pituitary surgery.[21] The relatively stereotyped nature of this procedure, the fact it is almost entirely performed under endoscopic vision (therefore is entirely recordable) and that endonasal video is not identifiable (therefore reduces governance concerns), makes this procedure an ideal application of AI workflow analysis.[22] In a pilot study using 50 videos of endoscopic pituitary adenoma resection annotated for surgical phases and steps, a model composed of a convolutional neural network (CNN) (trained to recognize steps and phases from a short temporal window of 1–5 frames) and a recurrent neural network (to improve temporal resolution and prediction consistency) was created.[21] Phase and step recognition was primarily evaluated using F1 scores—the harmonic mean between precision and recall. This was calculated per class and then summed across classes, weighted to the prevalence of the respective class. The pilot model achieved a 75% F1 score for step recognition and 90% for phase recognition.[21,23] Similarly, there have been numerous models developed for anatomy recognition in endoscopic pituitary surgery, dovetailing with the step recognition models in an effort to generate integrated automated workflow analysis. For example, PAINet, an encoder-decoder model with a convolution layer (based on EfficientNetB3 and UNet++) achieved an intersection-over-union (IoU) score of 66% for sella recognition after training on 640 endoscopic intra-sphenoid operative images.[24] The next iteration of this model, PitSurgRT, used HRNet and TensorRT to improve the sella IoU score to 70% and achieve real-time performance speeds.[25] Similarly, nasal anatomy (septum and turbinates) recognition models using a U-Net-based ANN have displayed promising performance compared with baseline models when trained on 367 endonasal images.[26] Further, 2023 saw the first neurosurgical CV challenge "PitVis," releasing 25 endoscopic pituitary adenoma resection videos annotated for surgical steps and instruments.[27] This generated multiple workflow analysis models from teams all around the globe—with instrument recognition models achieving F1 scores of up to 0.57 using a model leveraging ResNet152, EfficientNet B7 and SwinL.[27] This challenge also stimulated the creation of combined instrument and step recognition models, with modest F1 scores of 0.5.[27]

While AI-powered surgical workflow analysis has been largely pioneered in endoscopic pituitary surgery within neurosurgery, there are other notable examples of its development. Instrument detection using a dataset of 35 open-access microneurosurgery videos and a YOLOv5-based ANN achieved a precision of up to 93% for suction, ultrasonic aspirator, dissection forceps and bipolar forceps.[28] Otherwise, the only other published models currently use data from simulated models—for example, for tool detection in arachnoid dissection 3D-printed models and endoscopic endonasal carotid injury cadaveric simulators.[28,29]

All of the above workflow analysis AI models in neurosurgery are recent advances, having emerged over the last 5 years, and are all still preclinical phases of development. However, this is clearly a rapidly developing space, with each year bringing larger datasets, more sophisticated workflow ontologies and more advanced AI models—unlocking numerous avenues for clinical translation.[3,22]

APPLYING AI-DRIVEN WORKFLOW ANALYSIS TO NEUROSURGICAL PROBLEMS

The next decade of AI-driven workflow analysis will see this preclinical technology translated into the clinical domain with a variety of potential benefits.

First, this technology has the potential to augment surgical training and education.[17,21,22] In its most basic form, workflow analysis serves as a medium for indexing and time-stamping key steps of neurosurgical operative videos, which is a simple yet effective way to make otherwise unstructured videos easier to navigate and more interactive. This will improve the ease of contemporary surgical video review by surgeons, as part of routine reflective practice on one's surgical logbook. Building on this step recognition, the integration of action recognition including instrument segmentation will allow the generation of quantitative automated performance metrics, which can be fed back to surgeons.[30] This could form part of a surgical coaching program, akin to that pioneered by professional sports. Such programmes have shown benefits across surgical specialities, with AI-assisted surgical coaching programmes being pioneered by neurosurgeons (again, for endoscopic pituitary adenoma surgery)—showing improvements in surgical performance and surgical outcomes leveraging this technology.[30] Programmes such as this will be augmented by skill and error analysis which, at present, are largely derived through surrogate markers (e.g. instrument tracking metrics) rather than specific automated skill scoring systems or error detection models.[9]

Second, automated workflow analysis can be used to augment surgical audits. For example, automated performance metrics can be tracked over time, to identify cases with unexpected patterns of events or errors using a cumulative sum (CUSUM) approach, which could trigger case-based review and closer patient monitoring.[31] Additionally, the information derived from workflow analysis can be used to generate AI-assisted operative notes, which are standardized, with improved accuracy and comprehensiveness and reduced administrative burden when compared with traditional operative notes.[32] Again, this has been demonstrated in endoscopic pituitary adenoma surgery, with this structured data entry facilitating comparison across surgeries and more transparent governance review.[32]

Third, this technology can be used for clinical decision support intraoperatively and postoperatively. Intraoperatively, the output of workflow analysis models can be presented in real time to the surgical team using intraoperative displays. Displaying the current and predicted future surgical steps may improve operational efficiency during surgery, orchestrating the entire team to a common workflow—for example, highlighting the instruments needed next to the scrub technician or upcoming critical steps to the anesthetists.[20] This technology will likely synergize with other complementary technologies. For example, using augmented reality overlays of CV-based detection of anatomic structures (e.g. optic nerves or carotid arteries) during high-risk portions of the procedure could help with error avoidance, surgical guidance and education.[22]

This technology will also synergize with the analysis of the multimodal dataset of the wider neurosurgical patient pathway.[22] This will include preoperative data (e.g. patient factors, presentation, work-up including imaging), surgical video and postoperative data (e.g. outcomes, patient-reported metrics, imaging). This will allow numerous avenues of data-driven improvements to neurosurgical patient care. For example, leveraging this multimodal dataset using a combination of CV workflow analysis models and other AI algorithms could bolster our ability to predict outcomes that are otherwise currently challenging to predict (e.g. sodium disorders after pituitary adenoma resection).[3,22] For example, patients could be classified into high- and low-risk groups for a particular surgical complication.[33] High-risk groups may benefit from extended monitoring with closer attention to potential complications or prophylactic treatments, while low-risk groups may benefit from early discharge and fast-track protocols (sparing risks of nosocomial disease and streamlining resource allocation).[34,35] Further, a similar approach could be used to calculate a more personalized surgical risk score for patient selection and informed consent processes or to identify types or patterns of surgery associated with superior outcomes.[22]

CONCLUSION

Surgical workflow analysis, automated and made scalable through the use of AI, is a rapidly developing field. Neurosurgery is an ideal candidate to benefit from this technology, and interest is clearly mounting in its potential to facilitate more data-driven and personalized care to our patients. The next decade will see the expansion of neurosurgical multimodal multicentric datasets, the development of underpinning AI models, increasing synergy with complementary surgical technologies and translation into operating rooms of the future.

REFERENCES

1. Lalys F, Jannin P. Surgical process modelling: A review. *Int J Comput Assist Radiol Surg* 2014; 9(3): 495–511.
2. Sarker SK, Chang A, Albrani T, Vincent C. Constructing hierarchical task analysis in surgery. *Surg Endosc* 2008; 22(1): 107–11.
3. Maier-Hein L, Eisenmann M, Sarikaya D, et al. Surgical data science–from concepts toward clinical translation. *Med Image Anal* 2022; 76: 102306.
4. Meireles OR, Rosman G, Altieri MS, et al. Sages consensus recommendations on an annotation framework for surgical video. *Surg Endosc* 2021; 35(9): 4918–29.
5. Neumann J, Uciteli A, Meschke T, et al. Ontology-based surgical workflow recognition and prediction. *J Biomed Inform* 2022; 136: 104240.
6. van Amsterdam B, Clarkson MJ, Stoyanov D. Gesture recognition in robotic surgery: A review. *IEEE Trans Biomed Eng* 2021; 68(6): 2021–35.
7. Nyangoh Timoh K, Huaulme A, Cleary K, et al. A systematic review of annotation for surgical process model analysis in minimally invasive surgery based on video. *Surg Endosc* 2023; 37(6): 4298–314.
8. Béjar Haro B, Zappella L, Vidal R (eds). *Surgical Gesture Classification from Video Data*. Heidelberg: Springer; 2012.
9. Ma R, Ramaswamy A, Xu J, et al. Surgical gestures as a method to quantify surgical performance and predict patient outcomes. *NPJ Digit Med* 2022; 5(1): 187.
10. Birkmeyer JD, Finks JF, O'Reilly A, et al. Surgical skill and complication rates after bariatric surgery. *N Engl J Med* 2013; 369(15): 1434–42.
11. Senders JT, Arnaout O, Karhade AV, et al. Natural and artificial intelligence in neurosurgery: A systematic review. *Neurosurgery* 2018; 83(2): 181–92.
12. Panesar SS, Kliot M, Parrish R, et al. Promises and perils of artificial intelligence in neurosurgery. *Neurosurgery* 2020; 87(1): 33–44.
13. Marcus HJ, Khan DZ, Borg A, et al. Pituitary society expert Delphi consensus: Operative workflow in endoscopic transsphenoidal pituitary adenoma resection. *Pituitary* 2021: 24(6): 839–53.
14. Horsfall HL, Khan DZ, Collins J, et al. Generating operative workflows for vestibular schwannoma resection: A two-stage Delphi's consensus in collaboration with the British Skull Base Society. Part 2: The translabyrinthine approach. *J Neurol Surg B Skull Base* 2023; 84(05): 433–43.
15. Horsfall HL, Khan DZ, Collins J, et al. Generating operative workflows for vestibular schwannoma resection: A two-stage Delphi's consensus in collaboration with the British Skull Base Society. Part 1: The retrosigmoid approach. *J Neurol Surg B Skull Base* 2023; 84(05): 423–32.
16. Pangal DJ, Kugener G, Shahrestani S, et al. A guide to annotation of neurosurgical intraoperative video for machine learning analysis and computer vision. *World Neurosurg* 2021; 150: 26–30.
17. Garrow CR, Kowalewski K-F, Li L, et al. Machine learning for surgical phase recognition: A systematic review. *Ann Surg* 2021; 273(4): 684–93.
18. Lecuyer G, Ragot M, Martin N, et al. Assisted phase and step annotation for surgical videos. *Int J Comput Assist Radiol Surg* 2020; 15(4): 673–80.

19. Twinanda AP, Shehata S, Mutter D, et al. Endonet: A deep architecture for recognition tasks on laparoscopic videos. *IEEE Trans Med Imaging* 2016; 36(1): 86–97.
20. Luengo I, Grammatikopoulou M, Mohammadi R, et al. 2020 cataracts semantic segmentation challenge. arXiv:2110.10965, 2021.
21. Khan DZ, Luengo I, Barbarisi S, et al. Automated operative workflow analysis of endoscopic pituitary surgery using machine learning: Development and preclinical evaluation (ideal stage 0). *J Neurosurg* 2021; 137(1): 51–8.
22. Khan DZ, Hanrahan JG, Baldeweg SE, et al. Current and future advances in surgical therapy for pituitary adenoma. *Endocr Rev* 2023; 44(5): 947–59.
23. Das A, Bano S, Vasconcelos F, et al. Reducing prediction volatility in the surgical workflow recognition of endoscopic pituitary surgery. *Int J Comput Assist Radiol Surg* 2022; 17(8): 1445–52.
24. Das A, Khan DZ, Williams SC, et al. A multitask network for anatomy identification in endoscopic pituitary surgery. *MICCAI Conference Proceedings*, 2023.
25. Mao Z, Das A, Islam M, et al. Pitsurgrt: Real-time localization of critical anatomical structures in endoscopic pituitary surgery. *Int J Comput Assist Radiol Surg* 2024: 19(6): 1053–60.
26. Staartjes VE, Volokitin A, Regli L, et al. Machine vision for real-time intraoperative anatomic guidance: A proof-of-concept study in endoscopic pituitary surgery. *Oper Neurosurg* 2021; 21(4): 242–7.
27. Speidel S, Maier-Hein L, Stoyanov D, et al. Endoscopic Vision Challenge 2023. Available from: https://zenodo.org/records/8315050 (Accessed April 2026).
28. Ramesh A, Beniwal M, Uppar AM, et al. Microsurgical tool detection and characterization in intra-operative neurosurgical videos. *Annu Int Conf IEEE Eng Med Biol Soc* 2021; 2021: 2676–81.
29. Pangal DJ, Kugener G, Cardinal T, et al. Use of surgical video–based automated performance metrics to predict blood loss and success of simulated vascular injury control in neurosurgery: A pilot study. *J Neurosurg* 2021; 137(3): 840–9.
30. Khan DZ KC, Das A, Valetopolou A, et al. Video-based performance analysis in pituitary surgery—Part 2: AI-assisted coaching. *World Neurosurg* 2024; 190: e797–e808.
31. Biau DJ, Resche-Rigon M, Godiris-Petit G, et al. Quality control of surgical and interventional procedures: A review of the CUSUM. *BMJ Quality & Safety* 2007; 16(3): 203–7.
32. Das A, Khan DZ, Hanrahan J, et al. Automatic generation of operation notes in endoscopic pituitary surgery videos using workflow recognition. *Intell Based Med* 2023; 8: 100107.
33. Marcus AP, Marcus HJ, Camp SJ, et al. Improved prediction of surgical resectability in patients with glioblastoma using an artificial neural network. *Sci Rep* 2020; 10(1): 5143.
34. Lobatto DJ, Vliet Vlieland TPM, van den Hout WB, et al. Feasibility, safety, and outcomes of a stratified fast-track care trajectory in pituitary surgery. *Endocrine* 2020; 69(1): 175–87.
35. Hughes MA, Culpin E, Darley R, et al. Enhanced recovery and accelerated discharge after endoscopic transsphenoidal pituitary surgery: Safety, patient feedback, and cost implications. *Acta Neurochir (Wien)* 2020; 162(6): 1281–6.

11

The Mind–Machine Interface

BENJAMIN C. SHERMAN, PAUL M. HARARY, PRIYA BHANOT AND VIVEK P. BUCH

INTRODUCTION

Definition and purpose of brain–computer interfaces

Brain–Computer Interfaces (BCIs) represent a combination of technologies at the intersection of neuroscience, electrical engineering and computing. These interfaces facilitate a direct communication pathway between the brain's neural activity and external devices, circumventing conventional neuromuscular routes, or augmenting damaged neuronal or network functionality. This enables individuals to control computers, prosthetic limbs or other assistive devices via direct neural input, as well as directed stimulation to modulate individual neurons, groups of neurons or neural networks. The core objective of BCIs is to repair, augment or amplify human sensory-motor and potentially cognitive abilities. Through the precise interpretation and conversion of neural signals into actionable commands and via targeted neurostimulation, BCIs hold the transformative potential to restore functions lost due to various neuro- or neuromuscular pathologies. With continued advancements, particularly involving artificial intelligence (AI) in the computational domain, they may enhance human capabilities beyond natural biological limits in the future.

Historical context and evolution

The origin of BCI technology can be traced back to the pioneering work in electrophysiology by Hans Berger in 1924,[1] with the implementation of the first in-human electroencephalogram (EEG), and initial description of alpha and beta waves. After further characterization of electrophysiological neural activity throughout the mid-twentieth century, particularly via exploration of frequency bands (**Figure 11.1**), the foundational research and conceptualization of direct brain-to-machine communication was posited by Jacques Vidal at UCLA.[2] Beginning around the same time in the 1970s, significant technological leaps enabled the transition from theoretical models to practical applications. Initial explorations demonstrated the feasibility of using EEG signals for basic control tasks, setting the stage for a burgeoning field of research and development.[3–5]

Subsequent decades witnessed rapid advancements, propelled by breakthroughs in signal processing, microfabrication and, particularly, the advent of computational methods capable of analyzing complex neural data.[6–8] Key milestones include the development of invasive neurosensing techniques that provide detailed insights into brain activity, and the application of machine learning (ML) algorithms which significantly enhanced the decoding and interpretation of neural signals.[9,10]

The historical trajectory of BCI research reflects a multidisciplinary effort, drawing upon the expertise of neuroscientists, electrical engineers, computer scientists, psychiatrists, philosophers and ethicists. This collaboration has been instrumental not only in overcoming the technical and conceptual barriers to practical implementation of BCI technology, but also the individual and societal impact of such advancements. Chief among these developments, and particularly prescient in recent years, is the integration of AI. The use of AI to address computational requirements

DOI: 10.1201/9781003471165-11

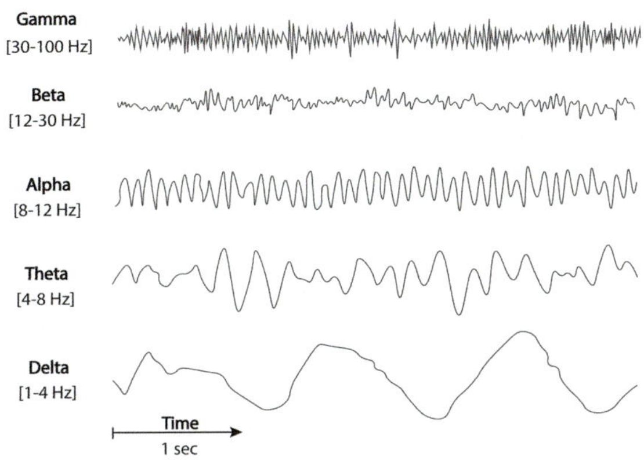

Figure 11.1 Electroencephalographic frequency bands. Representative waveforms of gamma (30–100 Hz), beta (12–30 Hz), alpha (8–12 Hz), theta (4–8 Hz), and delta (1–4 Hz) oscillations shown over time. Scale bar, 1 second.

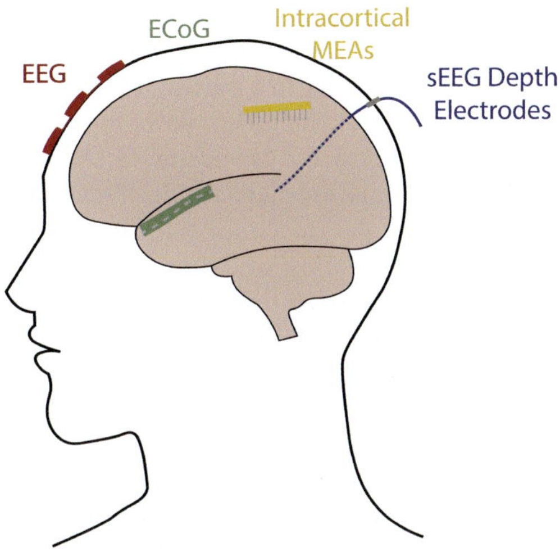

Figure 11.2 Electrophysiological approaches for recording neural activity. EEG electrodes are positioned on the scalp, electrocorticography (ECoG) electrodes on the cortical surface, intracortical microelectrode arrays (MEAs) within the cortex, and stereoelectroencephalography (sEEG) depth electrodes within deeper brain structures.

of BCIs marks a pivotal juncture, offering unprecedented capabilities in learning from, predicting, and adapting to the intricate and often personalized patterns of neural data.[7,11–13] AI's role in BCIs not only enhances the interfaces' accuracy and functionality but also broadens the spectrum of potential applications, from rehabilitation to cognitive augmentation.[14]

FUNDAMENTALS OF BRAIN–COMPUTER INTERFACES

Neuroscience

The basis of BCI development involves the translation of physiological data generated by brain tissue into computational information that can be interpreted by external systems. In closed-loop BCI systems, information is processed continuously in real time to create a bidirectional feedback loop between the brain and computer. Many closed-loop BCI systems also induce therapeutic brain modulation based on this neurofeedback. They do so by recording brain activity and identifying relevant neural signatures for the purpose of restoring a pathologic disconnect between a neural impulse

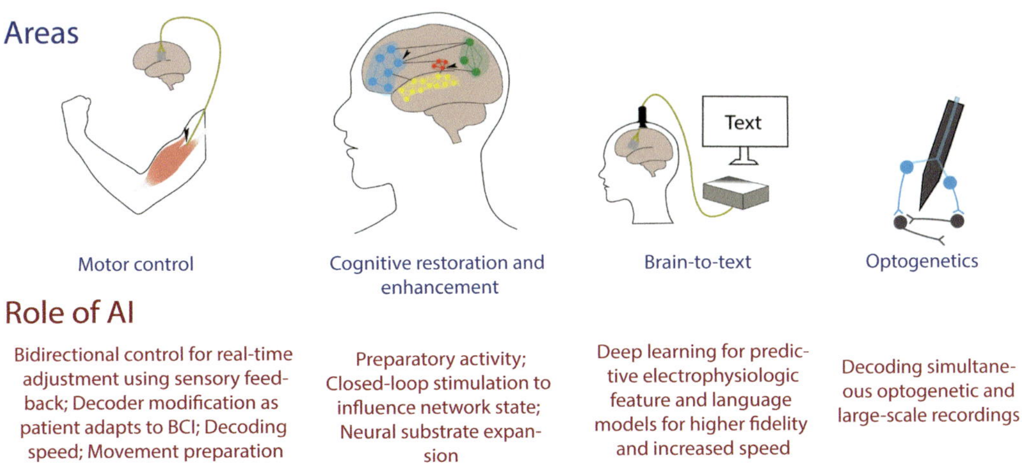

Figure 11.3 Applications of AI-integrated BCI.

and the corresponding action it should elicit or anticipating when a pathologic event may occur. Neural signatures refer to a pattern of brain activity that can predict a behavior, pathological event or cognitive process and is specific to the type of recording used, disease state and individual brain dynamics. Some parameters include neural oscillations, synchronization and functional connectivity patterns or evoked responses.

The current foci of BCI application include motor rehabilitation, speech decoding, seizure detection and prevention and, more recently, cognition. In motor function, something as simple as the decision to move a finger requires a cascade of signals that must pass through several structures from the premotor cortex to the M1 cortex, SMA, basal ganglia, thalamus and spinal cord before even reaching the motor end plates that actually initiate muscle contractions. As these signals propagate across the brain, they are filtered and contextualized with sensory input from systems such as vision or proprioception. When patients who have experienced stroke or other brain injury lose function in one or more of these areas, they also lose the ability to translate their motor intentions to concrete motor output. Neural signatures from residual tissue, however, can be recorded and decoded by computational models to characterize motor intention.[15,16] This information can then be used to stimulate the corresponding surviving downstream pathways[17] or integrated with external systems like prosthetics or computer cursors to restore some level of motor function.[18] Similarly, in patients with speech dysfunction, the ability to communicate a desired thought or message may be inhibited by neural or motor deficits, but neural signatures of intention can be extracted and translated artificially.[7,13] In patients suffering from epilepsy, analyzing seizure loci and individualized patterns of electrophysiological changes in the brain preceding or during seizure onset, enables clinicians to develop personalized neural signatures that predict when one may occur.[19,20] BCIs used in the treatment of cognitive impairment are still evolving, as these disease states involve global neural networks, but depend on the same essential concept in which specific neural signatures corresponding to different aspects of cognition such as decision-making or to disease states like depression can help guide rehabilitative modulation.[21,22]

While some BCIs are purely diagnostic or involve external output systems like prosthetics or computer cursors, many therapeutic BCIs involve some form of direct brain modulation. Modulation can induce changes in brain activity by directly electrically stimulating relevant neuronal networks and by promoting neuroplasticity. Neuroplasticity enhances the strength of certain neuronal pathways over others, allowing for neural circuits to change or form. This encourages functional recovery in damaged tissue and/or compensation by other neural networks.[23] As in any introduction of an external system into a biological one, seamless integration of the two is the fundamental goal and largest barrier to success. Neuroplasticity not only rehabilitates but also promotes the convergence of the BCI and the biological system.

Electrical engineering

Electrical engineering in BCI development is critical for signal acquisition and modulation. BCIs detect neural signatures through direct or indirect measurement of brain activity. Direct measurement involves the intake of the electrophysiological activity generated by individual neurons or groups of adjacent neurons within distinct brain regions, or axons connecting these regions.[24,25] The more invasive the recording method, the more signal strength can be achieved since the recording sensors are closer to the actual input source. However, more invasive recording also increases the standard surgical risks associated with implantation,[26] the cost of the procedure and the difficulty associated with replacing the BCI when indicated. In direct BCI systems, there are four main methods of collecting neural data:

1. Non-invasive electroencephalogram (EEG) recordings taken from the surface of the scalp.
2. Invasive electrocorticography (ECoG) recordings taken from the cortical surface.
3. Invasive intracortical microelectrode arrays.
4. Invasive subcortical depth electrode recordings.[26,27]

All of these methods involve the placement of biocompatible electrodes capable of detecting the electrical fields generated by the action potentials of neurons. Since these voltage differences are relatively small and susceptible to extraneous interference, amplifiers in the recording system filter and intensify these summative signals. These resultant signals then undergo feature extraction where neural signatures can be identified through frequency band, power and entropy analysis.[15–18]

EEG is the standard for most BCI recording because of its accessibility and noninvasive quality, but the layers of CSF, meninges, skin and scalp that the signal must travel through to reach the electrode limits its informational capacity.[26] ECoG provides better spatial and temporal resolution than EEG with a higher amplitude and frequency range, but is still limited to encoding broadscale synchronized activity of large neuron populations in defined cortical areas. Intracortical microelectrode arrays can be directly placed within the cerebral cortex and can measure local field potentials representing low-frequency signals from much smaller and more specific neural circuits. These local field potentials operate at a millisecond timescale and are particularly relevant in characterizing the functional connectivity of neuronal networks.[28] Depth electrodes can be placed subcortically in more centralized brain structures like the thalamus or hippocampus using stereotactic EEG (sEEG)—signals that cannot be acquired from more superficial recording methods.[27] Indirect BCI recording systems such as fMRI, magnetoencephalography (MEG) and near-infrared spectroscopy measure the peripheral effects of brain activity on other physiological properties like blood flow or oxygenation.[26]

As discussed previously, the most classic form of BCI neuromodulation is direct stimulation of brain tissue by focused applications of electric current. In the same way that common, standard-of-care recording methods in neurosurgery can be used by BCIs to input information within the system, common, standard-of-care stimulation methods like deep brain stimulation (DBS), transcranial magnetic stimulation, functional electrical stimulation or responsive neurostimulation (RNS) can be used to deliver an output. Because ECoG electrodes and microelectrode arrays used in intracortical recording connect directly with neural tissue, they can also be used to deliver cortical stimulation. Like naturally evoked brain signals, this stimulation can be controlled by its frequency, duration, strength or synchronization across different brain regions by an external pulse generator. Functional electrical stimulation involves neuromuscular excitation, so these electrodes would act upon the peripheral motor neurons innervating relevant muscle groups.[26,29] Recording electrodes communicate with a computational system processing the data and determining feedback course through several possible avenues that require consideration of either power management or transmission range. These include wires and connectors connected to an internal device implanted beneath the skin dependent on a battery or an external computational device separate from the body. Some BCI systems also facilitate wireless communication of electrodes with an external system through wireless transceivers within the implant that can both transmit and receive data through radiofrequency signals. Instead of providing neural stimulation, these external systems may instead deliver a feedback-driven output to prosthetics, computer screens or communication devices depending on the clinical need.[28]

Computation

Since many of these recording and stimulation methods are already being used in neurosurgery outside of BCI, the true innovation underlying this field lies in the computation that establishes the adaptive neurofeedback loop. Even in healthy patients, the brain operates in very personalized ways dependent on a person's situational input and specific experiences.[30] In neurologic disease states, the type and extent of neural damage or dysfunction is variable, so the more personalized the neural signature identification process is, the more clinically beneficial the BCI will be. However, increasingly contextualized and dynamic feedback systems have increasing computational demands from data load to recursive processing complexity to stimulation metrics that must be managed and interpreted efficiently for real-time processing. The most intricate machine in existence is the healthy human brain. When BCI feedback systems more closely mimic natural neural function, they will be more readily integrated with natural neural circuits. However, this requires the same type of computing capacity with more complexity than current AI utilizing layers of computerized neurons that are purely excitatory or inhibitory, just as our own diversity of neurotransmitters and respective circuits developed over billions of years of evolution.[31,32] The basis of AI was inspired by biological neural networks but may be further developed for optimized computational power and integration with biological neural networks.

Like the brain, the first step in creating a recursive artificial neural network is calibrating an initial fixed network. As more data become available from recording electrodes, the fixed neural network mimics the resting state of the brain and can be used as a standard for comparison to evoked neural signatures. In biological systems, experiences reinforce, depress or connect neural networks through Hebbian-plasticity. Artificial neural networks are similarly iteratively trained by experience in which supervised volitional or pathologic events are repeated so that patterns associated with these events emerge and establish themselves, providing the basis for neural signature characterization.[28,30,33] Eventually, the model is tested with new and unsupervised events that must be integrated with the existing computational framework and engage in a process of continuous recursive learning. Once the system begins output delivery either through stimulation or external application, the neural responses can be optimized by determining which parameters elicit the greatest therapeutic benefit. Interfaces are interactive, adaptive and constantly evolving whether they are between biological structures or biological and artificial ones. As our understanding of the brain's natural computation grows and recording apparatuses become more accurate and efficient, artificial computational performance will continue to improve and approach true autonomous intelligence.[30]

CURRENT AND FUTURE APPLICATIONS OF AI-INTEGRATED BCI

Historically, a major challenge in BCI development has been limitations in the spatial resolution with which cortex could be recorded and stimulated, particularly while minimizing damage to underlying tissue. This is further complicated by factors such as the topography and low mechanical modulus of the brain,[34] variation in cortical localization of function across individuals,[35,36] and risks associated with overcrowding the intracranial space.[37] In addition, the longevity of penetrating electrodes such as the Utah array, which was central to early examples of motor BCI,[9] may be limited at 6 months to 1 year. However, recent advances in neurosensing technologies represent significant progress toward addressing these limitations. For example, the development of flexible microelectrode arrays, capable of both recording and stimulating, has enabled neural recordings with higher spatial resolution and reliability than traditional ECoG grids.[9,10] In addition, the latest generation of linear probes such as Neuropixels, which enable simultaneous recording of up to 100 single units across cortical depth,[13] have facilitated basic research into cortical dynamics, allowing for more informed target selection for BCI. Collectively, these have enabled more sensitive large-scale recordings, providing larger quantities of electrophysiological data.[38,39] With improved access to electrophysiological data, issues such as data transfer, device power and decoding may represent new constraints in BCI. Rational decoding of these data may become a primary bottleneck, especially with regard to analyzing functional connectivity across large-scale networks.[14] In addition, optogenetic approaches, which may enable cell-type specificity and possibly neuromodulation without surgery, may move closer to clinical translation.[40]

AI will continue to be instrumental in rational decoding for guidance of BCI, particularly for testing network-level hypotheses. Currently, referencing, band-pass filtering, denoising, feature extraction and feature classification are largely based on AI. In addition, with the increasing focus on studying neuronal dynamics at the population-level, recurrent neural networks are likely to play a central role.[41,42] Here, we will discuss current applications of BCI and AI and how their further integration may support future developments across key application areas.

Motor brain–computer interfaces

Motor BCIs aim to replace or restore motor function by using neuronal activity from intact motor cortical circuitry to guide movement devices or directly stimulate a patient's muscles while circumventing damaged neural pathways, often in cases of spinal cord injury. By comparison, neurostimulator approaches such as functional electrical stimulation and spinal cord stimulation are based on external muscle movements or constant stimulation parameters, rather than being directly guided by brain signals. Of additional note, spinal cord stimulators have shown some evidence in enhancing functionality but are primarily for the purpose of mitigating neuropathic pain. While these are effective in many cases, they require a degree of intact independent movement capacity. Landmark studies by Georgopoulos and collaborators established proof-of-principle that population-level cortical dynamics can serve as a means to control motor prosthetics,[43,44] and Milekovic et al. have demonstrated proof of concept for a motor prosthesis for Parkinson's disease.[45] Major advances toward clinical translation were later made by Hochberg and the BrainGate collaboration.[46,47] Rapid progress in the field of ML has been closely linked with motor BCI development for both discrete and continuous movements. For example, real-time control of motor prosthetics has moved toward using recurrent neural networks (RNNs) and deep neural networks, particularly as electrophysiology data used in training sets have improved.[7,12]

Recently, there has been an increased focus on using network-inspired hypotheses to guide motor BCIs, with a key role for AI-based decoding. Initial BCI decoding pipelines prioritized directional signaling as a means to determine movement intent.[48] However, growing evidence indicates that preparatory activity may be a powerful means of decoding voluntary movement.[24,41] This spontaneous, "null-space" neural activity can be used to infer preparatory patterns associated with motor function memory formation and cognitive function.[24,49] As more sophisticated AI models are applied to these datasets, more accurate and rapid decoding may be achieved. This may facilitate development of more naturalistic motor BCIs. In addition, increased efficiency in decoding imaging-based BCIs may support less invasive motor prostheses.

Cognitive BCI

Cognitive BCIs aim to restore or enhance cognitive function using two broad strategies:

1. Optimization of intact neural circuitry.
2. Expansion of neural substrate through electronic means.

The first of these strategies generally attempts to use neurostimulation to push distributed networks which may be dysfunctional in neuropsychiatric or developmental disorders into a state of higher function.[50] Intracranial recordings may be used to assess functional connectivity and inform stimulation intensity and target areas. This is particularly true in the case of closed-loop stimulation, which adapts stimulation parameters based on real-time brain activity to optimize certain functions, such as cognitive control.[50] Further, recent investigations have underscored the role that white matter may play as a functional contributor to networks.[25,51] Electrophysiological data from intracranial recordings in natural environments, may be facilitated by progress in implantable devices. Of note, some degree of cognitive function must be intact for current BCI training protocols to be successful. This results in a functionally dependent rate of BCI illiteracy and may limit generalizability of BCI technology.[52] Consequently, a different approach may be necessary in BCI for patients with more extensive cognitive impairment or diffuse or profound neurological injury.

Expansion of neural substrate using neuroprosthetics entails going beyond neurostimulation to the addition of processing units. Perhaps the most well-known effort aimed at such cognitive enhancement is Neuralink.[53] However, earlier studies have similarly explored adding computational capacity. Berger and collaborators used a multi-input/multi-output nonlinear model to construct a prosthesis to enhance hippocampal function in a rodent model.[54] Subsequently, prostheses emulating primate prefrontal cortex[55] and cerebellar function[56] were developed. Although these studies established an intriguing foundation, they remain far from clinical translation. Modern AI and recording methods, however, may advance this field to a point where it may more realistically offer cognitive enhancement.

Brain-to-text

Speech BCIs use intracortical recordings to infer sentences from a subject based on previous recordings. Recently, there has been significant progress utilizing recordings from two distinct areas:

1. The speech cortex (Brodmann area 44 of Broca's area) directly.
2. The sensorimotor and ventral premotor cortex to interpret control of orofacial, glossal and pharyngeal muscles encoding speech.[7,8,12,13]

AI was central to these efforts, with machine-learning techniques used for word classification and language models used to increase speed and accuracy.

In milestone 2021 and 2023 studies by the BrainGate2 group, intracortical recordings were used to decode handwriting movements and orofacial movements, respectively.[7,12] Microelectrode arrays were placed in ventral premotor cortex and Brodmann area 44 to decode orofacial movement and attempted speech, resulting in a high degree of accuracy in language decoding. Separately, Metzger and collaborators were successful in achieving brain-to-text using broad-coverage, high-density ECoG to record from sensorimotor cortex, rather than penetrating electrodes.[13] A combination of DL models based on training data and predictive language models were used to achieve higher speed and accuracy. Advances in AI-based decoding are arguably just as responsible for the rapid rate of progress as advances in surgical and signal acquisition technologies, if not more. Studies by both teams, however, were performed in patients with motor dysfunction due to conditions such as bulbar-onset amyotrophic lateral sclerosis, high-level spinal cord injury or brainstem stroke. Consequently, while they had impairments in their ability to vocalize, they had otherwise intact and fully developed language centers. To this end, it was noted that neural substrates mediating language production were still intact after an extended period of anarthria. Given the investigational device exemption status of motor BCI and the single-participant nature of these investigations, it is not clear how much variation between studies may be due to underlying differences in patient disease severity rather than BCI devices themselves. In addition, further work is necessary to expand access to BCI technology to patient populations whose auditory or speech cortices did not undergo typical neurologic development during key stages of myelination and pruning, as well as those with productive or receptive aphasia, as is common in stroke.[51] Of note, the relationship between Broca's area and language production has recently been revealed to be more complex than traditionally believed.[57,58] This may be relevant to target selection for development of BCI for aphasic patients.

Significant progress in predictive language models, language decoding using noninvasive imaging,[59] and basic research into the cortical dynamics mediating language production[60] all indicate that the near future may hold rapid development in speech BCI.

Emerging optogenetic approaches to brain–computer interfaces

An area of significant interest for future BCI development is optical-neural interfaces, due to their potential to provide cell type specificity. Optogenetic approaches exploit light-sensitive genetically encodable opsins to manipulate specific cell populations with a high degree of temporal control, both *in vitro*[61] and in *in vivo*.[62] These tools have been used to demonstrate proof-of-principle of optically driven BCI platforms.[63] In addition, optical bidirectional systems may incorporate AI-guided adaptive stimulation intensity, representing a very high therapeutic ceiling. This type of closed-loop optogenetic-based BCI has made significant progress in rodent models and non-human primates.[64] Further, optical approaches to BCI offer the prospect of stimulation without intracranial surgery, through the use of transcranial photoactivation.[40] Notably, optical-based DBS has been explored for Parkinson's disease.[65] Hybrid bidirectional implants, which incorporate optogenetics and ECoG, have also been studied.[66] Further, recent developments in voltage-sensing optogenetic tools may provide both high temporal and high spatial resolution for BCI.[67] By comparison, implanted microelectrodes can provide high sensitivity but may only record from a small number of neurons at a time. This effectively limits the networks which may be captured and may also require a large number of electrodes to be implanted to measure distributed processes.

The field of BCI continues to demonstrate a rapid rate of progress. Advances in AI have been a major contributor, enabling increasingly sophisticated decoding of electrophysiological data. Increased integration of AI will likely be instrumental in finding solutions to current limitations in BCI. However, if AI accelerates BCI development as anticipated, new and even more complex challenges will quickly arise.

CHALLENGES AND LIMITATIONS

Technical challenges

Numerous technical challenges present themselves when considering the optimization of BCIs. Notably, the challenges today have shifted from basic signal interference to more intricate issues of integration, processing and application. Unlike initial concepts involving standard EEG where artifact interference was a significant concern, current invasive technologies have largely mitigated these issues through advanced filtering techniques and improved sensor design. The focus now is on enhancing the quality and specificity of neural data capture to achieve a granular, single-neuron resolution, understanding of electrophysiological signals without compromising the integrity of the neural tissue being monitored and stimulated. The advancement of microelectrode arrays by BrainGate2 and the introduction of technologies like Neuropixels illustrate significant strides in this domain.[7,12,68] However, challenges remain in optimizing these technologies for long-term stability and minimizing the invasiveness of neural interfaces that have broader coverage than a single cortical region.

The evolution of BCI technology is deeply intertwined with progress in hardware design, where size, power, efficiency and durability are crucial considerations. Achieving miniaturization while enhancing the biocompatibility of implantable devices is necessary for both patient safety and the long-term viability of BCIs. Innovations in materials science have introduced flexible substrates and bioresorbable electronics, promising to reduce the foreign body response and adapt more naturally to biological tissues.[34,38,66] Further, wireless energy transfer and battery technology are areas of intense research aimed at providing reliable power to BCI systems without frequent surgical interventions.[69] The integration of these advancements presents a complex engineering challenge.

With the advent of sophisticated signal acquisition methods from sEEG to ECoG and depth electrode recordings, BCI systems now generate vast amounts of complex neural data, necessitating unprecedented computational resources for real-time analysis and interpretation.[70,71] The challenge lies not only in managing this data deluge but also in developing decoding algorithms and ML models that can effectively translate neural patterns into precise, reliable outputs, and integrate more naturally with biological neural circuitry. As BCIs become more integrated with AI, these computational demands will likely only escalate. Developing hardware capable of supporting these computational needs, while maintaining efficiency and responsiveness is critical. This requires a concerted effort in computational neuroscience and computer engineering to devise new algorithms and architectures that can process high-dimensional datasets in real time, ensuring the seamless operation of BCI systems, with a parallel focus on development of sufficient hardware to support this logical architecture.[72]

Long-term viability and patient safety

The integration of BCIs into the healthcare ecosystem presents a transformative potential for patient care but also introduces significant challenges related to their long-term viability and safety. A prominent concern in the deployment of BCIs, as with any neurally invasive technology, is the risk of infection associated with implantable devices. The breach of the blood–brain barrier and the introduction of foreign materials into the body necessitates advanced materials and surgical techniques designed to minimize this risk.[37] Pre-planning depth and grid electrode placement with programs such as Brainlab (Brainlab, Chicago) and implanting them with a precise and patient customized coordinate system with stereotactic equipment or the ROSA robot (Zimmer Biomet, France) represent the current leading edge of advancement in ensuring minimal risk. Additionally, the stability and durability of neural implants pose significant challenges. Over time, the glial scarring and neovascularization in response to implanted devices can lead to new neurologic deficits and degradation in performance, requiring careful consideration of materials science and implant design to ensure long-term functionality.[34,37]

Further, the implications of adverse neural plasticity and dependency on BCI technologies are critical areas of study. The brain's ability to adapt to, and incorporate, BCI devices can lead to changes in neural circuit architecture and function, which, while often beneficial, can also pose risks of dependency or unexpected changes neuronal activity. Ongoing monitoring is essential to understand these effects fully and to develop strategies to mitigate any negative consequences as they arise.[73]

The ethical considerations surrounding the long-term use of BCIs are multifaceted, involving questions of autonomy, identity and the potential for cognitive enhancement or alteration. Ensuring that BCIs are used in ways that respect patient autonomy and personal identity requires ongoing ethical scrutiny. To address these challenges, robust regulatory frameworks are needed to guide the development, testing and deployment of BCIs. Such frameworks exist already in the FDA approval and clinical trial pipelines, but due to the magnitude of impact BCI technology can have on individuals and humanity, further ethical considerations are raised.

ETHICAL AND PRIVACY CONSIDERATIONS

The rapid advancement and integration of BCI technologies into various aspects of human life raise profound ethical and privacy concerns. At the heart of these concerns is the stewardship and commercialization of neural data, personal information that is unparalleled in its intimacy and sensitivity.

As BCIs bridge the gap between the human brain and digital worlds, they generate neural data that could offer unprecedented insights into an individual's thoughts, intentions and preferences. This raises critical questions about data ownership, privacy and consent. Who owns these data? How can they be used? and Who gets to decide? The development of comprehensive regulatory frameworks to address these questions is crucial. Such frameworks must ensure the secure collection, storage and analysis of neural data, safeguarding against unauthorized access and potential exploitation.[74] As has been demonstrated with arguably para-neural data, exquisitely detailed information on consumer habits and app interaction is being exploited to maximize social media advertising profits.[75] For the same to occur with direct neural data would be unthinkable.

The intersection of BCIs with private sector interests further complicates the ethical landscape. While the commercialization of BCI technology can drive innovation and accessibility, it also risks widening the gap between those who can afford advanced neurotechnologies and those who cannot. Ensuring equitable access to the benefits of BCIs is a pressing ethical challenge, raising questions about social justice and the digital divide in the context of neurotechnology.[76] If only the wealthy can afford technology to enhance cognitive function, will there ever be a chance for someone of low socioeconomic status to compete?

The potential for BCIs to affect or even alter an individual's cognitive and motor functions necessitates a reevaluation not only of private interest involvement, but also of patient autonomy and consent in a medical setting. The integration of AI-driven systems with the human brain introduces the possibility of influencing user intent, challenging traditional notions of autonomy and free will. Informed consent becomes complex in this context, as participants must understand, not only the immediate effects of BCI use, but also the long-term implications for their own personhood, autonomy and mental integrity.[77] This is a particularly critical evaluation for BCIs which influence cognition,[14] and necessitates the question—is this the same person who initially consented to a BCI?

Addressing these ethical and privacy considerations requires a multidisciplinary approach, bringing together experts from neuroscience, law, ethics, technology and public policy. Such a consortium is essential for navigating the complex moral landscape of BCI technologies, ensuring that they enhance human capabilities without compromising individual personhood, rights or societal values.[74] These ethical and privacy considerations surrounding BCI technology are as complex as they are critical. As we venture further into this frontier, the need for vigilant ethical oversight, robust regulatory frameworks, and ongoing multidisciplinary dialogue has never been more apparent. These efforts will be crucial in ensuring that BCI technologies develop in a manner that respects and enhances our shared human values.

CONCLUSION

BCIs represent the pinnacle of multidisciplinary progress from the fields of neuroscience, psychiatry, electrical engineering, philosophy and scientific computing. Should they reach their full potential, they will herald a new era in which the fusion of mind and machine can transcend biological limitations and restore lost functionalities. Through the lens of historical achievements and modern groundbreaking research, it is evident that BCIs have developed substantially since their theoretic conception to their nascent form as fully functional enhancements of damaged human capability.

However, as BCIs inch closer to mainstream adoption, they bring significant ethical considerations that demand meticulous attention. The stewardship of neural data, the implications of cognitive enhancement, and the equitable distribution of these technologies emerge as paramount concerns, underscoring the need for a collaborative, multidisciplinary approach to governance and ethical oversight.

As we look to the future, the promise of BCIs to augment human capabilities, restore lost functions and even explore new realms of network based cognitive enhancement is undeniably compelling. Yet, even with current advancements in neurosensing and stimulating technologies, the complete solution to integrating mind and machine lies behind numerous substantial biological, engineering and computational barriers. As scientists and clinicians collaborate to overcome these practical barriers, we must remain vigilant that the ethical dilemmas inevitably raised be handled with utmost care to preserve personhood, autonomy and humanity both within individuals and throughout society.

REFERENCES

1. Tudor M, Tudor L, Tudor KI. [Hans Berger (1873–1941)—the history of electroencephalography]. *Acta Med Croatica* 2005; 59(4): 307–13.
2. Vidal JJ. Toward direct brain-computer communication. *Annu Rev Biophys Bioeng* 1973; 2: 157–80.
3. Wolpaw JR, McFarland DJ. Multichannel EEG-based brain-computer communication. *Electroencephalogr Clin Neurophysiol* 1994; 90(6): 444–9.
4. Pfurtscheller G, Flotzinger D, Pregenzer M, et al. EEG-based brain computer interface (BCI). Search for optimal electrode positions and frequency components. *Med Prog Technol* 1995; 21(3): 111–21.
5. Birbaumer N, Kubler A, Ghanayim N, et al. The thought translation device (TTD) for completely paralyzed patients. *IEEE Trans Rehabil Eng* 2000; 8(2): 190–3.
6. Xu F, Yan Y, Zhu J, et al. Self-supervised EEG representation learning with contrastive predictive coding for post-stroke patients. *Int J Neural Syst* 2023; 33(12): 2350066.
7. Willett FR, Avansino DT, Hochberg LR, et al. High-performance brain-to-text communication via handwriting. *Nature* 2021; 593(7858): 249–54.
8. Moses DA, Metzger SL, Liu JR, et al. Neuroprosthesis for decoding speech in a paralyzed person with anarthria. *N Engl J Med* 2021; 385(3): 217–27.
9. Hochberg LR, Serruya MD, Friehs GM, et al. Neuronal ensemble control of prosthetic devices by a human with tetraplegia. *Nature* 2006; 442(7099): 164–71.
10. Kim SP, Simeral JD, Hochberg LR, et al. Neural control of computer cursor velocity by decoding motor cortical spiking activity in humans with tetraplegia. *J Neural Eng* 2008; 5(4): 455–76.
11. Deo DR, Willett FR, Avansino DT, et al. Brain control of bimanual movement enabled by recurrent neural networks. *Sci Rep* 2024; 14(1): 1598.
12. Willett FR, Kunz EM, Fan C, et al. A high-performance speech neuroprosthesis. *Nature* 2023; 620(7976): 1031–6.
13. Metzger SL, Littlejohn KT, Silva AB, et al. A high-performance neuroprosthesis for speech decoding and avatar control. *Nature* 2023; 620(7976): 1037–46.
14. Buch VP, Richardson AG, Brandon C, et al. Network brain-computer interface (nBCI): An alternative approach for cognitive prosthetics. *Front Neurosci* 2018; 12: 790.
15. Gannouni S, Belwafi K, Aboalsamh H, et al. EEG-based BCI system to detect fingers movements. *Brain Sci* 2020; 10(12): 965.
16. Lorach H, Galvez A, Spagnolo V, et al. Walking naturally after spinal cord injury using a brain-spine interface. *Nature* 2023; 618(7963): 126–33.
17. Bonizzato M, James ND, Pidpruzhnykova G, et al. Multi-pronged neuromodulation intervention engages the residual motor circuitry to facilitate walking in a rat model of spinal cord injury. *Nat Commun* 2021; 12(1): 1925.
18. Wang X, Lu H, Shen X, et al. Prosthetic control system based on motor imagery. *Comput Methods Biomech Biomed Engin* 2022; 25(7): 764–71.
19. Sopic D, Teijeiro T, Atienza D, et al. Personalized seizure signature: An interpretable approach to false alarm reduction for long-term epileptic seizure detection. *Epilepsia* 2023; 64 (Suppl 4): S23–3.

20. Khamis H, Mohamed A, Simpson S. Frequency-moment signatures: A method for automated seizure detection from scalp EEG. *Clin Neurophysiol* 2013; 124(12): 2317–27.
21. Klein-Flügge MC, Kennerley SW, Friston K, Bestmann S. Neural signatures of value comparison in human cingulate cortex during decisions requiring an effort-reward trade-off. *J Neurosci* 2016; 36(39): 10002–15.
22. Alagapan S, Choi KS, Heisig S, et al. Cingulate dynamics track depression recovery with deep brain stimulation. *Nature* 2023; 622(7981): 130–8.
23. Grosse-Wentrup M, Mattia D, Oweiss K. Using brain-computer interfaces to induce neural plasticity and restore function. *J Neural Eng* 2011; 8(2): 025004.
24. Buch VP, Bernabei JM, Ng G, et al. "Primed to Perform:" Dynamic white matter graph communicability may drive metastable network representations of enhanced preparatory cognitive control. *bioRxiv*, 2022.
25. Fields RD. White matter in learning, cognition and psychiatric disorders. *Trends Neurosci* 2008; 31(7): 361–70.
26. Kawala-Sterniuk A, Browarska N, Al-Bakri A, et al. Summary of over fifty years with brain-computer interfaces-a review. *Brain Sci* 2021; 11(1): 43.
27. Herff C, Krusienski DJ, Kubben P. The potential of stereotactic-EEG for brain-computer interfaces: Current progress and future directions. *Front Neurosci* 2020; 14: 123.
28. Obien ME, Deligkaris K, Bullmann T, et al. Revealing neuronal function through microelectrode array recordings. *Front Neurosci* 2014; 8: 423.
29. Han J, Jiang H, Zhu J. Neurorestoration: Advances in human brain–computer interface using microelectrode arrays. *J Neurorestoratol* 2020; 8(1): 32–9.
30. Olsen S, Zhang J, Liang KF, et al. An artificial intelligence that increases simulated brain-computer interface performance. *J Neural Eng* 2021; 18(4): 10.1088.
31. Moroz LL, Romanova DY, Kohn AB. Neural versus alternative integrative systems: Molecular insights into origins of neurotransmitters. *Philos Trans R Soc Lond B Biol Sci* 2021; 376(1821): 20190762.
32. Krogh A. What are artificial neural networks? *Nat Biotechnol* 2008; 26(2): 195–7.
33. Schwemmer MA, Skomrock ND, Sederberg PB, et al. Meeting brain-computer interface user performance expectations using a deep neural network decoding framework. *Nat Med* 2018; 24(11): 1669–76.
34. Budday S, Sommer G, Birkl C, et al. Mechanical characterization of human brain tissue. *Acta Biomater* 2017; 48: 319–40.
35. Fox PT, Huang A, Parsons LM, et al. Location-probability profiles for the mouth region of human primary motor-sensory cortex: Model and validation. *Neuroimage* 2001; 13(1): 196–209.
36. Branco DM, Coelho TM, Branco BM, et al. Functional variability of the human cortical motor map: Electrical stimulation findings in perirolandic epilepsy surgery. *J Clin Neurophysiol* 2003; 20(1): 17–25.
37. Chari A, Budhdeo S, Sparks R, et al. Brain-machine interfaces: The role of the neurosurgeon. *World Neurosurg* 2021; 146: 140–7.
38. Vazquez-Guardado A, Yang Y, Bandodkar AJ, Rogers JA. Recent advances in neurotechnologies with broad potential for neuroscience research. *Nat Neurosci* 2020; 23(12): 1522–36.
39. Glasser MF, Coalson TS, Robinson EC, et al. A multi-modal parcellation of human cerebral cortex. *Nature* 2016; 536(7615): 171–8.
40. Chen R, Gore F, Nguyen QA, et al. Deep brain optogenetics without intracranial surgery. *Nat Biotechnol* 2021; 39(2): 161–4.
41. Churchland MM, Shenoy KV. Preparatory activity and the expansive null-space. *Nat Rev Neurosci* 2024; 25(4): 213–36.
42. Wander JD, Blakely T, Miller KJ, et al. Distributed cortical adaptation during learning of a brain-computer interface task. *Proc Natl Acad Sci USA* 2013; 110(26): 10818–23.
43. Georgopoulos AP, Kalaska JF, Caminiti R, Massey JT. On the relations between the direction of two-dimensional arm movements and cell discharge in primate motor cortex. *J Neurosci* 1982; 2(11): 1527–37.
44. Georgopoulos AP, Schwartz AB, Kettner RE. Neuronal population coding of movement direction. *Science* 1986; 233(4771): 1416–19.

45. Milekovic T, Moraud EM, Macellari N, et al. A spinal cord neuroprosthesis for locomotor deficits due to Parkinson's disease. *Nat Med* 2023; 29(11): 2854–65.
46. Viventi J, Kim DH, Vigeland L, et al. Flexible, foldable, actively multiplexed, high-density electrode array for mapping brain activity in vivo. *Nat Neurosci* 2011; 14(12): 1599–605.
47. Ajiboye AB, Willett FR, Young DR, et al. Restoration of reaching and grasping movements through brain-controlled muscle stimulation in a person with tetraplegia: A proof-of-concept demonstration. *Lancet* 2017; 389(10081): 1821–30.
48. Taylor DM, Tillery SI, Schwartz AB. Direct cortical control of 3D neuroprosthetic devices. *Science* 2002; 296(5574): 1829–32.
49. Hesselmann G, Kell CA, Eger E, Kleinschmidt A. Spontaneous local variations in ongoing neural activity bias perceptual decisions. *Proc Natl Acad Sci USA* 2008; 105(31): 10984–9.
50. Basu I, Yousefi A, Crocker B, et al. Closed-loop enhancement and neural decoding of cognitive control in humans. *Nat Biomed Eng* 2023; 7(4): 576–88.
51. Ding Z, Huang Y, Bailey SK, et al. Detection of synchronous brain activity in white matter tracts at rest and under functional loading. *Proc Natl Acad Sci USA* 2018; 115(3): 595–600.
52. Jeunet C, Jahanpour E, Lotte F. Why standard brain-computer interface (BCI) training protocols should be changed: An experimental study. *J Neural Eng* 2016; 13(3): 036024.
53. Musk E, Neuralink. An integrated brain-machine interface platform with thousands of channels. *J Med Internet Res* 2019; 21(10): e16194.
54. Berger TW, Hampson RE, Song D, et al. A cortical neural prosthesis for restoring and enhancing memory. *J Neural Eng* 2011; 8(4): 046017.
55. Hampson RE, Gerhardt GA, Marmarelis V, et al. Facilitation and restoration of cognitive function in primate prefrontal cortex by a neuroprosthesis that utilizes minicolumn-specific neural firing. *J Neural Eng* 2012; 9(5): 056012.
56. Herreros I, Giovannucci A, Taub AH, et al. A cerebellar neuroprosthetic system: Computational architecture and in vivo test. *Front Bioeng Biotechnol* 2014; 2: 14.
57. Andrews JP, Cahn N, Speidel BA, et al. Dissociation of Broca's area from Broca's aphasia in patients undergoing neurosurgical resections. *J Neurosurg* 2023; 138(3): 847–57.
58. Flinker A, Korzeniewska A, Shestyuk AY, et al. Redefining the role of Broca's area in speech. *Proc Natl Acad Sci USA* 2015; 112(9): 2871–5.
59. Leonard MK, Gwilliams L, Sellers KK, et al. Large-scale single-neuron speech sound encoding across the depth of human cortex. *Nature* 2024; 626(7999): 593–602.
60. Tang J, LeBel A, Jain S, Huth AG. Semantic reconstruction of continuous language from non-invasive brain recordings. *Nat Neurosci* 2023; 26(5): 858–66.
61. Deisseroth K. Optogenetics. *Nat Methods* 2011; 8(1): 26–9.
62. Carter ME, de Lecea L. Optogenetic investigation of neural circuits in vivo. *Trends Mol Med* 2011; 17(4): 197–206.
63. Trautmann EM, O'Shea DJ, Sun X, et al. Dendritic calcium signals in rhesus macaque motor cortex drive an optical brain-computer interface. *Nat Commun* 2021; 12(1): 3689.
64. Zaaimi B, Turnbull M, Hazra A, et al. Closed-loop optogenetic control of the dynamics of neural activity in non-human primates. *Nat Biomed Eng* 2023; 7(4): 559–75.
65. Valverde S, Vandecasteele M, Piette C, et al. Deep brain stimulation-guided optogenetic rescue of parkinsonian symptoms. *Nat Commun* 2020; 11(1): 2388.
66. Cho M, Han JK, Suh J, et al. Fully bioresorbable hybrid opto-electronic neural implant system for simultaneous electrophysiological recording and optogenetic stimulation. *Nat Commun* 2024; 15(1): 2000.
67. Abdelfattah AS, Kawashima T, Singh A, et al. Bright and photostable chemigenetic indicators for extended in vivo voltage imaging. *Science* 2019; 365(6454): 699–704.
68. Chung JE, Sellers KK, Leonard MK, et al. High-density single-unit human cortical

recordings using the Neuropixels probe. *Neuron* 2022; 110(15): 2409–21.
69. Kim CY, Ku MJ, Qazi R, et al. Soft subdermal implant capable of wireless battery charging and programmable controls for applications in optogenetics. *Nat Commun* 2021; 12(1): 535.
70. Isaacs RE, Weber DJ, Schwartz AB. Work toward real-time control of a cortical neural prothesis. *IEEE Trans Rehabil Eng* 2000; 8(2): 196–8.
71. Belkacem AN, Jamil N, Khalid S, Alnajjar F. On closed-loop brain stimulation systems for improving the quality of life of patients with neurological disorders. *Front Hum Neurosci* 2023; 17: 1085173.
72. Fasi M, Higham NJ, Mikaitis M, Pranesh S. Numerical behavior of NVIDIA tensor cores. *PeerJ Comput Sci* 2021; 7: e330.
73. Carmena JM. Advances in neuroprosthetic learning and control. *PLoS Biol* 2013; 11(5): e1001561.
74. Yuste R, Goering S, Arcas BAY, et al. Four ethical priorities for neurotechnologies and AI. *Nature* 2017; 551(7679): 159–63.
75. Kramer AD, Guillory JE, Hancock JT. Experimental evidence of massive-scale emotional contagion through social networks. *Proc Natl Acad Sci USA* 2014; 111(24): 8788–90.
76. Kellmeyer P, Cochrane T, Muller O, et al. The effects of closed-loop medical devices on the autonomy and accountability of persons and systems. *Camb Q Healthc Ethics* 2016; 25(4): 623–33.
77. Ienca M, Andorno R. Towards new human rights in the age of neuroscience and neurotechnology. *Life Sci Soc Policy* 2017; 13(1): 5.

12

Neurosurgical Sub-Task Automation

HEATHER GRIMAUDO, JARED LAWSON, NIA BOLES, MICHAEL LONGO, NABIL SIMAAN AND ROHAN CHITALE

Introduction

Over the past five decades, automation has become a keyword synonymous with cutting-edge technological advancements. The manufacturing industry has represented the archetype for automation, where large robot arms have often replaced human operators on assembly lines, increasing the efficiency and precision of task execution. If one were to use this example directly in the context of surgery, it may incorrectly suggest that surgical automation could completely replace surgeons with robot arms. While this is not yet realized, there are repetitive tasks in surgery that demand time and care to successfully complete even by the highest-skilled operator. We believe that such tasks represent opportunities for surgical automation.

Automation in the surgical theater is an increasingly growing research domain in the surgical robotics and artificial intelligence (AI) communities. In parallel to self-driving cars, levels of surgical autonomy have been defined in a surgical context in multiple works.[1,2] These levels range from no autonomy (manual surgery) to full autonomy, in which a robot completes the procedure entirely. Beyond no autonomy, considered Level 0, the first level of autonomy considers robotic assistance, which leaves the surgeon in complete control but with intervention delivered physically through robotic manipulators and instruments. Level 2 considers task autonomy, in which specific brief, everyday aspects of the procedure can be completed autonomously under surgeon supervision, such as needle passing or knot-tying. Levels 3, 4 and 5 represent Conditional/Supervised Autonomy, High-Level Autonomy and Full Autonomy, respectively. These levels place increasing control onto the robotic system and ideally require decreasing oversight from the surgeon. While Levels 4 and 5 offer a look into the future, they still need to be realized with available robotic technology.[2] **Figure 12.1** shows each of these levels of autonomy (LoA) in the context of three neurosurgical procedures. An assumption underpinning each level of autonomy is that a surgical robotic system can deliver the surgical treatment of interest.

Robotics were first introduced to neurosurgery when an industrial robot arm was used to perform a CT-guided brain biopsy in 1985.[3] Since then, robots have been designed for various neurosurgical applications, from spinal fixation to endovascular aneurysm coiling. While many different architectures have been reviewed for different neurosurgical applications, they will not be extensively enumerated as they have been well reviewed in other works.[4] Instead, the scope of this work is to review the existing automation of neurosurgical tasks presented in the literature.

In the following two sections, automation in diagnostic imaging and within neurosurgical subspecialties including tumor, vascular, functional and spinal procedures, are reviewed to understand its impact in the full breadth of the discipline. In the "Future Opportunities" section, surgical subtask automation from different surgical domains are reviewed, based on their relevance to neurosurgery, as a means to motivate future applications

DOI: 10.1201/9781003471165-12

	Level 0: No autonomy	Level 1: Robot Assistance	Level 2: Task Autonomy	Level 3: Supervised Autonomy	Level 4: High-Level Autonomy	Level 5: Full Autonomy
Craniotomy	Handheld drills used without guidance or external stabilization	Robotic drill limits hand tremor for smoother operation	Robotic drill autonomously stabilizes the drill bit, or limits penetration of dura mater	Robotic drill sharing control with surgeon, who can intervene at any time	Autonomous drilling and removal of bone flap, should only require intervention in emergency	Autonomous full procedure, including drilling, bone flap removal, and flap closure without surgeon intervention
Tumor Resection	Manual instruments and no sensory information available	Surgeon telemanipulating robotic instruments, and/or provided some sensed information	Few aspects of the procedure are performed autonomously, such as margin identification	Surgeons plan resection and oversee autonomous execution of plan	Surgeons plan resection with full autonomous execution of plan, only intervention in emergency	Resection is autonomously planned and executed, with surgeon intervention only if necessary
Mechanical Thrombectomy	Passive catheters manually inserted under fluoroscopy	Teleoperated insertion of catheters, removing interventionalist from radiation field	Teleoperated insertion with automated steering to point the catheter away from the vessel walls	Automated navigation which can be corrected or stopped by the interventionalist at any time	Navigation is completely autonomous, interventionalist chooses when to extract thrombus and system performs	Full navigation and retrieval performed autonomously

Figure 12.1 Levels of Autonomy (LoA) defined in Haidegger[1] applied to three neurosurgical procedures.

for automation. Finally, the findings presented throughout the chapter are summarized, and an outlook is provided on the future of automation in neurosurgery.

AUTOMATION OF DIAGNOSTIC IMAGING

The accurate and efficient interpretation of diagnostic imaging is crucial across various medical specialties, with particular significance in neurosurgery. Sub-task automation can enhance both the efficiency and accuracy of diagnostic medical imaging. Current applications of automation include image acquisition, processing, registration and fusion and segmentation, each of which is elaborated upon below. This serves as a foundation for subsequent sections of this chapter.

With the advancement of medical imaging technology, an increasing amount of imaging data is being generated and processed in the digital imaging format. Secondary to this, is a tremendous burden of image acquisition and computer memory requirements for hospital systems. For example, the memory required to store 3D imaging data is significant. A high-resolution brain MRI containing >200 slices of 512×512 pixels each will contain more than 50 million voxels, and each pixel requires ~2 bytes, leading to over 100 megabytes.[5] Thus, the storage and visualization of such studies require large disk capacity, computer memory and even simple viewing operations like zooming and navigation require fast hardware. Modern hospital systems use a "Picture Archiving and Communication System," or PACS, to address these issues on a hospital-systems level.[5] With the PACS, images from several imaging modalities, different manufacturers, and often separate hospital buildings, are stored in a standardized format (e.g. Digital Imaging and Communications in Medicine or DICOM files) and can be retrieved and displayed by any in-network workstation.[5,6] In general, the PACS imaging acquisition system consists of the medical imaging system, a computer system that acquires the images from the imaging system, and an interface or software between the imaging system and the acquisition computer.[6]

Another layer of complexity is automated image analysis. In general, automation of medical imaging analysis is challenging, given the complexity of the shape and contour of anatomic structures, the wide biological variability between subjects, and the added complexity of pathologic tissue (e.g. tumor, edema, inflammation). Despite this, some strategies for basic automated imaging analysis exist. First of these are standardized display protocols that utilize gray-level transformations to optimize visualization of specific anatomic structures, such as "lung window" and "bone window."[5] For neurosurgical imaging, there are windows to optimize visualization of gray matter, white matter and ischemic stroke on CT, as well as acute stroke on diffusion MR imaging. Additionally, there are different filters to manipulate digital images, such as low-pass filters for averaging or blurring (e.g. Gaussian filter) and high-pass filters to extract edges or fine texture.[5] Further, there are automated pixel-based analysis methods that rely on local operators and heuristic pixel groupings, such as region growing, edge detection (Roberts, Pewit, Sobel operators), and pixel thresholding with methods of both supervised and unsupervised learning.[5,7] All of these methods allow for optimization of image analysis and interpretation for accurate clinical diagnosis.

Another critical sub-task automation within diagnostic imaging is imaging registration and fusion. In this analysis technique, any radiographic image is used as the prototype, and additional images are represented implicitly based on this image with simple deformations. Statistical methods for non-rigid image fusion are well described in prior texts and outwith the scope of this chapter.[5] This is important for fusing images of the same patient at different times or multiple imaging modalities (e.g. CT and MRI of the brain), which is essential for surgical planning. Image fusion is also crucial for intraoperative navigation, another automated sub-task based on point-matching that establishes a geometric correspondence between multiple preoperative images, the patient and surgical instruments. Based on the chosen anatomic landmarks or fiducials on the patient, an LED-based dynamic reference frame or markers, and the navigation software (e.g. Stealth), a 3D geometric transformation is performed from the imaging space, *I*, to the surgery space, *S*.[5] This registration and tracking of solid tissue, such as bone, is commonly used for cranial and spine procedures within neurosurgery, allowing for safer and more efficient navigation.

Finally, image segmentation is the most challenging sub-task automation within diagnostic medical imaging. As stated above, automatic segmentation of medical imaging is difficult given the complex shapes of normal anatomic structures (e.g. the gyri and sulci of the brain), the wide biological variability between subjects, and the added complexity of pathologic tissue (e.g. a tumor causing mass effect). Manual imaging segmentation is time-demanding and has large intra- and inter-rater variability.[5,8] Consequently, this remains an active area of research with several commonly used techniques, including atlas-based segmentation,[9] voxel-based morphometry,[10,11] pixel intensity-based segmentation (e.g. region growing, edge detection, clustering algorithms),[5] graph-based segmentation,[12,13] active contour models (or snakes),[14] and deep learning (DL)-based segmentation.[8,15,16] Automated imaging segmentation is utilized for normal structural segmentation for resident learning or surgical planning, tumor segmentation to analyze size and tumor boundaries on serial scans, and lesion detection and characterization, such as intracranial hemorrhage, infarctions, multiple sclerosis plaques and more.

Specific uses of automated sub-tasks within the different subspecialties of neurosurgery are discussed below.

AUTOMATION OF PROCEDURAL SUB-TASKS

Tumor

Sub-task automation within neurosurgery, specifically tumor surgery, can significantly enhance planning, surgical precision, surgical safety and outcome analysis.

First, as outlined in the preceding section, automation plays a critical role in imaging analysis, co-registration and 3D reconstruction, which are essential for devising an optimal surgical strategy. While the specifics of these processes will not be reiterated here, their importance in ensuring safe surgical planning and effective tumor resection cannot be overstated.

A crucial component of procedural automation in tumor surgery is intraoperative imaging guidance, also known as image-guided neuronavigation. In this process, the brain is conceptualized as a geometric volume delineated into axial, sagittal and coronal planes within Cartesian coordinates.[17] Based on specified anatomic landmarks or fiducials on the patient, the preoperative imaging is registered to the actual landmarks, and the navigation software (e.g. Stealth) references the 3D Cartesian coordinates of the anatomic space to the 3D-imaging data based on a geometric transformation.[5,17] Image guidance facilitates the planning of the craniotomy and approach, the accurate trajectory to the lesions (most crucial for smaller lesions), the delineation of eloquent areas of the brain, and lastly, helps define the tumor margins and limits of surgical resection.[17] More recent research has focused on the potential use of augmented reality (AR) for intraoperative guidance, with the surgeon's ability to see and interact with the images in the microscope to provide anatomic guidance.[18] For oncologic lesions, AR can be used to superimpose images of the tumor and surrounding neurovascular structures to better understand their relationship of what cannot be seen directly throughout tumor resection.[18] Both of these guidance techniques facilitate safer surgical planning and surgical tumor resection.

Another promising area of procedural automation in tumor surgery is robotic assistance. Advanced surgical robots, such as the Da Vinci® Surgical System and the ROSA ONE® Brain stereotactic robot, are now routinely employed to perform tasks including cutting, suturing, tissue manipulation, surgical instrument handling, device implantation and biopsies. Recent research has particularly emphasized the use of robots for tumor biopsy and resection. For instance, a study by Minchev et al. details the development of a novel tubular instrument set used by the iSYS-1 robotic device to conduct stereotactic robot-guided tumor biopsies.[19] This innovation aims to enhance diagnostic accuracy, improve cosmetic outcomes, and reduce operative time.[19] Similarly, Sutherland and colleagues describe the first-time clinical use of an image-guided robot called NeuroArm, which gives the surgeon novel feedback during glioma resection, such as augmented force feedback, haptic high-force warning and tool-tissue interaction forces, to help improve surgical safety and outcome (**Figure 12.2**).[20] And finally, others have investigated the use of robots for endoscopic skull base surgery. Pangal et al. performed a systematic review of 22 articles demonstrating the use of robotic instrumentation in endoscopic transoral skull base surgery.[21] Although these various applications remain largely investigational and are not

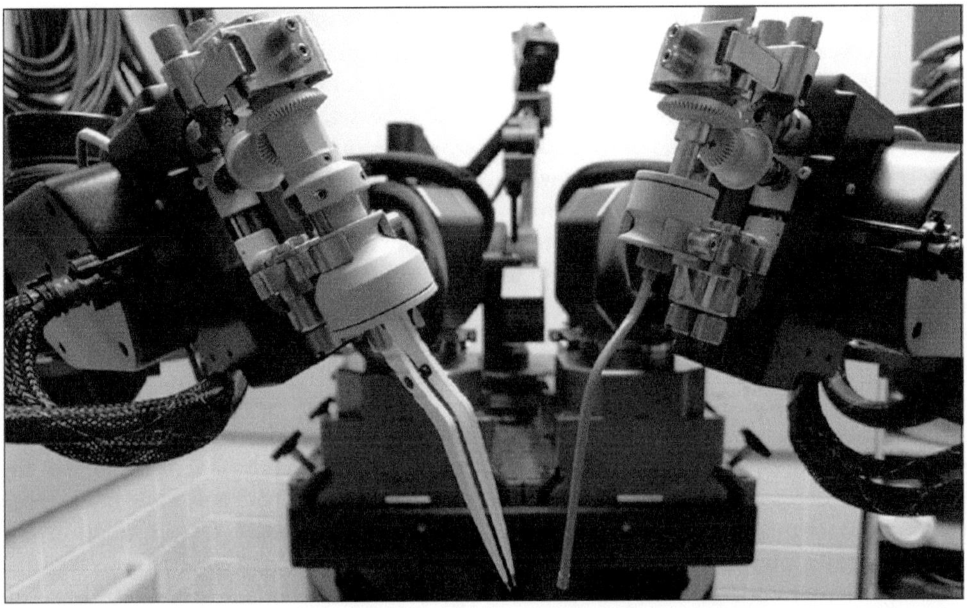

Figure 12.2 NeuroArm providing the surgeon with augmented force feedback from tool-tissue interaction forces. (Reproduced from Sutherland et al., 2015.[20])

yet the standard of care, they hold the potential to significantly enhance target accuracy, reduce operating time and improve cosmetic outcomes through smaller incisions.

Currently, the largest applications of robotic automation for tumor treatment is in radiation therapy. The use of robotics and computer-aided radiation therapy allows the robot to manipulate a radiation source to allow focusing the radiation at the target tumor location while minimizing focused radiation to surrounding tissues. Procedures using GammaKnife and CyberKnife allow the radiation of inoperable tumors and the GammaKnife alone has been used for more than 400,000 cases worldwide.[22]

Lastly, integrating AI-based automation in the review of surgical records and outcomes can significantly enhance patient care. Advanced AI techniques such as machine learning (ML), predictive analytics, DL and natural language processing can analyze extensive electronic health records to evaluate postoperative outcomes, develop clinical prediction models and guide clinical decision-making.[23,24] Although this approach is not limited to tumor surgery, the precise selection of patients to inform postoperative decisions including chemoradiation, represent some of the most complex challenges in managing these patients effectively.

VASCULAR

Automation in vascular neurosurgery is complex due to the intricate and delicate nature of neurovascular structures. Recently, significant progress has been made in using ML and robotics for the diagnosis and treatment of cerebrovascular pathologies.

First, AI-based DL algorithms have proven effective in interpreting diagnostic imaging, thereby aiding clinical decision-making and triage.[25] DL algorithms have demonstrated the ability to diagnose and triage urgent neurosurgical imaging conditions such as intracranial hemorrhage, stroke, large vessel occlusion (LVO) and hydrocephalus—more quickly and accurately than human radiologists.[25] Second, studies indicate that AI-based models can accurately analyze CT/CTA images of patients with suspected LVO, significantly reducing the door-to-groin puncture time for thrombectomy procedures.[26] Subsequently, several comprehensive stroke centers have begun implementing AI-based triage systems for the management of LVO stroke with hopes of reducing the time from patient presentation to intervention.[27] There is significant potential for applying these automated technologies to the radiographic diagnosis of various pathologies.

In addition to diagnostic potential, more recent research efforts have focused on automation with robotic integration in endovascular procedures. The first study to showcase robotic-assisted neurovascular treatment was conducted in 2020 on a single patient with a large saccular aneurysm originating from the basilar artery. The CorPath GRX® Robotic System, previously approved for use in the percutaneous coronary and peripheral vascular intervention (PCI and PVI), was used for stenting and coiling both the posterior cerebral and basilar arteries (**Figure 12.3**).[28] In a subsequent study performed at the same institution, the CorPath system was used to perform robotically assisted embolization utilizing a combination of stent plus coil or stent-only techniques for large neck saccular aneurysms of the basilar, posterior communicating and paraophthalmic internal carotid arteries.[29] In line with this, a recent review article by Beaman and colleagues summarized the use of robotics in neuroradiology and automated maneuvers to reduce procedural time and variability.[30] This described the CorPath robotic system's attempts to provide procedural assistance through robotic automation of specific maneuvers, such as "Rotate on Retract," which is a rotational maneuver of the wire to select a new vessel, "Spin," "Wiggle" and "Dotter" to cross a lesion or stenosis.[30] This integration of both robotics and ML to advance robotic interventional neuroradiology has the potential to benefit the surgeon and patient by reducing exposure to ionizing radiation, as well as increasing the efficiency of procedures.

Functional

Throughout the years, the field of functional neurosurgery has broadened due to increased knowledge of the pathophysiology of neurocognitive disorders. Deep brain stimulation (DBS) is a widely used approach in the treatment and management of movement, psychiatric and complex pain disorders. Several studies have shown that using robotics for precise electrode implantation during DBS surgery is safe and efficient. In addition to DBS surgery, some of the earliest applications of robotics in functional neurosurgery include the Surgiscope system for image-guided placement of depth electrodes for the localization of epileptogenic zones.[31]

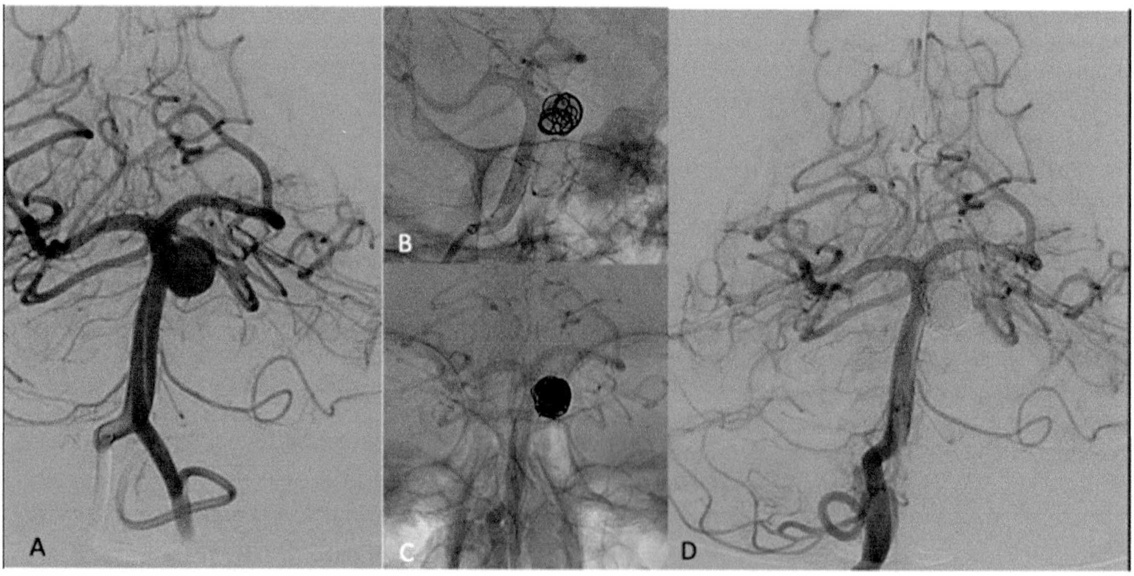

Figure 12.3 Robot-assisted endovascular aneurysm coiling performed in a human with the Corindus GRX system. (Reproduced from Pereira et al., 2020.[28])

Since then, systems such as the Mazor™ Renaissance robot[32] have demonstrated increased precision in electrode placement for asleep DBS procedures (**Figure 12.4**). The ROSA robotic stereotactic assistance system has been used for bilateral subthalamic nucleus electrode placement to treat Parkinson's disease, as well as for other DBS procedures.[33] In those DBS surgeries, when compared with conventional frame-based mechanical devices, the ROSA system was shown to be more accurate and efficient.[34]

SPINE

Automation is most readily applied to the diagnostic aspect of spine surgery, wherein AI and ML methods may be used to bolster efficiency and accuracy. The literature offers several examples of precedent for automatic image interpretation, such as algorithms that quantify the severity of spinal stenosis,[35] and severity of disc degeneration.[36] This extends to the direct evaluation of implants, as *in vitro* models demonstrate good prediction of screw pullout strength.[37] Presently, automation in imaging interpretation and outcome prediction plays an important role in spine surgery.[38]

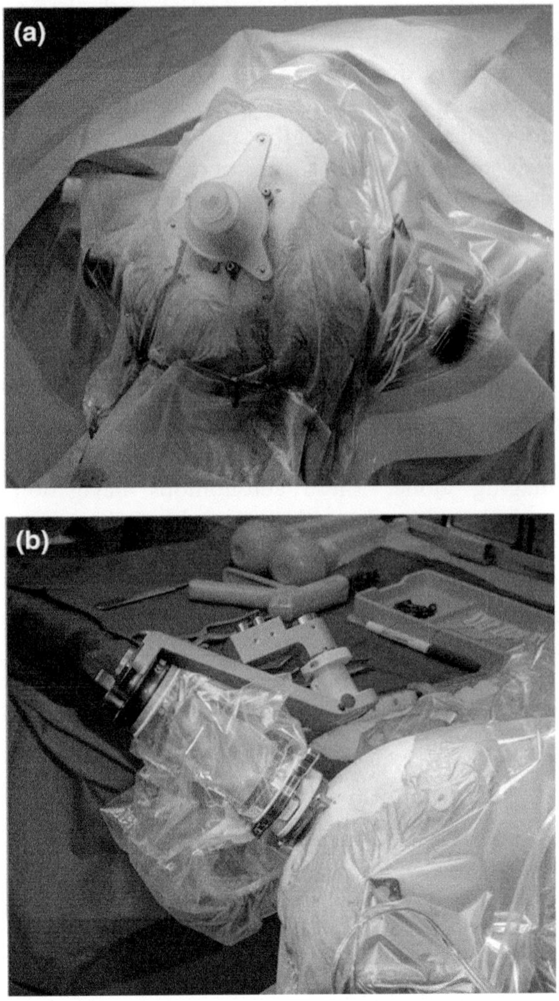

Figure 12.4 The set up of the fiducial frame (a) and the mounted Mazor Renaissance robot (b) for electrode placement in a DBS procedure. (Reproduced from VanSickle et al., 2019.[32])

When considering the role of robotics in automatic processes, such advancements are partly responsible for improving spine surgery outcomes. The literature offers level 1 evidence that the use of neuronavigation improves pedicle screw placement accuracy, reduces operative time, and lessens radiation exposure in deformity surgery when compared to freehand techniques.[39] Since the first spine robot, Mazor SpineAssist (Medtronic), received FDA approval in 2004, several others have received FDA approval and are currently in use by spine surgeons, such as Mazor X (Medtronic), ROSA ONE Spine (Zimmer Biomet) and ExcelsiusGPS™ (Globus Medical).[40] Broadly, these robots function as a means to augment surgeon skills with implant placement, and increase accuracy and reduce operative times. While the autonomy level is low and there is a learning curve for surgeons to use these machines efficiently, robots have a well-established and fundamental role in modern spine surgery.

FUTURE OPPORTUNITIES FOR AUTOMATION IN NEUROSURGERY

Neurosurgery is a technically demanding surgical domain that spans diseases from vascular malformations (VMs) to malignant tumors. While covering such a broad range of neurological diseases and corresponding interventions, the techniques employed by neurosurgeons are often found to be shared with surgeons in other clinical domains. Neurosurgical tasks such as bone drilling, suturing and soft tissue grasper manipulation are found in orthopedic, general and minimally invasive surgery, respectively. It may help some neurosurgeons to be aware that some of these domains have received significant research in sub-task automation. To that end, this section reviews sub-task automation, which has been reported in other clinical domains that may, however, represent opportunities for use in neurosurgery.

HARD TISSUE

Whether treating the spine or preparing for any open intracranial procedure, interacting with and manipulating bone is a frequent, if not daily, task for neurosurgeons. Techniques from osteotomy and screw fixation are standard not only for neurosurgeons but also for orthopedic surgeons treating hips, knees and other bone-related ailments. Autonomous drilling was performed for 500 patients receiving knee reconstruction, where the orthopedic surgeon planned the drilling path on preoperative CT.[41] Similarly, automated osteotomy far outperformed the accuracy of manual osteotomy with standard guides for dental procedures.[42] Mastoidectomy and cochleostomy have been the subject of much research in surgical robotics and automation. Sensory-guided and robotic drills were proposed to detect different bone properties to control drill insertion for fully autonomous drilling.[43]

Although the risks to the patient are different between osteotomies performed for knee reconstruction, inner ear access and intracranial access, technologically, these procedures include the tasks of collecting preoperative imaging and planning and carrying out the osteotomy with either manual (LoA 0) or fully autonomous (LoA 5) drilling. While these works don't guarantee that the same technology can be used for neurosurgery, the methods they present may motivate future directions in the field.

SOFT TISSUE

Bone and other rigid tissues are ideal candidates for task automation, as preoperative imaging and planning can closely match the intraoperative surgical environment. However, soft tissues deform intraoperatively with instrument interactions and patient motion, further complicating robotic assistance and task automation. There has been a significant interest in equipping surgical robotic systems with sensing and instrumentation to automate common but technically demanding soft tissue sub-tasks, such as suturing. The current state of research in autonomous suturing was recently reviewed in Ostrander et al.,[44] which includes many clinical applications, such as laparoscopic and ophthalmic surgery. Some works propose implementing novel imaging techniques, modalities and instruments for a more technological suturing approach,[45] while other works implement motion primitives based on the manual suturing techniques to seamlessly integrate with standard end-effector designs.[46] The most enormous scale clinical application has performed suturing or anastomosis of the bowel, which is not relevant to the scale for neurosurgery. However, many works have focused on more precise procedures such as keratoplasty. Automation at this small scale shows promise for the application of these techniques for small neurosurgical tasks, including duraplasty and small cerebral vessel anastomoses.

VASCULAR/INTERVENTIONAL

Interventional procedures are becoming more and more common for the treatment of endovascular disease throughout the body, including the heart, periphery and brain. Although this treatment approach is desirable in significantly minimizing the impact of surrounding tissue, it becomes more difficult to control the small, flexible devices navigated throughout the body. Additionally, interventionalists perform the procedure without direct visibility or sensation of their tools, as they can only rely on interventional imaging modalities (i.e. fluoroscopy) to visualize anatomy and devices. These challenges have motivated the work of robotic catheter navigation. Automation of this navigation aids the technical demand for traversing vessels and the cognitive demand of interpreting 3D anatomy and contact forces from imaging alone. These autonomous navigation works have been recently reviewed in Robertshaw et al.[47] Autonomous navigation to a selected vessel endpoint has only been conducted in phantom models leveraging single imaging or motion planes.[48] Other works aim to sensorize catheters with electromagnetic trackers at their tip for compliant control.[49] These related works may not be well suited for the navigation of small, tortuous cerebral vessels, where catheters must be smaller than 2 mm in outer diameter and must be tracked with biplane imaging. These technical limitations make neuroendovascular navigation difficult to automate, though ongoing research will aim to overcome such obstacles.

CONCLUSION

Although fully autonomous surgery is a future prospect, aspects of autonomy can be found within particular sub-tasks of neurosurgery. Within the many subspecialties of neurosurgery, automation of critical sub-tasks has been found in both the research and clinical literature, indicating not only the technical capability but also acceptance of such developments. Throughout tumor, vascular, functional and spine procedures, the most common automated sub-tasks are related to preoperative image analysis, including segmentation and registration. Intraoperative automation is still nascent for many of these disciplines, however, the ongoing development and acceptance of surgical robotics has created a pathway for automation of intraoperative sub-tasks.

Outside of neurosurgery, there have been many research efforts into automation of surgical tasks which may be relevant or shared in neurosurgery. Autonomous osteotomy has been explored for use in oral surgery and cochleostomy, with some efforts indicating improved performance compared to manual drilling. For soft tissue tasks related to suturing, including needle passing and knot-tying, autonomous robotic systems have been deployed to work on *ex vivo* samples. For interventional procedures, autonomous robotic catheter navigation has only been tested, so far, in benchtop models. Each of these developments represent solutions for autonomous tasks found in neurosurgery, although their current embodiments may not be at a suitable scale to translate to the neurosurgical theater. Additionally, the risk of such techniques need to be considered in the context of the surrounding anatomy.

The literature reviewed throughout this chapter tends to represent automation between levels of autonomy (LoA) 1 and LoA 2, where the neurosurgeon maintains close control and oversight of the procedure. As higher levels of autonomy are sought for development, the ethical considerations of taking control away from the neurosurgeon must be weighed. Among such ethical considerations include legal and regulatory standards which have been proposed in the literature.[50]

Although neurosurgical automation may seem like a futuristic undertaking, it is already present within sub-tasks of common procedures. Going forward, further research to improve enabling technologies, such as more advanced robotics, imaging and sensing, will make further automation possible. In doing so, it is imperative to measure the impact of these advancements in terms of patient care and positive outcomes.

REFERENCES

1. Haidegger T. Autonomy for surgical robots: Concepts and paradigms. *IEEE Trans Med Robot Bionics* 2019; 1(2): 65–76.
2. Lee A, Baker TS, Bederson JB, Rapoport BI. Levels of autonomy in FDA-cleared surgical robots: A systematic review. *NPJ Digit Med* 2024; 7(1): 1–8.
3. Kwoh YS, Hou J, Jonckheere EA, Hayati S. A robot with improved absolute positioning accuracy for CT guided stereotactic brain surgery. *IEEE Trans Biomed Eng* 1988; 35(2): 153–60.
4. Marcus HJ, Payne CJ (eds). *Neurosurgical Robotics*. New York: Springer; 2021.
5. Suetens P. *Fundamentals of Medical Imaging*. Cambridge: Cambridge University Press; 2017.
6. Lou SL, Wang J, Moskowitz M, et al. Methods of automatically acquiring images from digital medical systems. *Comput Med Imaging Graph* 1995; 19(4): 369–76.
7. Jing J, Liu S, Wang G, et al. Recent advances on image edge detection: A comprehensive review. *Neurocomputing* 2022; 503: 259–71.
8. Magadza T, Viriri S. Deep learning for brain tumor segmentation: A survey of state-of-the-art. *J Imaging Sci Technol* 2021; 7(2): 19.
9. Cabezas M, Oliver A, Lladó X, et al. A review of atlas-based segmentation for magnetic resonance brain images. *Comput Methods Programs Biomed* 2011; 104(3): e158–77.
10. Whitwell JL. Voxel-based morphometry: An automated technique for assessing structural changes in the brain. *J Neurosci* 2009; 29(31): 9661–4.
11. Penny WD, Friston KJ, Ashburner JT, et al. *Statistical Parametric Mapping: The Analysis of Functional Brain Images*. London: Elsevier; 2011.
12. Parisot S, Duffau H, Chemouny S, Paragios N. Graph-based detection, segmentation & characterization of brain tumors. In: 2012 *IEEE Conference on Computer Vision and Pattern Recognition*. IEEE; 2012, pp. 988–95.
13. Kong Y, Chen X, Wu J, et al. Automatic brain tissue segmentation based on graph filter. *BMC Med Imaging* 2018; 18(1): 9.

14. Veeramalla SK, Hindumathi V, Reddy TV, et al. Segmentation of MRI images using a combination of active contour modeling and morphological processing. *J Mech Med Biol* 2023; 23(4): 2340002.
15. Jyothi P, Singh AR. Deep learning models and traditional automated techniques for brain tumor segmentation in MRI: A review. *Artif Intell Rev* 2023; 56(4): 2923–69.
16. Sharma M, Miglani N. Automated brain tumor segmentation in MRI images using deep learning: Overview, challenges and future. In: Dash S, Acharya BR, Mittal M, et al. (eds). *Deep Learning Techniques for Biomedical and Health Informatics*. Cham: Springer International Publishing; 2020, pp. 347–83.
17. Ganslandt O, Behari S, Gralla J, et al. Neuronavigation: Concept, techniques and applications. *Neurol India* 2002; 50(3): 244–55.
18. Contreras López WO, Navarro PA, Crispin S. Intraoperative clinical application of augmented reality in neurosurgery: A systematic review. *Clin Neurol Neurosurg* 2019; 177: 6–11.
19. Minchev G, Kronreif G, Ptacek W, et al. A novel robot-guided minimally invasive technique for brain tumor biopsies. *J Neurosurg* 2019; 132(1): 150–8.
20. Sutherland GR, Maddahi Y, Gan LS, et al. Robotics in the neurosurgical treatment of glioma. *Surg Neurol Int* 2015; 6(Suppl 1): S1–8.
21. Pangal DJ, Cote DJ, Ruzevick J, et al. Robotic and robot-assisted skull base neurosurgery: Systematic review of current applications and future directions. *Neurosurg Focus* 2022; 52(1): E15.
22. UVA Health. Gamma Knife, 2015. Available from: https://med.virginia.edu/neurosurgery/services/gamma-knife/for-physicians/comparison-gamma-knife-to-cyberknife/ (Accessed May 2026).
23. Panesar SS, Kliot M, Parrish R, et al. Promises and perils of artificial intelligence in neurosurgery. *Neurosurgery* 2020; 87(1): 33–44.
24. Senders JT, Staples PC, Karhade AV, et al. Machine learning and neurosurgical outcome prediction: A systematic review. *World Neurosurg* 2018; 109: 476–86.e1.
25. Tripathy P. Artificial intelligence in cerebrovascular surgery: A brief review. *J Cerebrovasc Sci* 2023; 11(1): 27–9.
26. Martinez-Gutierrez JC, Kim Y, Salazar-Marioni S, et al. Automated large vessel occlusion detection software and thrombectomy treatment times: A cluster randomized clinical trial. *JAMA Neurol* 2023; 80(11): 1182–90.
27. Morey JR, Zhang X, Yaeger KA, et al. Real-world experience with artificial intelligence-based triage in transferred large vessel occlusion stroke patients. *Cerebrovasc Dis* 2021; 50(4): 450–5.
28. Pereira VM, Cancelliere NM, Nicholson P, et al. First-in-human, robotic-assisted neuroendovascular intervention. *J Neurointerv Surg* 2020; 12(4): 338.
29. Cancelliere NM, Lynch J, Nicholson P, et al. Robotic-assisted intracranial aneurysm treatment: 1 year follow-up imaging and clinical outcomes. *J Neurointerv Surg* 2022; 14(12): 1229–33.
30. Beaman CB, Kaneko N, Meyers PM, Tateshima S. A review of robotic interventional neuroradiology. *AJNR Am J Neuroradiol* 2021; 42(5): 808–14.
31. Spire WJ, Jobst BC, Thadani VM, et al. Robotic image-guided depth electrode implantation in the evaluation of medically intractable epilepsy: Technical note. *Neurosurg Focus* 2008; 25(3): E19.
32. VanSickle D, Volk V, Freeman P, et al. Electrode placement accuracy in robot-assisted asleep deep brain stimulation. *Ann Biomed Eng* 2019; 47(5): 1212–22.
33. Vadera S, Chan A, Lo T, et al. Frameless stereotactic robot-assisted subthalamic nucleus deep brain stimulation: Case report. *World Neurosurg* 2017; 97: 762.e11–762.e14.
34. Neudorfer C, Hunsche S, Hellmich M, et al. Comparative study of robot-assisted versus conventional frame-based deep brain stimulation stereotactic neurosurgery. *Stereotact Funct Neurosurg* 2018; 96(5): 327–34.
35. Huber FA, Stutz S, de Martini IV, et al. Qualitative versus quantitative lumbar spinal stenosis grading by machine learning supported texture analysis—Experience from the LSOS study cohort. *Eur J Radiol* 2019; 114: 45–50.

36. Huang J, Shen H, Wu J, et al. Spine explorer: A deep learning based fully automated program for efficient and reliable quantifications of the vertebrae and discs on sagittal lumbar spine MR images. *Spine J* 2020; 20(4): 590–9.
37. Varghese V, Krishnan V, Kumar GS. Evaluating pedicle-screw instrumentation using decision-tree analysis based on pull-out strength. *Asian Spine J* 2018; 12(4): 611.
38. DelSole EM, Keck WL, Patel AA. The state of machine learning in spine surgery: A systematic review. *Clin Spine Surg* 2022; 35(2): 80.
39. Rajasekaran S, Vidyadhara S, Ramesh P, Shetty AP. Randomized clinical study to compare the accuracy of navigated and non-navigated thoracic pedicle screws in deformity correction surgeries. *Spine* 2007; 32(2): E56.
40. Gajjar AA, Huy Dinh Le A, Lavadi RS, et al. Evolution of robotics in spine surgery: A historical perspective. *Interdiscip Neurosurg* 2023; 33: 101721.
41. Chandrashekar P, Babu KA, Nagaraja HS, et al. Intra-operative safety of an autonomous robotic system for total knee replacement: A review of 500 cases in India. *Indian J Orthop* 2023; 57(11): 1800–8.
42. He J, Zhang Q, Wang X, et al. In vitro and in vivo accuracy of autonomous robotic vs. fully guided static computer-assisted implant surgery. *Clin Implant Dent Relat Res* 2024; 26(2): 385–401.
43. Du X, Assadi MZ, Jowitt F, et al. Robustness analysis of a smart surgical drill for cochleostomy. *Int J Med Robot* 2013; 9(1): 119–26.
44. Ostrander BT, Massillon D, Meller L, et al. The current state of autonomous suturing: A systematic review. *Surg Endosc* 2024; 38(5): 2383–97.
45. Shademan A, Decker RS, Opfermann JD, et al. Supervised autonomous robotic soft tissue surgery. *Sci Transl Med* 2016; 8(337): 337ra64.
46. Amirshirzad N, Sunal B, Bebek O, Oztop E. Learning medical suturing primitives for autonomous suturing. In: *2021 IEEE 17th International Conference on Automation Science and Engineering* (CASE). IEEE; 2021, pp. 256–61.
47. Robertshaw H, Karstensen L, Jackson B, et al. Artificial intelligence in the autonomous navigation of endovascular interventions: A systematic review. *Front Hum Neurosci* 2023; 17: 1239374.
48. Jayender J, Azizian M, Patel RV. Autonomous image-guided robot-assisted active catheter insertion. *IEEE Trans Robot* 2008; 24(4): 858–71.
49. Wu D, Ha XT, Zhang Y, et al. Deep-learning-based compliant motion control of a pneumatically-driven robotic catheter. *IEEE Robot Automat Lett* 2022; 7(4): 8853–60.
50. Yang GZ, Cambias J, Cleary K, et al. Medical robotics—Regulatory, ethical, and legal considerations for increasing levels of autonomy. *Science Robotics* 2017; 2(4): eaam8638.

13

Artificial Intelligence for Simulation and Neurosurgical Training

ANDRE A. PAYMAN AND ROBERTO RODRIGUEZ RUBIO

NEUROSURGICAL SIMULATION AND TRAINING BEFORE AI

Neurosurgical simulation traditionally relied on cadaveric and animal models supervised by experienced neurosurgeons. This allowed trainees to practice surgical procedures on real tissue, providing an invaluable understanding of anatomic variability, spatial relationships of structures and tactile feedback. However, these training modalities have limitations due to the global availability of donors, variability in postmortem quality of the anatomy, the need for a specialized space to conduct simulations, limited repetitive practice opportunities, and ethical concerns.

Synthetic physical models emerged, allowing repetitive practice but lacking human tissue realism and anatomic complexity. Technological advancements introduced virtual reality (VR)-based simulations, offering risk-free surgical practice environments. These systems evolved to include physics simulation of anatomy and haptic feedback, creating realistic, interactive 3D models of the human brain and spine.

Effective simulators require reliability and validity across several levels: face, content, construct and predictive. Face validity is the degree to which a procedure appears effective regarding its stated goal. Content validity is the ability to represent all facets of a given construct. Construct validity refers to the ability to distinguish between subjects with varying levels of experience. Predictive validity is the correlation between measured performance and technical ability *in vivo*. Ideal simulators accurately replicate surgical tasks, distinguish experience levels, and ensure skill transfer to patient care.[1]

Historically, trainee performance assessment was manual, relying on senior neurosurgeons' direct observation, introducing feedback quality. Basic performance metrics such as speed, accuracy and completion of surgical tasks were manually recorded and analyzed, providing rudimentary quantitative assessment to complement the subjective evaluations. Modern simulators use complex algorithms to provide immediate and quantifiable feedback with score reports based on a variety of metrics. These simulators objectively evaluate the progress and skill levels of trainees.

A systematic review examined VR simulators for neurosurgical skill assessment, using major automated performance metrics (APM), including distance to target, force, kinematics, time, blood loss or volume of resection. The following examples illustrate the various findings of the studies reviewed. The distance between an implanted device's final placement and the intended target has been used to assess performance during VR pedicle screw and ventricular catheter placements. Repetition improved performance irrespective of training level, but deskilling occurred if spaced far apart. The time to complete a surgical task or phase of surgery was studied, finding that residents conducted simulated ventriculostomies faster after practice and instruction. Kinematic measures include instrument movement and position, including velocity, acceleration and jerk. Experts

DOI: 10.1201/9781003471165-13

made fewer regular movements, indicating that they are more effective with each motion without the need for repetition. Force APMs include maximum force applied and summation of forces used. The variability in psychomotor performance between a novice resident and an expert neurosurgeon was examined through force pyramids and force histograms. These metrics were able to differentiate between an expert neurosurgeon and a junior resident. Volume of resection was calculated to determine the success of resection and the efficiency of surgical maneuvers.[2]

Conventional neurosurgical training faced challenges, including limited exposure to complex and rare surgical cases, and lack of scalable, tactile feedback. While technological enhancements such as VR and haptic simulation helped bridge some of these gaps, assessment methods remained largely manual.

Manual assessments are limited by subjectivity and interrater variability, while traditional metrics such as task completion time or accuracy often fail to capture the nuanced psychomotor and cognitive skills that define surgical expertise. Further, the absence of scalable methods for continuous, individualized feedback limits trainees' ability to identify weaknesses and track progress objectively. These gaps created the need for AI integration—tools capable of analyzing complex, high-dimensional data to provide objective, real-time feedback and to accelerate skill acquisition in ways not possible with conventional methods.

THE USE OF AI IN SURGICAL SKILLS ASSESSMENT

With the advent and integration of AI into the medical field, a viable application of the new technology was seen within surgical simulation and skills assessment. The current main application of AI in neurosurgical simulation is to analyze surgical skill metrics produced by various simulators and then classify the users by skill level. However, there are additional studies described in this section that utilize more creative metrics to classify user skill level.

VIRTUAL REALITY SUBPIAL TUMOR RESECTION SKILL ANALYSIS

AI models have been used to analyze metrics from the NeuroVR simulator, a virtual surgical simulation station developed by the National Research Council of Canada, designed to recreate the visual and haptic experience of resecting a cortical tumor through an operative microscope. Various studies have used machine learning (ML) algorithms to determine skill levels, monitor bimanual surgical expertise, assess learning curves and provide automated feedback on performance.

To examine the operative factors that ML algorithms select to classify participants by expertise level, 50 participants (i.e. neurosurgeons, neurosurgical fellows, senior residents, junior residents and medical students) performed five simulated subpial tumor resections. Data on instrument handling, tissue removal volume, blood loss and instrument contact with tissue were compiled. Four classifier algorithms were trained: k-nearest neighbor (KNN), Naïve Bayes (NB), discriminant analysis and SVM. The KNN algorithm classifies data based on how its neighbors are classified by identifying the nearest data points and assigning the most common class among them. The NB algorithm calculates the probability of each class for a data point given the feature values and predicts the class with the highest probability. Discriminant analysis algorithms model the distribution of each class and estimate the likelihood of a data point belonging to a class. The SVM constructs a plane to maximize the margin between different classes. The KNN achieved 90% accuracy, classifying 45 of 50 participants correctly, followed by NB (84%), discriminant analysis (78%), and SVM (76%). Beyond reporting classifier accuracies, this study demonstrated how complex psychomotor performance can be quantified and distilled into discriminative metrics. The NeuroVR simulator recorded raw signals every 20 minutes, including tool tip position, orientation, force application, bleeding rates and tumor and normal tissue removal. These signals generated 270 candidate features, which were then reduced to 122 and iteratively optimized for each classifier. The KNN ultimately achieved 90% accuracy using six key metrics spanning domains of instrument kinematics, applied force, tissue handling and bleeding control.[3]

One study utilized deep learning (DL) to classify between skilled (i.e. neurosurgeons and senior residents) and novice (i.e. junior residents and medical students) participants. This larger study expanded both the dataset and analytic pipeline. The participants included 23 skilled neurosurgeons and senior residents, as well as 92 novices, who completed 18 tumor resections across six scenarios with varying tactile and visual properties. The simulator recorded kinematic and force data, from which 150 motion- and force-based features were extracted, including velocity, acceleration, jerk, applied forces and derivatives. Statistical filtering reduced this set to 68 discriminative features, followed by forward feature selection to identify the 15–30 features most useful for classification. Among these, force-derived features were disproportionately represented, underscoring their importance in differentiating expertise. The SVM demonstrated the best performance with 86–89% accuracy, identifying position, force, position derivative and force derivative features as crucial for classification.[4]

Another study developed the Intelligent Continuous Expertise Monitoring System (ICEMS) to make continuous assessments of psychomotor skills during surgery. Data from participants at different training stages was used to train a long short-term memory (LSTM) network, which evaluates each time point in a surgical video in relation to previous time points, giving the ability to consider movement sequences. The neurosurgeons were considered experts, while the medical students were considered novices, fellows and senior residents were considered seniors and junior residents were considered juniors. Sixteen performance metrics were extracted from the simulation data and input into the LSTM to quantify expertise level as a score from expert level (1.00) to novice level (−1.00). The expert group scored significantly higher than the seniors, and juniors scored significantly higher than the novices. The ICEMS also differentiated between surgical trainee groups. This can be applied to provide continuous, personalized feedback that helps trainees modify their movements and identify areas for improvement, thereby mitigating errors.[5]

Data from NeuroVR was used to generate learning curves, providing insights into technical skill acquisition over time. Participants included neurosurgeons, neurosurgical fellows, residents and medical students performing the subpial tumor resection task. Six performance metrics were analyzed over five trials, utilized by the KNN algorithm to classify individuals into four levels of expertise. The first trial was considered the participants' baseline level of performance. Learning curves were generated and assessed by comparing performance for each group between the first and fifth trials for each metric. Five of the six metrics showed significant changes between groups. Only the medical student group had a significantly decreased mean instrument distance between trials 1 and 5. Neurosurgeon, senior and junior groups showed a significant increase in median aspirator change in force between trials 1 and 5. Neurosurgeon and junior groups had significantly higher aspirator median velocity when comparing trials 1 and 5. Neurosurgeon, senior and junior groups showed a significant increase in mean aspirator force during tumor resection between trials 1 and 5. Neurosurgeon and junior groups showed an increase in mean aspirator velocity between trials 1 and 5. Learning curves created with AI-derived metrics enhance the precision of expertise classification during tumor resection and provide insight into technical skill acquisition.[6]

The virtual operative assistant

The virtual operative assistant (VOA) was constructed using data from the NeuroVR simulator and provides users with automated feedback on surgical performance metrics.

Data from 50 participants, divided into skilled (i.e. neurosurgeons, neurosurgical fellows and senior residents) and novice (i.e. junior residents and medical students) groups, were used to construct and validate the VOA. Four final metrics were selected to train an SVM algorithm. Cross-validation accuracy was 92%. The VOA provided metric-wise assessment of performance depending on the weight of each metric. The model was composed of four metrics, including two safety and two movement metrics. A metric whose corresponding weight has a larger magnitude will play a greater role in the algorithm's decision-making process.

The ML algorithm initially computes classification as skilled vs novice. Then, the metric-wise assessment occurs—with safety metrics first. The feedback reinforces user's positive behaviors where competency was achieved, while also addressing metrics where the user performed less well. The summary incorporates automated auditory and video-based instruction specific to the psychomotor metric issues identified. The VOA establishes a foundation for integrating AI and VR simulation into surgical and medical education.[7]

The VOA was then used to measure performance outcomes of participants after receiving personalized feedback from the VOA and to compare surgical skill acquisition after feedback from the VOA as compared to an expert instructor.

A retrospective analysis compared surgical skill acquisition between a VOA group and a control group. Skilled attendings established expert benchmarks, and medical students were randomized into two groups to perform five simulated tumor resections with or without instructions from the AI-enhanced curriculum. The intervention for the VOA group involved receiving post-hoc audiovisual instructions on four learning objectives based on the learners' lack of competency. Participants in the VOA group responded successfully to performance feedback and achieved expert benchmarks in the curriculum's learning objectives. The results showed that the VOA group had significant improvements in 42 metrics during the entire procedure and 20 metrics during tumor resection, compared to 10 and 0 metrics, respectively, in the control group. By the end of training, the VOA participants' tumor resection technique resulted in significantly less damage to the surrounding brain compared with the control group. The VOA group achieved a significantly lower instrument divergence compared with the control group and achieved expert benchmarks. The change in maximum bipolar force during tumor resection was reduced considerably in the VOA group and not in the control group. By the end of the AI curriculum, students performed with significantly lower velocity and acceleration in their dominant hand compared to the control group. The VOA group had a substantially lower rate of tumor resection compared with no intervention.[8]

A randomized controlled trial involved 70 medical students performing five practice simulated tumor resections, followed by feedback (intervention) or no feedback (control), and then completing one realistic tumor resection simulation to evaluate learning and technical skill transfer. The feedback received and progress toward learning objectives were monitored by either the VOA or an instructor. The effect of feedback on surgical performance improvement over time was measured by the ICEMS expertise score: the mean of expertise predictions (range from −1 to 1, reflecting novice to expert rating) computed by a DL algorithm using an LSTM network with input performance metrics. Another outcome was learning and skill retention, evaluated based on realistic tumor resection performed by the ICEMS. The VOA feedback group achieved a difference of 0.66 points higher compared with the instructor group and 0.65 points higher compared with the control group. Learners performed significantly better than baseline after AI tutoring feedback. VOA feedback was more effective in enhancing metric scores compared with expert instruction. The VOA group achieved significantly higher expertise scores in the realistic subpial resection than the instructor and control groups. Compared with the control group, feedback significantly improved participants' respect for tissue and economy of movement. Expert instruction significantly enhanced instrument handling. Performing simulated brain tumor resection was more effective with input from an AI tutor compared with learning from expert instruction.[9]

Virtual reality spine surgery skills analysis

AI has been employed in VR simulations for spine surgery, including anterior cervical discectomy and fusion (ACDF) and lumbar hemilaminectomy, to analyze and classify surgical skill metrics.

In one study, 27 participants performed VR ACDF using the Sim-Ortho platform, divided into post-resident, senior and junior groups. Simulation steps include cutting the annulus to gain disc access, discectomy, posterior osteophyte removal and posterior longitudinal ligament (PLL) excision. Sixteen significant metrics were selected, and an artificial neural network (ANN) was then trained, achieving an accuracy of 83.3%. Key metrics included contacts with dura and force applied to the PLL. A decrease in contact with the dura increases the likelihood of being classified in the post-resident group. A larger force application increases the probability of post-resident or senior classification. Overall, this study successfully employed an ANN to classify participant skill levels based on significant performance metrics.[10]

Another study categorized ACDF simulation participants into post-resident, senior and junior resident groups. Six metrics were selected, and an ANN was trained with 80% accuracy in training and 83.3% in testing. The metrics and their corresponding connection weight products (CWPs) for each group revealed two patterns of learning: continuous and discontinuous. Continuous learning involves a progressive and sequential change in which learning occurs in incremental stages. The CWP associated with the average force applied to the C5 vertebra illustrated a continuous learning pattern. The results showed an increased likelihood of being classified as a senior resident, if the participant applied less force on the C5 vertebra, while even less force applied, increased the possibility of being classified as a post-resident. A discontinuous learning pattern is a variable and inconsequential modification of skills learning as residents progress in training, such as when participants were classified as senior rather than post-resident or junior if that participant had increased contact numbers on the spinal dura with an active burr. This ANN methodology was able to identify the metrics most important for surgical skill acquisition in ACDF surgery, and the learning patterns associated with these metrics.[11]

A study focused on the transverse box incision step, exposing the disc annulus in ACDF, with 23 participants comprising post-resident, senior resident and junior resident groups. A multi-layer perceptron ANN was trained, achieving an accuracy of 80% in the testing set. The most impactful metrics that distinguish the level of surgical performance between junior, senior and post-resident groups are the C4 vertebra contact length and time, as well as the maximum velocity in the z-direction. The ANN successfully highlights the relevant aspects of expertise and performance for assessment and training.[12]

A study using the NeuroVR simulator for a left L3 hemilaminectomy divided participants into senior (PGY4 and above) and junior (PGY3 and below) groups. SVM, KNN, linear discriminant analysis (LDA), NB and decision-tree algorithms were trained to assess whether selected metrics could achieve accuracy. Twelve metrics related to tool motion, safety, efficiency and coordination were identified. The study found that the maximum force applied to the dura is lower in the senior group. The amount of time spent while simultaneously using the burr and suction instruments was higher for senior participants. Senior participants touched adjacent structures more with their suction instrument while removing L3 with the burr. Senior participants displayed slower deceleration overall and exhibited less variance in the pitch angle of the burr when they removed L3. The SVM algorithm achieved the highest accuracy at 97.6%, followed by KNN (92.7%), LDA (87.8%), decision tree (70.7%) and NB (65.9%). Overall, this study further demonstrated the potential for ML algorithms to assess surgical skill levels in spine procedures.[13]

A study utilized simulated cadaveric durotomy repair to construct a surgical video dataset (SOSpine) for training AI models. Task outcomes and demographic data were recorded, and YOLOv4, an object detection algorithm, was trained to detect surgical instruments. This approach demonstrated the potential for using surgical video datasets to enhance AI applications in neurosurgical simulation and education.[14]

The integration of AI into surgical skills assessment has revolutionized neurosurgical training, offering unprecedented objectivity in characterizing performance metrics. AI models provide detailed analyses of surgical proficiency, capturing nuances often overlooked in manual assessments. These metrics not only objectively evaluate performance but also reveal intricate patterns in learning, enabling a tailored educational approach for each trainee.

Advancements in hard- and software technologies, including realistic real-time rendering, sophisticated physics simulations and immersive clinical scenario simulations, significantly enhance the realism and efficacy of training environments. These improvements elevate the quality of simulations and yield richer datasets, facilitating the development and refinement of AI applications. Consequently, trainees can engage in more accurate and varied practice scenarios, leading to better skill acquisition and retention.

AI for skill analysis has been applied to the clinical setting. For example, a study used a mask R-CNN to identify instrument movements and characterize microscope usage from microsurgical video.[15] This application of AI shows promise for further integration and should be explored in more detail.

Despite these advancements, the broad adoption of AI-enhanced educational models faces challenges. High costs and the necessity for customized solutions tailored to specific academic needs pose significant barriers. However, the development of standardized, out-of-the-box products could mitigate these issues, promoting wider acceptance and integration of AI-based simulators in residency programs across various medical institutions.

Currently, the main application of AI in surgical simulation focuses on the analysis and classification of surgical skills. AI models, through detailed performance metrics, offer precise and actionable feedback, fostering continuous improvement in surgical training. This marks a pivotal shift in neurosurgical education, moving from subjective evaluations to data-driven, objective assessments, ultimately enhancing the overall quality of surgical training and patient care.

OTHER USES OF AI WITHIN NEUROSURGICAL SIMULATION AND TRAINING

AI applications have been explored in various neurosurgical training settings beyond tumor resection and spine surgery simulators.

A study used videos from expert, intermediate and novice surgeons performing arachnoid dissection to train a CNN for tool segmentation, tool motion analysis and skill level classification. Using a 3D-printed brain model, surgeons had to perform an arachnoid dissection to locate an aneurysm. A mask R-CNN tracked instrument tips and extracted instrument coordinates. A prediction accuracy of 84.21% was achieved. The AUROC curve measurement was 0.9773, indicating a high, true separability between experts and novices. Experts had a lower mean dissector velocity, fewer jerks and a lower percentage of frames with no tools present compared to novices. Experts were also more likely to use bimanual handling of surgical tools than novices. The dissector working area was significantly greater in experts compared with novices. There was a significant reduction in the inter-tool tip distance observed for experts compared to novices. This study developed a computer vision (CV) framework for automated technical skill assessment in microneurosurgery using annotated videos.[16]

Another study analyzed videos of simulated vessel dissection and microsuturing in an *ex-vivo* model using a CV model to evaluate training improvement. A group of junior residents, senior residents and a cerebrovascular neurosurgeon performed a human placenta vessel dissection, arteriotomy and microsuture. The PRIME (Proficiency Index in Microsurgical Education) model counted surgical maneuvers by recognizing color-labeled surgical instruments. Feedback endpoints included total time to execute tasks and the number of hand movements. The success of the procedure was verified by flow without leak. Reduced procedure time and instrument motion range improved the PRIME score. Senior residents and the neurosurgeon showed nonsignificant improvements, but junior residents did not improve. This proof-of-concept study demonstrated PRIME's potential for providing continuous feedback in microsurgical training.[17]

A study used Shannon Entropy (ShEn) and DL to predict hemorrhage control success in endoscopic endonasal carotid artery laceration repair. The YOLOv4 algorithm was trained to detect surgical instruments using the Simulated Outcomes after Carotid Artery Laceration (SOCAL) video dataset. Instrument detection created precision-recall curves and calculated average precision (AP) for each instrument using the area under the curve (AUC). The normalized ShEn was used to generate a logistic regression classification model, with internal carotid artery injury control success as the binary outcome. Successful and unsuccessful hemorrhage control attempts demonstrated different patterns in tool usage across trial progression. Among successful trials, surgeons used instruments in a varied pattern, while the unsuccessful attempts displayed less varied instrument use. The surgical instrument detection model had a mean precision of 0.594 for all instruments and 0.743 for metallic instruments. The ShEn automated performance metric can enable automated assessment of surgeons in real time.[18]

Some studies used physiological metrics to analyze surgical skill performance and classify surgical expertise using ML. A study used EEG data from 24 participants performing a tumor resection on the NeuroVR simulator. Neurosurgeons and senior residents formed the skilled group, junior residents and medical students formed the less skilled group. Mean spectral power per tumor was calculated for the relevant EEG bandwidths. Theta/beta ratios (TBRs), associated with cognitive processing capacity, was calculated. An ANN provided high accuracy, finding significantly higher values of low alpha, overall beta, beta 1 and beta 2 in the skilled group. A considerably lower TBR was found for the skilled compared to the less skilled group. The ANN model could predict the levels of expertise of both skilled and less-skilled participants based on EEG recordings with high fidelity during the performance of VR-simulated brain tumor resection.[19]

A study used a force myography (FMG) band to measure volumetric arm muscle changes during a craniotomy simulator with 3D-printed bone. The study comprised 22 subjects, including neurosurgeons, senior residents and junior residents. The performance of NB, LDA, SVM and decision-tree classifiers in classifying surgical skills into expert, intermediate and novice categories was evaluated. The NB classifier (90%) achieved the highest accuracy, followed by the decision tree (86.2%) and LDA (81.9%). This study highlighted FMG band analysis as a viable method for classifying surgical skill levels.[20]

Few simulators use actual patient datasets—a concept described as "surgiality," which adapts models for specific interventions. Neuro-fuzzy systems, combining neural network architecture and fuzzy logic, have been developed for VR applications in neurosurgery. These systems create viscoelastic objects for simulation using real-world data. A vectorized recurrent neural network defines physical models with two neuron groups representing the mass and viscoelastic nodes, incorporating external forces on the objects. The fuzzy system assigns physical parameters, including viscosity, spring constant and friction. The RNN improves the model's appearance using these parameters. ROBO-SIM, an advanced simulation tool, uses this technology to simulate an endoscopic approach to the ventricles of the brain. The procedure involves defining the entry and target points, planning the surgical track and performing a virtual burr hole. Evaluated using MRI datasets from 38 patients, the ROBO-SIM showed high accuracy in visualizing anatomic structures. Overall, ROBO-SIM effectively uses patient neuroanatomy datasets, simulating both outer and inner surfaces with high realism, enhanced by neuro-fuzzy systems that adapt parameters interactively or based on real object measurements.[21]

Overall, these studies highlight the diversity in the applications of AI in neurosurgical simulation and training. These various uses of ML technology provide a glance at potential future opportunities for research and application to clinical and educational settings.

CONCLUSION

The integration of AI into neurosurgical training and simulation marks a significant advancement in the education and skill development of neurosurgeons. AI-enhanced simulators have transformed the landscape that initially consisted of cadaveric dissection, animal models, synthetic models and simple VR programs. These advanced systems now provide highly realistic, interactive 3D models with immediate, quantifiable feedback, capable of differentiating skill levels, monitoring learning curves and providing personalized feedback, thereby enhancing the training process.

Despite these advancements, challenges remain. The computational demands of real-time simulations using actual patient datasets are significant, and integrating AI into training programs requires careful validation to ensure reliability and accuracy. Moreover, while AI can enhance technical skills, it cannot replace the nuanced decision-making and problem-solving abilities developed through real-life surgical experience.

Future directions for AI in neurosurgical training should focus on improving the realism and responsiveness of simulations, integrating more comprehensive datasets and ensuring that AI systems can adapt to the evolving needs of trainees. Ongoing research into AI-driven feedback mechanisms will be crucial for developing more effective and efficient training programs.

In conclusion, the incorporation of AI into neurosurgical training and simulation offers tremendous potential for improving surgical education. By providing detailed, data-driven feedback and highly realistic practice environments, AI can help prepare neurosurgeons for the complexities of real-world procedures. As technology continues to evolve, so will the capabilities of AI-driven simulators, promising even greater advancements in neurosurgical training.

REFERENCES

1. Konakondla S, Fong R, Schirmer CM. Simulation training in neurosurgery: Advances in education and practice. *Adv Med Educ Pract* 2017; 8: 465–73.
2. Chan S, Conti F, Salisbury K, Blevins NH. Virtual reality simulation in neurosurgery: Technologies and evolution. *Neurosurgery* 2013; 72(Suppl 1): 154–64.
3. Winkler-Schwartz A, Yilmaz R, Mirchi N, et al. Machine learning identification of surgical and operative factors associated with surgical expertise in virtual reality simulation. *JAMA Netw Open* 2019; 2(8): e198363.

4. Siyar S, Azarnoush H, Rashidi S, et al. Machine learning distinguishes neurosurgical skill levels in a virtual reality tumor resection task. *Med Biol Eng Comput* 2020; 58(6): 1357–67.
5. Yilmaz R, Winkler-Schwartz A, Mirchi N, et al. Continuous monitoring of surgical bimanual expertise using deep neural networks in virtual reality simulation. *NPJ Digit Med* 2022; 5(1): 54.
6. Ledwos N, Mirchi N, Yilmaz R, et al. Assessment of learning curves on a simulated neurosurgical task using metrics selected by artificial intelligence. *J Neurosurg* 2022; 137(4): 1160–71.
7. Mirchi N, Bissonnette V, Yilmaz R, et al. The virtual operative assistant: An explainable artificial intelligence tool for simulation-based training in surgery and medicine. *PLoS One* 2020; 15(2): e0229596.
8. Fazlollahi AM, Yilmaz R, Winkler-Schwartz A, et al. AI in surgical curriculum design and unintended outcomes for technical competencies in simulation training. *JAMA Netw Open* 2023; 6(9): e2334658.
9. Fazlollahi AM, Bakhaidar M, Alsayegh A, et al. Effect of artificial intelligence tutoring vs expert instruction on learning simulated surgical skills among medical students: A randomized clinical trial. *JAMA Netw Open* 2022; 5(2): e2149008.
10. Mirchi N, Bissonnette V, Ledwos N, et al. Artificial neural networks to assess virtual reality anterior cervical discectomy performance. *Operative Surg* 2020; 19(1): 65–75.
11. Reich A, Mirchi N, Yilmaz R, et al. Artificial neural network approach to competency-based training using a virtual reality neurosurgical simulation. *Oper Neurosurg* 2022; 23(1): 31–9.
12. Alkadri S, Ledwos N, Mirchi N, et al. Utilizing a multilayer perceptron artificial neural network to assess a virtual reality surgical procedure. *Comput Biol Med* 2021; 136: 104770.
13. Bissonnette V, Mirchi N, Ledwos N, et al. Artificial intelligence distinguishes surgical training levels in a virtual reality spinal task. *J Bone Joint Surg Am* 2019; 101(23): e127.
14. Balu A, Kugener G, Pangal DJ, et al. Simulated outcomes for durotomy repair in minimally invasive spine surgery. *Sci Data* 2024; 11(1): 62.
15. Deepika P, Deepesh KVV, Vadali PS, et al. Computer assisted objective assessment of micro-neurosurgical skills from intraoperative videos. *IEEE Open J Eng Med Biol* 2023; 4: 11–20.
16. Davids J, Makariou SG, Ashrafian H, et al. Automated vision-based microsurgical skill analysis in neurosurgery using deep learning: Development and preclinical validation. *World Neurosurg* 2021; 149: e669–86.
17. Oliveira MM, Quittes L, Costa PHV, et al. Computer vision coaching microsurgical laboratory training: PRIME (Proficiency Index in Microsurgical Education) proof of concept. *Neurosurg Rev* 2022; 45(2): 1601–6.
18. Natheir S, Christie S, Yilmaz R, et al. Utilizing artificial intelligence and electroencephalography to assess expertise on a simulated neurosurgical task. *Comput Biol Med* 2023; 152: 106286.
19. Singh R, Godiyal AK, Chavakula P, Suri A. Craniotomy simulator with force myography and machine learning-based skills assessment. *Bioengineering* 2023; 10(4): 465.
20. Balu A, Pangal DJ, Kugener G, Donoho DA. Pilot analysis of surgeon instrument utilization signatures based on Shannon entropy and deep learning for surgeon performance assessment in a cadaveric carotid artery injury control simulation. *Oper Neurosurg* 2023; 25(6): e330–7.
21. Radetzky A, Nürnberger A. Visualization and simulation techniques for surgical simulators using actual patient's data. *Artif Intell Med* 2002; 26(3): 255–79.

14

Computer Vision in Neurosurgery

JAY J. PARK, MICHAEL LEE, NEHAL DOIPHODE, AARYAN SHAH, TOMASZ JAN ZALUSKA, AUDREY H. LIMB, ADVAIT PATIL, MANUEL REBOL, SIMON LEVINSON AND VIVEK P. BUCH

INTRODUCTION

Computer vision (CV) is a field within artificial intelligence (AI) that enables computers to process and interpret visual data in a manner akin to human vision and cognition. With the rise of the internet, online image platforms and image benchmark datasets,[1,2] the paradigm of recognizing and learning from data patterns through machine learning (ML) became the most successful method for image processing in CV. Nowadays, deep artificial neural networks in AI achieve the best results in CV benchmarking. In this chapter, we dive into the key fundamentals of CV within the context of neurosurgery. We begin by exploring the applications of CV in preoperative settings. We introduce the term Intraoperative CV (iCV) to refer specifically to CV used during surgical procedures. Much like Intraoperative AI (iAI), iCV encompasses CV computations within the operating room (OR) setting. This distinction is crucial, as CV in surgery includes broad applications, many intersecting with radiology (primarily for diagnostic purposes). iCV mainly involves numerous models that directly impact surgical procedures in real time. This chapter will trace the development of CV in neurosurgery, from its applications in neuroimaging, surgical training, to use in the OR (**Figure 14.1**).

Computer vision fundamentals

COMPUTER VISION TASKS

CV tasks involve image acquisition, processing and understanding of recorded visual information. The primary CV tasks related to image understanding are shown in **Table 14.1**.

COMPUTER VISION–ARTIFICIAL NEURAL NETWORK ARCHITECTURES

Artificial neural networks (ANNs) are an AI method based on biological neural networks. The ANN architectures that typically achieve the highest accuracy in neurosurgical CV involve deep learning (DL) architectures designed to analyze medical imaging and video data and assist in surgical procedures (**Table 14.2**). DL architectures that are trained for a specific CV task are referred to as models. The training process involves the learning of patterns in the data by processing image samples.

- *Convolutional Neural Networks (CNNs)* are a type of ANN specifically designed for processing structured grid data, such as pixels in an image. CNNs are extensively used for image/video analysis due to their ability to learn spatial hierarchies from input images. They are characterized by their ability to learn spatial hierarchies of features from input

DOI: 10.1201/9781003471165-14

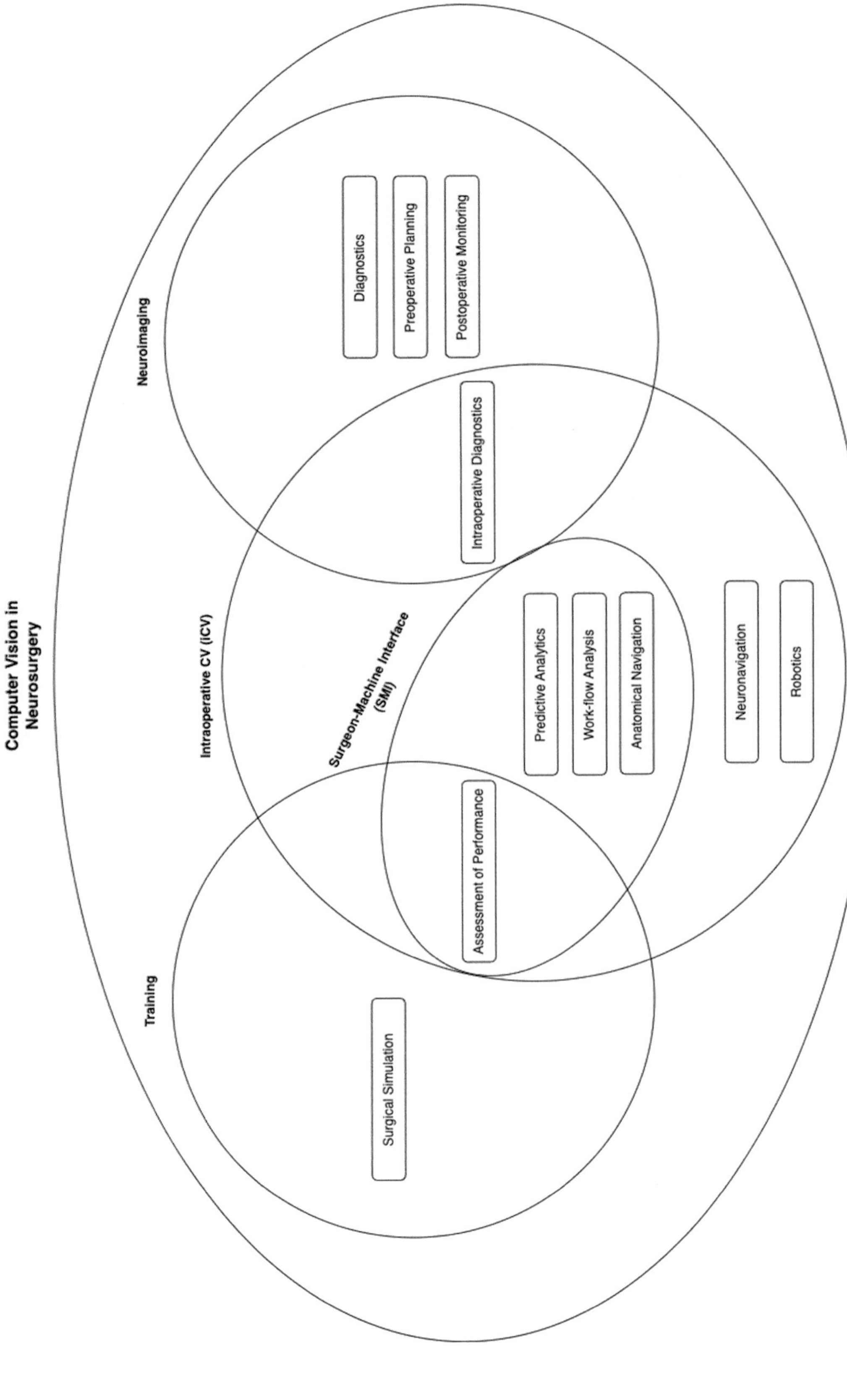

Figure 14.1 Venn diagram defining computer vision in neurosurgery.

Table 14.1 Computer vision tasks and examples

Tasks	Definition	Examples in neurosurgery
Image classification	Assigning a label to an entire image	Classifying MRI images of tumors into different types (i.e. gliomas, meningiomas, metastases)
Object detection	To identify and locate objects within an image using bounding boxes	Foreign body detection in the brain parenchyma using ultrasound[3]
Object tracking	Tracking spatial movement and position of an object in a video sequence	Monitoring the position and movement of tools to prevent unintended tissue damage
Semantic segmentation	Classifying each pixel in an image to a particular class	Segmentation of brain tumors in MRI scans for planning and guiding surgical resection
Instance segmentation	Identifies and separates individual objects within the same class in an image	Individual surgical tool and anatomy segmentation in endoscopic surgeries
Panoptic segmentation	Combines both semantic segmentation and instance segmentation to provide a comprehensive understanding of the scene	Segmentation of all nerves, blood vessels, brain tissue, cerebrospinal fluid and blood in surgical videos
Scene reconstruction	Constructs a 3D model from 2D images	3D Brain reconstruction for surgical training and planning
Video motion analysis	Involves processing and interpretation of video data to understand and quantify the movement of objects, people, or features within the frames	Analyzing the motion captured in surgical videos to assess
Image restoration	Refers to the process of enhancing or recovering the quality of a degraded or corrupted image to improve its visual appearance and fidelity	Detect and correct artifacts in MRI images
Video object segmentation	Task of segmenting objects of interest across frames in a video sequence	Identify and segment critical structures (i.e. tumors, blood vessels, or functional areas) within the surgical field
Video instance segmentation	Detects and segments multiple objects in a video sequence, distinguishing between different instances of the same class. It extends instance segmentation from static images to dynamic video data, offering detailed and context-aware insights into moving scenes	Real-time segmentation of multiple critical anatomical structures in intraoperative video feeds

data through the application of convolutional filters, which are pixel windows that slide over an image.

- *Recurrent Neural Networks (RNNs)* are a type of ANN designed for processing sequential data (temporal analysis of brain scans, predicting disease progression and monitoring postoperative recovery). RNNs have state vectors and connections that form directed cycles, allowing them to maintain a "memory" of previous inputs. This makes them well-suited for tasks where the context or temporal order of inputs is important.
- *U-Net* is a fundamental CNN encoder-decoder architecture for medical image analysis, particularly effective in neurosurgery segmentation tasks such as brain tumor delineation.[4] Its strengths include combining contextual understanding with fine detail, making it ideal for precise segmentation of complex structures such as tumor sub-regions in MRI scans. A notable example of its success is the BraTS Challenge,[5] where U-Net excels in accurately identifying enhancing tumors, tumor cores and edema.
- *Transformer-Based Architectures*, such as Vision Transformers (ViTs),[6] excel in handling long-range dependencies that traditional CNN models struggle to capture. This is particularly useful for medical images, which often come in sequences, whether multimodal, 3D (slices), or video (temporal). Transformer-based models help distinguish between similar-looking regions that are spatially distant but contextually different, improving segmentation accuracy. ViTs facilitate global context understanding through a self-attention mechanism that considers relationships between all pairs of image patches, which is crucial for accurately segmenting interconnected and complex anatomic structures in neurosurgery. Hybrid models combining CNNs and ViTs further enhance results, such as glioma segmentation in brain MRI, by leveraging both local and global feature extraction capabilities.[7]

Table 14.2 Structures of commonly used CV architectures in neurosurgery

CNN	Convolutional layers	Apply filters (kernels) to the input to create feature maps, highlighting various aspects and capturing spatial relationships through local connectivity between neurons of adjacent layers
	Pooling layers	Reduce the spatial dimensions of the feature maps while retaining important information. This down-sampling helps reduce computational cost and control overfitting
	Fully connected layers	Final layers of the CNN, have full connections to all activations in the previous layer, as seen in traditional neural networks. These layers are responsible for combining the learned features to make predictions
RNN	Recurrent layers	Where each neuron has a connection to itself in the next time step. This feedback loop enables the network to retain information across time steps
	LSTM	Type of RNN designed to overcome the vanishing gradient problem with memory cells that retain information over time. They use input, forget and output gates to manage information flow and learn long-term dependencies
U-Net based deep convolutional networks	Symmetric U-Shape	U-Net consists of a contracting path to capture context and a symmetric expanding path that enables precise localization. This is crucial in neurosurgery where the accurate delineation of anatomical structures and pathological regions is necessary

(Continued)

Table 14.2 (*Continued*) Structures of commonly used CV architectures in neurosurgery

U-Net based deep convolutional networks (*continued*)	Skip connections	These connections allow the network to combine high-resolution features from early layers with the contextual information from deeper layers. This maintains spatial accuracy and preserves small, fine details, which is crucial in neurosurgical contexts
Transformer architectures	Patch embedding and positional encoding	The input image is split into fixed-size patches, flattened and converted into vectors, turning 2D data into a 1D sequence for transformers. Positional encodings are added to these path embeddings to preserve spatial information, helping the model understand the position of each patch
	Transformer encoder	Primary building block of transformer architectures. It processes input data through a series of layers, each consisting of two main sub-layers: the multi-head self-attention mechanism and the feed-forward network
	Multi-head self-attention	One of the sub-layers within the transformer encoder. It computes attention scores between all pairs of input tokens (e.g. image patches), allowing the model to weigh the importance of each token relative to others. By using multiple attention heads, the model can capture various types of relationships and patterns in different subspaces
	Feed-forward network	Second sub-layer within the transformer encoder that applies multi-layer perceptron (MLP) to each token. It helps in learning complex representations by transforming the input through nonlinear activations

COMPUTER VISION IN NEUROIMAGING

The initial applications of CV in neurosurgery, like most medical specialties, involve imaging—including diagnostics, preoperative planning and outcome prediction.

Diagnostics

CV models facilitate expert-level diagnostics via recognition, segmentation and classification of neurological conditions, enabling time-sensitive diagnoses and recognition of subtle radiological features.[8]

In cases of infarcted brain tissue and large-vessel occlusions in CT angiograms, CV models facilitate rapid management of stroke-related pathologies.[9] Additionally, CNNs identify subtle features that predict outcomes and treatments for intracranial hemorrhage, where diagnosis relies on volume and expansion measurements, mitigating high interrater variability and over-approximation with irregular hematomas.[10] Brain tumors shape and size are heterogeneous; ML segmentation algorithms improve brain tumor localization, grading and postoperative prognostication (*see* Prognostics and Prediction of Outcomes).[8] Biologically informed ANNs such as BioNet[11] adapt parts of the DL process, such as the pre-training of the model, the design of the ANN architecture, and the learning objective function to reflect the biological task. DeepGlioma[12] uses a separate stimulated Raman histology image and genetic encoder for the task of molecular classification.

Advanced motion correction algorithms use DL (e.g. CNNs or generative adversarial networks [GANs]), to remove artifacts and enhance image quality. MRI artifacts can arise from patient movement, hardware imperfections or external electromagnetic interference. These images can be retrospectively adjusted to correct positions, providing a true representation of a tumor's location and size.[13]

Accurate 3D reconstruction of the brain from medical imaging data significantly improves diagnosis, particularly in cerebrovascular disorders where visualizing blood vessels is critical for understanding pathology. CNN-based reconstruction algorithms provide 3D understanding from 2D angiographies, forming an alternative to the traditional 3D rotational angiography (3DRA).[14] This approach aids in identifying abnormalities such as aneurysms, arteriovenous malformations (AVMs), stenosis and other vascular pathologies. Additionally, it permits image rotation and multi-angle vasculature views, facilitating comprehensive lesion assessment.

Preoperative planning and postoperative monitoring

SURGICAL PLANNING

Navigating optimal surgical pathways is crucial for preoperative planning. CV algorithms accurately localize and classify neuroanatomical features, identifying surgical targets in specific brain regions. They generate proposed pathways based on risk minimization and feasibility.[15,16]

Once targets and eloquent brain regions are identified, numerous pathways must be evaluated. Reinforcement learning (RL) algorithms are particularly useful for this task, exploring various pathways, receiving feedback and learning to avoid undesired actions. Examples in neurosurgery include Q-learning and the SurgiNav platform, which optimize trajectories by calculating scores based on intrusiveness to neighboring tissue and ranking pathways to identify the lowest-risk and least-invasive options.[15,16] While AI aids in mapping and suggesting pathways, human judgment is crucial for informed surgical decisions and final selection and execution must be performed by the neurosurgeon. Additionally, the substantial computational cost and time to produce multiple pathways present practical challenges,[15,16] highlighting the need for advancements.

PROGNOSTICS AND PREDICTION OF OUTCOMES

CV enables radiomics (extracting quantitative features from neuroimaging with data-characterization algorithms). Combined with clinical variables, predictive models can forecast survival, functional and surgical outcomes for conditions such as brain tumors, epilepsy and vascular and spine disorders.

CNNs and graph neural networks (GNNs) identify connectivity patterns in preoperative diffusion-weighted MRI, predicting outcomes like language impairment and seizure recurrence in epileptic patients.[17] CNNs also assess endovascular treatment (EVT) efficacy for ischemic stroke by analyzing CT angiography images with RNNs, predicting reperfusion without annotated images.[18] When adapted with DL techniques such as autoencoders and structured receptive fields, this model can accurately predict good reperfusion following EVT and does not require annotated images.[18,19] For spinal stenosis, DL models on preoperative MRI scans determine endoscopic decompression success,[20] while SVMs handle recovery prognosis when DL methods overfit due to small datasets, streamlining treatment planning.[21]

CNNs trained for brain tumor segmentation generate radiomic features from multimodal MRI of glioblastoma patients, enhancing survival prognosis, especially when combined with clinical factors.[22,23] Both preoperative[22] and postoperative MRI[24] improve prognostic value for overall and progression-free survival in high-grade glioma patients.

Postoperative treatment response is monitored by imaging-based algorithms evaluating tumor pseudoprogression risk after resection and chemoradiation, with spatial maps identifying infiltrating tissue.[25] Long short-term memory (LSTM) models paired with CNNs recognize spatial sequences and outperform random forest (RF) models in predicting pseudoprogression and progression.[26] CNNs also predict brain-wide metastasis post-stereotactic radiosurgery, computing the probability of response with high sensitivity and specificity.[27] This informs prognosis preoperatively and can be updated postoperatively to guide treatment decisions and patient counseling.[27]

Current tools and practices

Neuroimaging products incorporating CV technology have received FDA approval for applications including detecting neurodegenerative diseases, automated radiological image processing, and stroke detection and triage (**Table 14.3**).

Table 14.3 Examples of commercialized products with CV technology

Clinical/ Technological task	Description	Tool
Automated radiological image processing	Automated processing of radiological images enhances the efficiency and accuracy of diagnostic procedures	**ANDI by Imeka**: This tool uses reinforcement learning with proprietary CV architecture to automate the processing of diffusion-weighted radiological images to map white matter tracts, aiding in the detailed analysis of brain connectivity and structural integrity
Stroke detection and triage	CV technologies can help assist in timely stroke detection and triage	• **360 e-ASPECTS (Brainomix)**: Segments scans to generate an Alberta Stroke Program Early CT Score, classifying regions as ischemic or normal to assess stroke severity and guide treatment • **Rapid NCCT Stroke (RapidAI)**: Analyzes CT images to detect intracranial hemorrhages and large vessel occlusions, providing quick diagnostic support in emergencies • **Annalise Enterprise CTB Triage Trauma (Annalise.AI)**: Provides computer-aided triage and notifications for various CT brain findings, improving detection and management of traumatic brain injuries
Deep learning super-resolution (DLSR)	DLSR techniques are used to enhance the resolution of medical images, allowing for more detailed visualization of anatomic structures without the need for additional imaging scans	**SubtleMR (Subtle Medical)** use DL algorithms to improve MRI image quality and resolution[28]
3D reconstruction and visualization	Advanced 3D reconstruction technologies enable the creation of detailed 3D models of the brain from 2D imaging data, aiding in surgical planning and intraoperative navigation	**OsiriX** software provides advanced 3D visualization tools that are widely used for surgical planning[29]
Machine learning-based image registration	Image registration techniques align images from different modalities (e.g. MRI, CT) to provide a comprehensive view of the brain's structure and function	**Elastix** is an open-source image registration software that uses ML algorithms for accurate image alignment[30]

COMPUTER VISION IN NEUROSURGICAL TRAINING

Evaluating a surgeon's proficiency is challenging, with traditional methods often failing to provide accurate assessments. Common metrics like operative durations, outcomes, complication rates and trainer feedback do not always accurately reflect surgeons' skills.[31] CV offers a solution by enabling objective, consistent, detailed assessments of neurosurgical skills. Video recordings of surgical procedures can be evaluated for performance aspects including instrument handling, precision and adherence to surgical protocols. CV algorithms can also enhance surgical simulations, reducing reliance on evaluations from experienced neurosurgeons.[32]

Postoperative video analysis

Traditional neurosurgical skill assessment and training rely on direct observation, which is subjective and prone to bias, reproducibility issues and limited availability of expert raters.[33] Checklist-based methodologies, while more objective, still require human experts and face subjectivity issues.[34] CV technology improves training and skill assessment in postoperative surgical video analysis, providing a more objective perspective on surgeons' skill and dexterity without the need for human evaluators.

CV accurately identifies surgical tools in videos, revealing experience and skill levels based on tool handling. Tool segmentation and tracking using advanced models like Mask R-CNN provide raw measurements and assess skill through metrics such as velocity, acceleration, jerk, tool distance, instrument collisions and tool presence in frames.[35–37]

These measurements stratify surgeons by skill level, often classifying them as "novice" or "expert." Combining CNNs or ViTs for segmentation with motion metrics and classifying with linear classifiers, SVMs and RF algorithms, performance is stratified using OSATS and GEARS references.[38] Trends like lower velocity, acceleration rates and increased bimanual tool usage indicate higher proficiency.[37] CV technology can differentiate surgeons by experience and dexterity, standardize trainee evaluation, provide near real-time feedback, and aids in developing individualized training plans as it advances.

Surgical simulation

Augmented Reality (AR) and Virtual Reality (VR) create immersive environments for surgical education, allowing surgeons to visualize and practice procedures in a risk-free setting. Improvements in virtual simulation across surgical scenarios are increasingly being explored as a low-risk environment for neurosurgical training.[37]

Although 3D rendering does not require ML, deep 3D approaches using CV enhance the quality and experience of 3D simulations. CNNs convert 2D images into 3D, aided by 3D segmentation and labeling.[39] They improve training by reducing sensory input latency through pre-rendering scenes based on the user's gaze.[39] GANs create hyperrealistic overlays on simulator video feeds, enhancing physical phantoms with intricate visual details.[40] This immersion offers a more realistic and effective training environment.[41]

Like postoperative video analysis, ML algorithms can be integrated into surgical simulations to assess and classify surgical skills by tracking various performance metrics over time. NeuroVR, a VR platform for training neurosurgeons, automatically extracts numerous objective metrics from virtual surgical tasks. These metrics can be processed by an SVM to classify discrete skill levels.[42]

INTRAOPERATIVE COMPUTER VISION

The primary distinction of iCV from other CV applications in surgery is its need to operate in (near) real time, requiring higher computational power and optimized algorithms. iCV technologies address clinical needs such as diagnostics, navigation and intraoperative decision support.

Intraoperative diagnostics

Integrating CV algorithms with intraoperative diagnostics like spectroscopy, histology, microscopy and imaging enhances time-sensitive diagnosis and diagnostic accuracy in neurological disorders. Advanced DL architectures, including CNNs, perform well in identifying tumor boundaries, maximum safe resection and classification.[43,44] RFs can integrate data types for robust predictions in medical imaging, aiding in accurate registration of preoperative MRI and intraoperative ultrasound (iUS) for improved tissue deformation calculations and neuroanatomical positioning.[45]

iCV involves various training methods that can adapt large-scale models for specialized tasks in medical diagnostics. Transfer learning (TL) reuses models developed for other tasks, leveraging large datasets like ImageNet to improve classification by fine-tuning for medical images. TL with Google Brain's EfficientNet aids in detecting tumor boundaries and diagnosing gliomas from intraoperative fluorescence imaging.[43] However, TL effectiveness varies; medical images differing from datasets like ImageNet may limit improvements.[44] Training solely on medical imaging, though computationally expensive, may avoid pretrained dataset biases. For CNS tumor prediction with stimulated Raman histology imaging, TL did not improve performance due to domain differences.[44] Testing TL versus training from scratch and exploring broader imaging modalities with extensive datasets (intraoperative surgical cameras, CT and MRI) is essential for iCV efficacy.

Navigation

NEURONAVIGATION

The standard for surgical guidance in neurosurgery has been stereotaxic neuronavigation, using preoperative imaging to align structural data with a patient's 3D anatomy through a tracing probe. Integrating CV improves neurosurgical accuracy and safety by offering real-time visual feedback, crucial for identifying neuroanatomical structures and assessing brain shifts.[46]

Stereotaxic and camera-based registration use preoperative MRI and CT scans to map neuroanatomical structures. Stereotaxic registration relies on tracing probes, while camera-based registration uses real-time cameras to capture images of the surgical site. CV tasks include volumetric reconstructions from preoperative imaging and object detection and localization.[45] By combining annotated structures and markers from pre- and intraoperative images, systems like Zeta's Snap-Surface algorithm convert CT scans into a 3D mesh, aligning it with real-time camera data.[47]

Ultrasound-based navigation offers real-time imaging without preoperative registration. iUS supports registration using preoperative MRI and CT scans and tracks dynamic changes during surgery. This enables CV tasks like tissue differentiation and segmentation, improving neuronavigation capabilities.[48]

Current stereotaxic methods are rigid and fixed, limiting their use, and procedures like external ventricular drain placement rely on freehand interpretation of anatomic landmarks. iCV-based registration can provide real-time guidance, improving accuracy and safety.[49]

Surgeon–machine interface

The confluence of the increased volume of minimally invasive surgery (MIS), videoscopic technology and CV has catalyzed the emergence of the field of surgical video analysis. Specialties such as general surgery, urology and ophthalmology have been at the forefront of adopting CV in surgery, driven by the emphasis on diagnostics, the simplicity and volume of certain laparoscopic procedures and the early adoption of robotics. However, the extensive use of videoscopic technology in neurosurgery, with approximately 10 million microscopic neurosurgical cases globally per year, alongside endoscopic procedures, has led to an increasing exploration of CV applications in neurosurgical videos.

Across all surgical specialties, the ultimate goal of integrating CV is to improve surgical outcomes by augmenting the surgical paradigm with machine intelligence. The term Surgeon–Machine Interface (SMI) has been introduced to collectively define this concept. SMI describes the intersection between surgeons and intelligent machine models to inform and enhance surgical procedures in real time (**Figure 14.2**). It is derived from the principle of the Human–Machine Interface (HMI) but is specifically tailored to AI interactions within the surgical field. SMI encompasses the system of both hardware and software through which a surgeon experiences augmented interaction, facilitating data-driven decisions, improved outcomes and greater precision in surgery. While SMI ultimately utilizes the fundamentals of multimodal AI, CV is a critical component in establishing the machine's understanding of a surgical operation, akin to an expert surgeon. We will be reviewing key components of SMI and the enablement of this technology in a neurosurgical context (**Figure 14.3**).

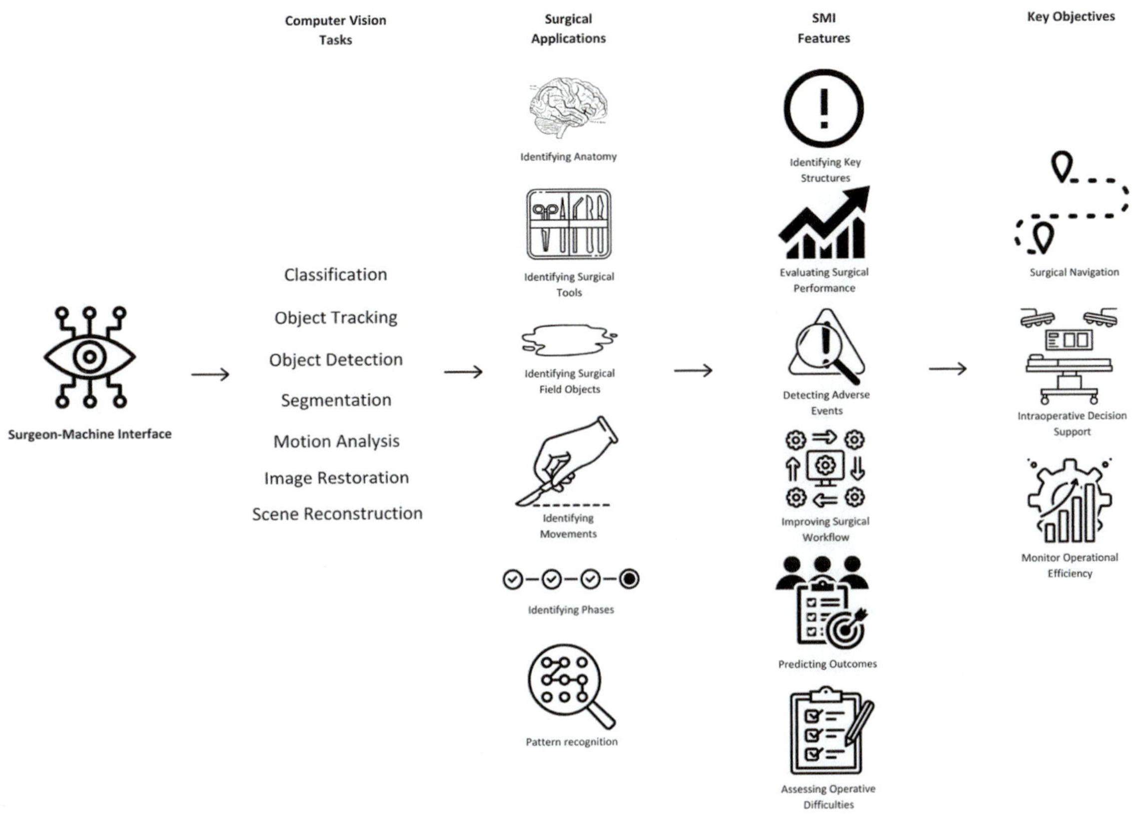

Figure 14.2 A flow diagram of Surgeon–Machine Interface and its role in surgery.

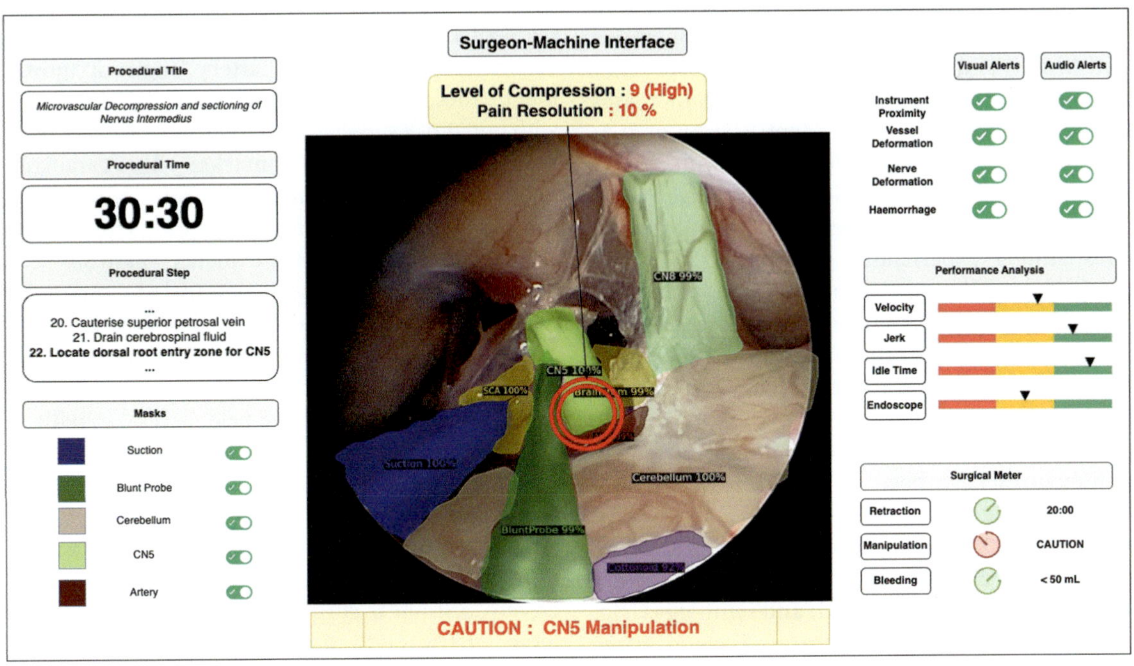

Figure 14.3 A mockup display of a Surgeon–Machine Interface.

OPERATIVE WORKFLOW ANALYSIS

Surgical phase recognition (SPR), or surgical workflow analysis, is foundational to enabling SMIs to understand surgical context.[47,48] Early work explored kinematic data recorded from sensors or robotic trajectories.[49] The focus has shifted to surgical videos, eliminating the need to introduce new devices into the standard surgical workflow. CV models are trained on labeled surgical video data to recognize various phases and steps. Early approaches used ML techniques like SVM, dynamic time warping (DTW) and HMM for workflow modeling.[50,51] While effective, these methods faced issues with scalability, complexity and overfitting. These problems have been addressed with CNNs and RNNs, which offer better accuracy, generalizability, efficiency, and importantly, real-time processing.[52]

Instead of classifying all surgical phases, methods now focus on critical phases or anatomic features. ViTs can detect aneurysms without explicit object detection or segmentation, reducing annotation burdens (highlighted in "Anatomical Guidance") while alerting the surgical team to high-risk phases like aneurysm rupture.[49]

ANATOMICAL GUIDANCE

SMI enhances traditional neuronavigation, which struggles with real-time brain deformation and shifts, reducing accuracy While intraoperative MRI (iMRI) and CT (iCT) address this issue, they are costly and time-consuming, and iUS increases cognitive load.[54,55] Real-time identification of anatomic objects and tools provides a viable alternative or supplement to improve navigation. Given variability in interrater agreement on anatomic structures among experienced surgeons,[56] SMIs are crucial for predicting critical structures and identifying eloquent areas in complex surgical scenes, even with significant neuroanatomic distortion.

The use of CV in anatomic scenes has evolved from simple object detection to complex panoptic segmentation tasks. In neurosurgery, various CNN architectures have been adapted for segmenting neuroanatomy in cranial, endonasal, spinal and endoscopic skull-base procedures.[57–59] These models address challenges posed by abundant non-rigid (e.g. blood, cerebrospinal fluid) and semi-rigid (e.g. nerves, blood vessels) structures. Beyond complete object segmentation, clinical applications include localization of bleeding origins to establish hemostasis.[60] While early CNNs and ViTs require substantial training and computational resources, ViTs' ability to capture global context in cluttered scenes offers promise for future anatomic segmentation advancements.

PERFORMANCE ASSESSMENT

Surgical skill assessments from video recordings offer insights for training, but real-time psychomotor evaluations provide immediate benefits. Metrics such as tool handling (on-off time, velocity, trajectory, idle time, jerk) and microscope handling can help operators make prompt adjustments,[37] with correlations to surgical outcomes enabling tailored feedback.[38] However, motion analysis alone does not fully capture surgical skills.[61] While detecting and segmenting neurosurgical instruments is key for automated analysis, using the anatomic landmark knowledge discussed in "Anatomical Guidance", surgical performance can be evaluated based on the presence or absence of anatomical structures or the completion of surgical tasks.[61]

REAL-TIME PREDICTIVE ANALYTICS

The core value of SMIs is their ability to provide real-time outcome predictions. By visually understanding anatomic objects in the surgical field, their interactions with surgical tools can be characterized qualitatively or quantitatively. For example, pixel-wise segmentation of surgical objects allows the measurement of attributes like artery length or movement. These characterizations must be correlated with outcomes and validated for accuracy to develop metrics, **surgical video biomarkers**. This paradigm creates a novel data stream of **videomics**, where multimodal AI can be utilized to enhance the predictive accuracy and capabilities of evidence-based surgical decisions. Early-stage examples include capturing the level of compression of the trigeminal nerve in Microvascular Decompression (MVD) surgery and manipulation and retraction of brain tissue. To further advance this innovative field, several initiatives exist. The SMART (Surgeon–Machine interface for Analytics in Real Time) Surgeon Collaborative led by the Surgical Innovation & Machine Interfacing (SIMI) Laboratory from Stanford University is a multicenter, global initiative aimed to transform data-driven decisions in surgical practice. The objective of these initiatives is to combine resources between surgical centers, especially data to train neural networks to succeed at complex neurosurgical imaging tasks.

Not all predictive techniques require explicit CV tasks including object detection or segmentation; some can utilize CNNs for feature extraction. Relevant features from input frames can train a CNN to learn hierarchical features such as edges and patterns within an image. It can also be trained on a dataset where each of the frames are labeled as a certain category (e.g. bleeding present / absent). By incorporating an RNN into the CNN architecture, temporal relationships between frames can be captured. This combined model has been shown to predict outcomes and amount of blood loss in simulated internal carotid artery injury control surgeries.[62]

CHALLENGES AND FUTURE DIRECTIONS

In this chapter, we covered a wide range of CV applications, from static neuroimaging to real-time computation using neurosurgical videos. Key barriers to CV advancement and potential future applications in neurosurgery are detailed in **Tables 14.4** and **14.5**. High-quality datasets are needed to train neural networks for complex neurosurgical tasks. Similar to the neurosurgeon's holistic understanding of the patient history, anatomy and the surgical procedure, holistic multi-model datasets are needed with well-annotated ground-truth samples, architectures and objective functions for supervised learning. In order for a holistic neural network to support real-time surgical decision-making, temporal visual context, the interpretability of the situation in natural language, and the patient's clinical data points relevant for the procedure are necessary components. These individual components need to be fed under supervision during the training process. At the annotation stage, clinical experts need to provide their deep knowledge in the form of text and visual labels, such that models will learn how experts reason about their clinical decisions. Annotation formats include pixel or voxel labels, (3D) bounding boxes, activity and action descriptions, time stamps and unstructured open-ended captions. The main challenge for supervised learning lies in acquiring all these annotation formats for the full surgery, analogous to the human surgeon's sensory input and resulting thoughts during the operation. The acquisition of these rich multimodal datasets can be improved by increasing the amount of data capture, e.g. additional sensors such as cameras, eye/hand tracking, pressure, microphones during neurosurgeries, and by automating the annotation process with AI-assisted systems.

Table 14.4 Major barriers to CV development in neurosurgery

Barrier	Description	Problems
Dataset availability	Effective CV models depend on large, diverse datasets of imaging and video data to minimize algorithmic bias	• There is a scarcity of publicly available imaging and surgical video datasets • Obtaining and curating surgical videos can be costly, often requiring specialized commercial products • Datasets are siloed, making it difficult to share information across different academic and clinical centers • Surgeons may not prioritize recording procedures due to perceived lack of value, forgetfulness, the labor-intensive nature of managing large data volumes, and concerns about medicolegal implications • No consensus on how to create surgical video datasets, leading to variability in training data that may affect model generalizability
Annotation burden	High-quality imaging and surgical video datasets need expert annotations for training, testing and validating CV models	• Expert annotation is costly and time-consuming • Even experts exhibit variability in annotations, necessitating stringent quality control measures • Annotation tools lack compatibility storage systems, complicating the workflow

(Continued)

Table 14.4 (*Continued*) Major barriers to CV development in neurosurgery

Barrier	Description	Problems
Data operations	Developing effective CV models for neurosurgery demands a seamless DataOps workflow, encompassing data acquisition, transfer, annotation, curation and utilization	• There is no comprehensive end-to-end solution for processing data in neurosurgical settings; existing tools often address only one stage of the DataOps pipeline and lack interoperability • Establishing a DataOps pipeline across academic and clinical centers requires substantial time and effort, often necessitating dedicated personnel to ensure consistent data preparation • Adapting solutions from other industries is limited, due to issues such as patient data de-identification and compliance with hospital-specific and country-specific regulations
Adherence to reporting guidelines	For CV models in neurosurgery to be effectively compared and evaluated, studies must adhere to detailed and standardized reporting guidelines	• Efforts to establish standardized reporting metrics for CV models are still evolving, leading to inconsistencies in how model details have been reported so far[63] • Clear and comprehensive details about datasets used—such as the number of frames, object types, ontology, video specifics, and limitations—are often lacking, making it difficult to compare model performance
Ethical concerns	There are universal ethical concerns regarding CV in medical imaging, which is also pertinent in the context of neurosurgery[64]	• Ownership of de-identified data is unclear and often involves multiple parties, including hospitals, surgeons and patients • Technological advancements increase the risk of re-identifying previously anonymized data • Balancing the need for large, diverse datasets to build effective CV models with concerns about data sharing and privacy remains a significant challenge

Table 14.5 Future areas of research and development for CV in neurosurgery

Research areas	Description
Zero-shot segmentation of surgical scenes	Future research should develop zero-shot panoptic segmentation models that can accurately segment 2D and 3D images and videos with neurosurgical expertise. These models, similar to the Segment-Anything Model (SAM; Meta Inc.), should be versatile across different pathologies, videoscopes and surgical scenes. Improvements should focus on inference time, sample efficiency and accuracy to ensure reliable guidance. The aim is for CV models to achieve a visual understanding comparable to that of a neurosurgeon, akin to how self-driving car models match the proficiency of an average driver
Federated learning models	Federated learning models address challenges of data availability, ownership and privacy in developing CV systems for neurosurgery. They enable the training of a global CV model while keeping data decentralized, thus tackling issues of data fragmentation and privacy. By allowing multiple institutions to collaborate without sharing sensitive information, federated learning enhances model robustness and generalizability, advancing the development of safe and broadly applicable CV models in neurosurgery[64]

Table 14.5 (*Continued*)

Research areas	Description
Contextual and multimodal understanding of surgery	A thorough visual understanding of medical images or surgical videos requires contextual knowledge. Future CV models in neurosurgery should integrate data from multiple sources to gain a multidimensional understanding of the patient, pathology, surgery and surgeon. This approach will enhance model capabilities for automating diagnoses, improving training and providing real-time predictions to guide surgical decisions
Generation of synthetic datasets	GANs have been used to generate high-quality synthetic neuroimaging data, augmenting training datasets and improving model robustness. Similar techniques should be applied to create synthetic video datasets to advance real-time CV models for use in the OR. Incorporating synthetic datasets into training, testing and validation should become standard practice for developing CV models in neurosurgery
Depth perception and 3D reconstruction of surgical scenes	Most CV applications focus on 2D segmentation, but using 3D neuroanatomy can greatly improve simulation, navigation and predictions in neurosurgery. Enhancing depth perception and speeding up 3D model reconstruction are key. Models like Neural Radiance Fields (NeRFs) should be optimized to lower computational demands and accurately reconstruct 3D models from monoscopic views or limited imaging slices
Implementation of SMI to drive neurosurgical robotics	Robotics in neurosurgery is currently limited to tasks like stereotactic biopsies, endovascular procedures, spine instrumentation and SEEG electrode insertion. The NeuroArm (IMRIS Inc.) is the only image-guided robotic system in use, though robotics is expanding into endoscopic transnasal operations. Integrating SMI, which enhances visualization, quantification and algorithm-driven outcomes, into robotic systems could improve their precision and effectiveness by enabling them to interpret the surgical scene and make expert-level decisions

REFERENCES

1. Ronneberger O, Fischer P, Brox T. U-Net: Convolutional Networks for Biomedical Image Segmentation. In: Navab N, Hornegger J, Wells WM, Frangi AF (eds). *Medical Image Computing and Computer-Assisted Intervention—MICCAI 2015*. Cham: Springer International Publishing; 2015, pp. 234–41.
2. Dong H, Yang G, Liu F, et al. Automatic Brain Tumor Detection and Segmentation Using U-Net Based Fully Convolutional Networks. In: Valdés Hernández M, González-Castro V (eds). *Medical Image Understanding and Analysis*. Cham: Springer International Publishing; 2017, pp. 506–17.
3. Dosovitskiy A, Beyer L, Kolesnikov A, et al. An image is worth 16x16 words: Transformers for image recognition at scale. *arXiv:2010.11929v2*, 2020.
4. Zeineldin RA, Karar ME, Elshaer Z, et al. Explainable hybrid vision transformers and convolutional network for multimodal glioma segmentation in brain MRI. *Sci Rep* 2024; 14(1): 3713.
5. Wagner DT, Tilmans L, Peng K, et al. Artificial intelligence in neuroradiology: A review of current topics and competition challenges. *Diagnostics* 2023; 13(16): 2670.
6. Shafaat O, Bernstock JD, Shafaat A, et al. Leveraging artificial intelligence in ischemic stroke imaging. *J Neuroradiol* 2022; 49(4): 343–51.
7. Patel A, Schreuder FHBM, Klijn CJM, et al. Intracerebral haemorrhage segmentation in non-contrast CT. *Sci Rep* 2019; 9(1): 17858.

8. Lim A, Lo J, Wagner MW, et al. Motion artifact correction in fetal MRI based on a generative adversarial network method. *Biomed Signal Process Control* 2023; 81: 104484.
9. Wu S, Kaneko N, Mendoza S, et al. 3D Reconstruction from 2D Cerebral Angiograms as a Volumetric Denoising Problem. In: Bebis G, Ghiasi G, Fang Y, et al. (eds). *Advances in Visual Computing*. Cham: Springer Nature Switzerland; 2023, pp. 382–93.
10. Dundar TT, Yurtsever I, Pehlivanoglu MK, et al. Machine learning-based surgical planning for neurosurgery: Artificial intelligent approaches to the cranium. *Front Surg* 2022; 9: 863633.
11. Marcus HJ, Vakharia VN, Sparks R, et al. Computer-assisted versus manual planning for stereotactic brain biopsy: A retrospective comparative pilot study. *Oper Neurosurg Hagerstown Md* 2020; 18(4): 417–22.
12. Banerjee S, Dong M, Lee MH, et al. Deep relational reasoning for the prediction of language impairment and postoperative seizure outcome using preoperative DWI connectome data of children with focal epilepsy. *IEEE Trans Med Imaging* 2021; 40(3): 793–804.
13. Hilbert A, Ramos LA, Van Os HJA, et al. Data-efficient deep learning of radiological image data for outcome prediction after endovascular treatment of patients with acute ischemic stroke. *Comput Biol Med* 2019; 115: 103516.
14. Hamann J, Herzog L, Wehrli C, et al. Machine-learning-based outcome prediction in stroke patients with middle cerebral artery-M1 occlusions and early thrombectomy. *Eur J Neurol* 2021; 28(4): 1234–43.
15. Lewandrowski KU, Muraleedharan N, Eddy SA, et al. Artificial intelligence comparison of the radiologist report with endoscopic predictors of successful transforaminal decompression for painful conditions of the lumber spine: Application of deep learning algorithm interpretation of routine lumbar magnetic resonance imaging scan. *Int J Spine Surg* 2020; 14(S3): S75–85.
16. Jin R, Luk KD, Cheung JPY, Hu Y. Prognosis of cervical myelopathy based on diffusion tensor imaging with artificial intelligence methods. *NMR Biomed* 2019; 32(8): e4114.
17. Choi Y, Nam Y, Jang J, et al. Radiomics may increase the prognostic value for survival in glioblastoma patients when combined with conventional clinical and genetic prognostic models. *Eur Radiol* 2021; 31(4): 2084–93.
18. Feng X, Tustison NJ, Patel SH, Meyer CH. Brain tumor segmentation using an ensemble of 3D U-Nets and overall survival prediction using radiomic features. *Front Comput Neurosci* 2020; 14: 25.
19. Han W, Qin L, Bay C, et al. Deep transfer learning and radiomics feature prediction of survival of patients with high-grade gliomas. *Am J Neuroradiol* 2020; 41(1): 40–8.
20. Rathore S, Akbari H, Doshi J. Radiomic signature of infiltration in peritumoral edema predicts subsequent recurrence in glioblastoma: Implications for personalized radiotherapy planning. *J Med Imaging* 2018; 5(2): 1.
21. Jang BS, Jeon SH, Kim IH, Kim IA. Prediction of pseudoprogression versus progression using machine learning algorithm in glioblastoma. *Sci Rep* 2018; 8(1): 12516.
22. Cha YJ, Jang WI, Kim MS, et al. Prediction of response to stereotactic radiosurgery for brain metastases using convolutional neural networks. *Anticancer Res* 2018; 38(9): 5437–45.
23. Lam K, Chen J, Wang Z, et al. Machine learning for technical skill assessment in surgery: A systematic review. *NPJ Digit Med* 2022; 5(1): 24.
24. Titov O, Bykanov A, Pitskhelauri D. Neurosurgical skills analysis by machine learning models: Systematic review. *Neurosurg Rev* 2023; 46(1): 121.
25. Shah J, Darzi A. Surgical skills assessment: An ongoing debate. *BJU Int* 2001; 88(7): 655–60.
26. Hackney L, O'Neill S, O'Donnell M, Spence R. A scoping review of assessment methods of competence of general surgical trainees. *Surgeon* 2023; 21(1): 60–9.
27. Buyck F, Vandemeulebroucke J, Ceranka J, et al. Computer-vision based analysis of the neurosurgical scene—A systematic review. *Brain Spine* 2023; 3: 102706.

28. Davids J, Makariou SG, Ashrafian H, et al. Automated vision-based microsurgical skill analysis in neurosurgery using deep learning: Development and preclinical validation. *World Neurosurg* 2021; 149: e669–86.
29. Deepika P, Deepesh KVV, Vadali PS, et al. Computer assisted objective assessment of micro-neurosurgical skills from intraoperative videos. *IEEE Open J Eng Med Biol* 2023; 4: 11–20.
30. Lee D, Yu HW, Kwon H, et al. Evaluation of surgical skills during robotic surgery by deep learning-based multiple surgical instrument tracking in training and actual operations. *J Clin Med* 2020; 9(6): 1964.
31. Chan J, Pangal DJ, Cardinal T, et al. A systematic review of virtual reality for the assessment of technical skills in neurosurgery. *Neurosurg Focus* 2021; 51(2): E15.
32. Park JJ, Tiefenbach J, Demetriades AK. The role of artificial intelligence in surgical simulation. *Front Med Technol* 2022; 4: 1076755.
33. Engelhardt S, De Simone R, Full PM, et al. Improving Surgical Training Phantoms by Hyperrealism: Deep Unpaired Image-to-Image Translation from Real Surgeries. In: Frangi AF, Schnabel JA, Davatzikos C, et al. (eds). *Medical Image Computing and Computer Assisted Intervention—MICCAI 2018*. Cham: Springer International Publishing; 2018, pp. 747–55.
34. Wang DD, Qian Z, Vukicevic M, et al. 3D printing, computational modeling, and artificial intelligence for structural heart disease. *JACC Cardiovasc Imaging* 2021; 14(1): 41–60.
35. Mirchi N, Bissonnette V, Yilmaz R, et al. The Virtual Operative Assistant: An explainable artificial intelligence tool for simulation-based training in surgery and medicine. *PLoS One* 2020; 15(2): e0229596.
36. Shen B, Zhang Z, Shi X, et al. Real-time intraoperative glioma diagnosis using fluorescence imaging and deep convolutional neural networks. *Eur J Nucl Med Mol Imaging* 2021; 48(11): 3482–92.
37. Hollon TC, Pandian B, Adapa AR, et al. Near real-time intraoperative brain tumor diagnosis using stimulated Raman histology and deep neural networks. *Nat Med* 2020; 26(1): 52–8.
38. Nitsch J, Klein J, Dammann P, et al. Automatic and efficient MRI-US segmentations for improving intraoperative image fusion in image-guided neurosurgery. *Neuroimage Clin* 2019; 22: 101766.
39. Chartrain AG, Kellner CP, Fargen KM, et al. A review and comparison of three neuronavigation systems for minimally invasive intracerebral hemorrhage evacuation. *J Neurointerv Surg* 2018; 10(1): 66–74.
40. Chiurillo I, Sha RM, Robertson FC, et al. High-accuracy neuro-navigation with computer vision for frameless registration and real-time tracking. *Bioengineering* 2023; 10(12): 1401.
41. BrainLab. Available from: https://www.brainlab.com/surgery-products/overview-neurosurgery-products/cranial-navigation/ (Accessed May 2026).
42. Robertson FC, Sha RM, Amich JM, et al. Frameless neuronavigation with computer vision and real-time tracking for bedside external ventricular drain placement: A cadaveric study. *J Neurosurg* 2022; 136(5): 1475–84.
43. Ramesh S, Dall'Alba D, Gonzalez C, et al. Multi-task temporal convolutional networks for joint recognition of surgical phases and steps in gastric bypass procedures. *Int J Comput Assist Radiol Surg* 2021; 16(7): 1111–19.
44. Jumah F, Raju B, Nagaraj A, et al. Uncharted waters of machine and deep learning for surgical phase recognition in neurosurgery. *World Neurosurg* 2022; 160: 4–12.
45. Zappella L, Béjar B, Hager G, Vidal R. Surgical gesture classification from video and kinematic data. *Med Image Anal* 2013; 17(7): 732–45.
46. Lalys F, Riffaud L, Morandi X, Jannin P. Automatic Phases Recognition in Pituitary Surgeries by Microscope Images Classification. In: Navab N, Jannin P (eds). *Information Processing in Computer-Assisted Interventions*. Berlin: Springer; 2010, pp. 34–44.
47. Lalys F, Riffaud L, Morandi X, Jannin P. Surgical Phases Detection from Microscope Videos by Combining SVM and HMM. In: Menze B, Langs G, Tu Z, Criminisi A (eds). *Medical Computer Vision Recognition Techniques and Applications in Medical Imaging*. Berlin: Springer; 2011, pp. 54–62.
48. Khan DZ, Luengo I, Barbarisi S, et al. Automated operative workflow analysis of endoscopic pituitary surgery using machine

learning: Development and preclinical evaluation (IDEAL stage 0). *J Neurosurg* 2022; 137(1): 51–8.
49. Zhou J, Muirhead W, Williams SC, et al. Shifted-windows transformers for the detection of cerebral aneurysms in microsurgery. *Int J Comput Assist Radiol Surg* 2023; 18(6): 1033–41.
50. Golby A (ed). *Image-Guided Neurosurgery.* London: Academic Press; 2015.
51. Zhang J, Chen X, Zhao Y, et al. Impact of intraoperative magnetic resonance imaging and functional neuronavigation on surgical outcome in patients with gliomas involving language areas. *Neurosurg Rev* 2015; 38(2): 319–30.
52. Mascagni P, Vardazaryan A, Alapatt D, et al. Artificial intelligence for surgical safety: Automatic assessment of the critical view of safety in laparoscopic cholecystectomy using deep learning. *Ann Surg* 2022; 275(5): 955–61.
53. Park JJ, Doiphode N, Zhang X, et al. Developing the surgeon-machine interface: Using a novel instance-segmentation framework for intraoperative landmark labelling. *Front Surg* 2023; 10: 1259756.
54. Staartjes VE, Volokitin A, Regli L, et al. Machine vision for real-time intraoperative anatomic guidance: A proof-of-concept study in endoscopic pituitary surgery. *Oper Neurosurg* 2021; 21(4): 242–7.
55. Witten AJ, Patel N, Cohen-Gadol A. Image segmentation of operative neuroanatomy into tissue categories using a machine learning construct and its role in neurosurgical training. *Oper Neurosurg* 2022; 23(4): 279–86.
56. Tang J, Gong Y, Xu L, et al. Bleeding contour detection for craniotomy. *Biomed Signal Process Control* 2022; 73: 103419.
57. Oropesa I, Escamirosa FP, Sánchez-Margallo JA, et al. Interpretation of motion analysis of laparoscopic instruments based on principal component analysis in box trainer settings. *Surg Endosc* 2018; 32(7): 3096–107.
58. Pangal DJ, Kugener G, Zhu Y, et al. Expert surgeons and deep learning models can predict the outcome of surgical hemorrhage from 1 min of video. *Sci Rep* 2022; 12(1): 8137.
59. Abramson HG, Curry EJ, Mess G, et al. Automatic detection of foreign body objects in neurosurgery using a deep learning approach on intraoperative ultrasound images: From animal models to first in-human testing. *Front Surg* 2022; 9: 1040066.
60. Chaudhari AS, Fang Z, Kogan F, et al. Super-resolution musculoskeletal MRI using deep learning. *Magn Reson Med* 2018; 80(5): 2139–54.
61. Rosset A, Spadola L, Ratib O. OsiriX: An open-source software for navigating in multidimensional DICOM images. *J Digit Imaging* 2004; 17(3): 205–16.
62. Klein S, Staring M, Murphy K, et al. elastix: A Toolbox for Intensity-Based Medical Image Registration. *IEEE Trans Med Imaging* 2010; 29(1): 196–205.
63. Maier-Hein L, Reinke A, Godau P, et al. Metrics reloaded: Recommendations for image analysis validation. *arXiv:2206.01653v8*, 2022.
64. Esteva A, Chou K, Yeung S, et al. Deep learning-enabled medical computer vision. *NPJ Digit Med* 2021; 4(1): 5.
65. McMahan HB, Moore E, Ramage D, et al. Communication-efficient learning of deep networks from decentralized data. *arXiv:1602.05629v4*, 2016.
66. Deng J, Dong W, Socher R, et al. ImageNet: A large-scale hierarchical image database. In: *2009 IEEE Conference on Computer Vision and Pattern Recognition.* Miami: IEEE; 2009, pp. 248–55.
67. Krizhevsky A, Sutskever I, Hinton GE. ImageNet classification with deep convolutional neural networks. *Adv Neural Inf Process Syst* 2012; 25: 1097–105.
68. Wang H, Argenziano MG, Yoon H, et al. Biologically informed deep neural networks provide quantitative assessment of intratumoral heterogeneity in post treatment glioblastoma. *NPJ Digit Med* 2024; 7: 292.
69. Hollon T, Jiang C, Chowdury A, et al. Artificial-intelligence-based molecular classification of diffuse gliomas using rapid, label-free optical imaging. *Nat Med* 2023; 29(4): 828–32.

15

Large Language Models in Neurosurgery

SUMEDHA RAI AND ERIC K. OERMANN

EMERGENCE OF ARTIFICIAL INTELLIGENCE IN NEUROSCIENCE AND NEUROSURGERY

In recent years, the term "Artificial Intelligence" (AI) has gone beyond the spheres of just technology and computer science to become a familiar concept even in everyday conversations. Today, AI is not just a buzzword; it is a potent force that is reshaping industries, with healthcare at the forefront of this revolution. Although AI's rise to prominence seems recent, its roots in medical research and its application in neuroscience go back several decades, setting the stage for pioneering and innovative advancements in brain science and surgical procedures.

The first significant step toward artificial neural networks was made in 1943 when Warren McCulloch, a neurophysiologist, and Walter Pitts, a young mathematician, developed the first models of neural networks. This work laid the groundwork for using AI to model and understand brain functions. Their paper, titled "A Logical Calculus of the Ideas Immanent in Nervous Activity,"[1] proposed a model of artificial neurons capable of performing simple logical functions. This work was groundbreaking as it combined neuroscience with computational theories, establishing an important link between brain function and artificial computation.

The introduction of backpropagation in 1970, a method that became widely recognized in the 1980s, subsequently made it practical to train deep neural networks by enabling gradient descent in multi-layer structures. Backpropagation allowed the computation of the gradient of the loss function concerning each weight and adjusted them to minimize errors after each iteration, thereby optimizing the network for more accurate results. These deep learning (DL) architectures became capable of dynamically adjusting the weights of the connections between the neurons in the network. This backpropagation process thus enabled the networks to improve their performance iteratively, making complex tasks such as image and speech recognition not only possible but also remarkably accurate.[2,3]

In parallel to these advances, data analysis in brain structure and function was being conducted as early as 1994 using statistical parametric mapping and voxel-based analysis methods.[4] However, the early 2000s saw the integration of powerful machine learning (ML) methods into neuroimaging studies, enabling practitioners to develop imaging signatures for brain function and structure. support vector machines (SVMs) and random forests (RFs) became popular techniques.[5–7]

SVMs gained broad popularity around this time due to their robustness and flexibility in handling different types of data through the use of various kernel functions, which allow them to efficiently capture complex patterns. On the other hand, ensemble methods such as RFs also became widely adopted because they effectively minimize prediction errors by aggregating the outputs of multiple models. These

DOI: 10.1201/9781003471165-15

models are constructed using random subsets of features and samples, which enhances the overall accuracy and generalization ability of the system by reducing the risk of overfitting and capturing diverse aspects of the data.

By the early 2010s though, neural networks and other DL techniques gained widespread adoption because they could learn complex features hierarchically, eliminating the need to construct the right features upfront. Moreover, DL architectures were capable of building highly nonlinear decision boundaries, which was also an advantage over some other ML methods. Convolutional neural networks (CNNs) and even ensembles of these DL structures became cornerstones of neuroimaging for critical applications such as accurate brain lesion segmentation and functional MRI (fMRI) analysis. Today, deep neural networks such as CNNs are used in a wide range of neuroimaging applications. These algorithms can process MRI scans to estimate cortical thickness, an important biomarker for various neurological conditions, including neurodegenerative diseases. Additionally, DL is being used for "brain age prediction" based on neuroimaging data.[8] This prediction serves as an indicator of brain health and helps in studying age-related diseases such as Alzheimer's.

AI has also been instrumental in analyzing complex neuroscience datasets to uncover patterns of neural activity and plan ahead for neurosurgeries. With the advent of AI, neurosurgery has entered a new era of enhanced precision and decision-making support, potentially reducing the invasiveness of some procedures. For instance, AI and ML algorithms can now analyze brain and spine imaging with greater accuracy, reducing the need for exploratory surgeries in certain cases. AI is helping medical practitioners understand a patient's brain structure, identify critical areas and predict the impact surgeries may have on important biomarkers, thereby allowing surgeons to approach procedures with a level of preparation and foresight that was previously unattainable.

NATURAL LANGUAGE PROCESSING AND THE USE OF TEXT IN NEUROSURGERY

In a field as critical as neurosurgery, extensive documentation is essential for almost every aspect of patient care. Detailed records are maintained for patients who have undergone or are being considered for neurosurgical procedures, encompassing a comprehensive account of their medical history, including prior surgeries, medications, allergies and even family medical histories. Hospitals meticulously document patient visits, hospital stays, future appointments and interactions with insurance providers, wherever required.

Neurosurgeons and doctors maintain crucial notes on their first impressions, diagnoses and prognoses of patients' conditions. They also document prescriptions, guidance for their staff, notes to patients and detailed accounts of surgical procedures. This documentation covers every phase of the process, including preoperative, intraoperative and postoperative notes. Nursing staff contribute by recording additional details about patient care and observations during hospital stays. Following surgery, progress notes are updated to reflect the patient's status, observations and highly personalized care plans crafted by neurosurgeons and other healthcare providers. When a patient is discharged, a comprehensive discharge summary is provided, detailing the care given, final diagnosis, follow-up treatment and instructions for future care. If any complications arose during surgery, these are carefully documented for future reference and as a resource for handling similar cases. Efforts are always underway to enhance these documentation practices using technology and other practices due to their significant impact on patient care and hospital costs.[9,10]

The neurosurgical field also involves the documentation of a vast array of diagnostic and follow-up tests. Radiology reports provide interpretations of MRIs and CT scans by radiologists, often in text form. Detailed descriptions and pathology reports capture the results of biopsies and other specimen tests. Additionally, neurological planning is supported by meticulous documentation of medical imaging tests and the patient's condition. Casey et al.[11] review the use of natural language processing (NLP) to automate clinical understanding of radiology reports, while Ghosh et al.[12] developed a pre-trained language model using a corpus of 500 K radiology reports, demonstrating its effectiveness in tasks like named entity recognition and classifying reports as normal or abnormal based on the presence of pathologies.

Before and after procedures, patients are often asked to complete surveys and questionnaires

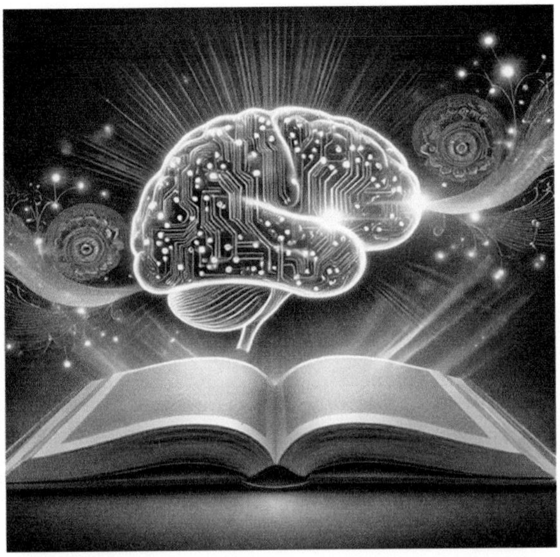

Figure 15.1 Use of natural language processing in neurosurgery. (Image generated using DALL-E, by ChatGPT [OpenAI].)

regarding their symptoms, quality of life, satisfaction with care and other demographic information. Text data may also be gathered directly from patients, such as from their pain diaries, notes of symptom tracking, and data from medical wearable devices. Kim et al. assess the performance of large language models (LLMs) (detailed in the next section) in health-related inferences using public datasets of user surveys and wearable data. [13]

Beyond patient care, the neurosurgical domain generates a wealth of text data through ongoing research and development. This includes journal articles and peer-reviewed research papers on new neurosurgical techniques, clinical trials and their outcomes. Renowned neurosurgeons and practitioners share their findings in conference papers, discussion documents and presentations at neurosurgery symposiums and conferences worldwide. Details of individual patient conditions, particularly those with rare or complex cases, offer valuable insights and are shared with the neurosurgical community as case reports. Esteemed databases and journals such as PubMed, the *Journal of Neurosurgery*, *World Neurosurgery*, to name a few, house millions of research papers, providing a rich repository of reliable textual data related to neurosurgery.

Researchers analyze studies over time to understand what doctors wrote, the diseases of the era and how research evolved. For instance, Mir et al. reviewed publications from 1902 to 2023 to track advancements in pediatric spine surgery and the evolution of its terminology.[14]

Fundamentally and importantly, the field of neurosurgery amasses a vast repository of textual data, which is critically essential for powering the advancing branch of AI called NLP. NLP models can ingest these extensive and reliable data, generating insightful models that enable medical practitioners and neurosurgeons to interact with and interpret vast amounts of text data more effectively. For neurosurgeons, using NLP models trained on these extensive data can provide access to a broader range of information and opinions from experts worldwide, far beyond their immediate professional network. Incorporating this valuable information into predictive models can revolutionize our understanding of neurosurgery through the lens of AI.

NLP in neurosurgery has begun to harness these large, critical textual data sources in neurosurgery both for research as well as patient care. NLP techniques can facilitate the conversion of these documents into tabular datasets for subsequent analysis, as well as to make predictive models of events ranging from the clinical to the educational.[15–17] While traditional NLP technologies built around treating text as a "bag of words" and subsequently applying models such as SVMs to simple features obtained from frequency counts or topic models has been utilized, the recent explosion in neurosurgical NLP has been driven by both the increasing availability of these text datasets, as well as the accessibility of LLMs.

LARGE LANGUAGE MODELS AND BEYOND

In the winter of 2022, on November 30, a generative AI chatbot called ChatGPT was released to the public. This large language model (LLM), GPT-3.5, was released by a company called OpenAI, a leading AI research organization (now backed by Microsoft), and is what is called an LLM. LLMs are NLP models that have already been fed and "trained" on vast amounts of publicly available text data. They are called "large" because they process and learn from billions of words and sentences, enabling them to understand the nuances of language that make sense both grammatically and semantically. Moreover, these models acquire knowledge of specialized terminology and business jargon used across different industries. This comprehensive understanding of both language rules and business terms allows LLMs to serve as a "foundation" for a wide variety of applications even if they haven't been explicitly trained on those data. Many AI models that require some understanding of text or semantic processing can be built upon these foundational models for different purposes across various industries. This versatility makes foundational models incredibly useful and widely applicable, but also very powerful, as a significant portion of AI architecture now depends on the smooth and correct functioning of these models. Just as a building will collapse if it has a faulty foundation, so will all models that are deployed on these foundational LLMs stop working, or have errors in deployment, if something were to go wrong with these models.

LLMs such as ChatGPT are based on a transformer architecture that was first introduced in 2017 by Vaswani et al.[18] The architecture is composed of a neural network, which, while inspired by biological neural networks, functions differently from the human brain. This neural network learns to represent various attributes or qualities of the input text through a process of forward and backward propagation of signals. Through this process, it adjusts variables called weights to encode information accurately within the network. The "largeness" of the neural network is determined by the number of parameters, which includes the weights that it uses to model its understanding of language. These parameters are adjusted during the training process to capture complex patterns and relationships in the data. In the case of LLMs, these parameters can number in the hundreds of billions, allowing for a deep and extensive understanding of language across different contexts and usage. For instance, OpenAI's GPT-3.5 had 175 billion parameters,

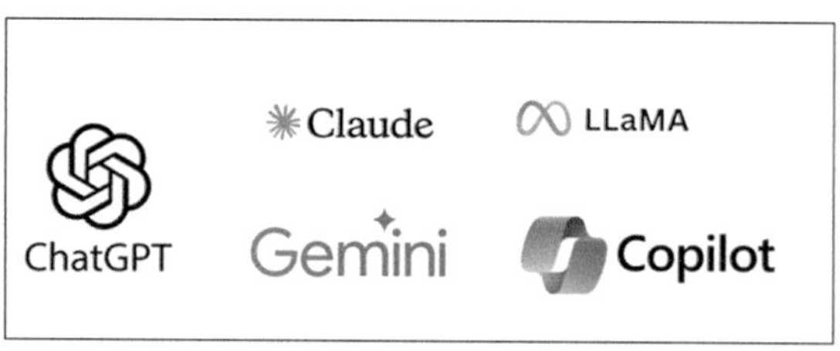

Figure 15.2 Large language models released by big technology companies.

Anthropic's Claude Sonnet was reported to have 100 billion parameters and although the exact number was not disclosed, OpenAI's GPT-4 was speculated to have been trained using trillions of parameters.

When asked about its medical and neurosurgical knowledge sources, ChatGPT-4 responded:

> My knowledge of medicine and neurosurgery comes from extensive training on a vast corpus of medical literature, textbooks, research papers, and other reputable sources up until my knowledge cutoff in October 2023. This includes information from established medical databases, academic journals, and expert-reviewed content across various medical fields.

Some key sources, where it draws its medical knowledge from, mentioned by GPT-4 include PubMed, and popular books such as *Gray's Anatomy*, and *Schmidek and Sweet: Operative Neurosurgical Techniques*, among others. This extensive knowledge base means that medical practitioners, including neurosurgeons, can potentially use these models as quick reference tools, accessing a wealth of information from highly regarded medical journals and trusted sources. This capability could significantly aid in research and reduce the time needed to look up important information. The conversational, human-like format of LLM responses and the ability to ask follow-up questions within the context of the conversation make these tools particularly user-friendly.

Some key applications of LLMs in neurosurgery include summarization of both clinical or scientific documents. A recent work demonstrates this capability by combining traditional bibliometric methods to select scientific articles, and then an LLM to summarize them and extract information about the natural history of disease.[19] This same capability can also be utilized to generate comprehensive hospital course summaries, detailing a patient's medical journey using the wealth of data available in the hospital's system. This can include both structured and unstructured information such as medical notes, diagnostic results, exam findings, recommendations and other relevant documents. Hartman et al. demonstrated this potential by fine-tuning BERT and BART models using electronic healthcare record (EHR) data from patients admitted to the neurology unit of an academic medical center.[20] They developed an automated method for generating the "hospital course" section of clinical notes using encoder-decoder sequence-to-sequence transformer models. Their goal was to reduce physician burnout by automating these time-consuming tasks. In a blind evaluation, two board-certified physicians rated 62% of the automated summaries as meeting the standard of care, suggesting that this method could be valuable in a clinical setting. Similarly, Jiang et al. utilized NLP techniques to train an LLM with unstructured clinical notes.[21] They developed an LLM-based system capable of integrating into clinical workflows to predict critical metrics such as 30-day all-cause readmission, in-hospital mortality and length of stay. These metrics, while crucial in all fields of medicine, are particularly significant in neurosurgical units for monitoring patient outcomes and optimizing care.

In another study titled *neuroGPT-X: Toward a Clinic-Ready Large Language Model*, Edward Guo et al. compared the performance of a context-enriched LLM with that of international neurosurgical experts on questions regarding the management of vestibular schwannoma.[22] The responses from the LLM were rated as not significantly different from those of human experts in terms of accuracy and coherence. In many cases, the LLMs' responses were rated significantly higher. The authors also developed neuroGPT-X, a chat-based platform designed to provide point-of-care clinical support while addressing the limitations of human memory. Their system incorporated features like in-text citations and references to deliver accurate and relevant information in real-time. It's important to emphasize that LLMs are not a replacement for expert opinions. Rather, they serve as powerful tools to augment the expertise of medical professionals. By surfacing relevant literature and diverse perspectives instantaneously, LLMs can help clinicians make better-informed decisions. Think of them as an expert assistant, combined with a dynamic, real-time literature database, enabling physicians to deliver even more effective care.

FUTURE OF LARGE LANGUAGE MODELS AND THEIR ROLE IN NEUROSURGERY

Despite the remarkable progress of AI and LLMs, their applications in clinical medicine is still in its infancy and their transformative impact on healthcare is just starting to unfold. With new advancements emerging daily, the development of LLMs has accelerated dramatically. Many models are being trained on increasingly larger and more diverse datasets to enhance their accuracy and reliability across various types and formats of text data. Simultaneously, efforts are underway to increase the context that an LLM can understand in a single conversation, enabling more coherent and contextually aware interactions. OpenAI, the organization behind ChatGPT, introduced their "reasoning" model, o1, in September 2024, which is designed to enhance problem-solving by allocating more time to deliberate and logically reason through a problem before responding to a user's prompt. Institutions are making efforts to ensure that LLMs produce outputs that are not just linguistically sophisticated but also analytically and logically robust. These advancements are driven, in part, by unprecedented access to computational resources, such as more powerful graphical processing units (GPUs) and tensor processing units (TPUs), and innovations in chip technology that enable faster and more efficient model training.[23]

The interplay of cutting-edge AI research and parallel developments in the hardware industry fosters an environment of relentless progress. As competition among researchers and companies intensifies, the boundaries of AI capability are being redefined at a rapid pace. This momentum suggests that breakthroughs in LLMs will continue to emerge, reshaping industries and pushing the limits of what AI can achieve. OpenAI is not the only company to develop an LLM; major tech players, such as Google, Meta and Anthropic, to name a few, have launched comparable models, with ongoing releases of improved versions.

In addition to general-purpose LLMs, significant strides are being made in developing domain-specific models. While obtaining accurate and extensive datasets in critical areas such as neurosurgery and neurology poses challenges, progress is evident. Domain-specific models tailored for healthcare, finance and legal applications are already surfacing.[24,25] As more data are curated and processed in specialized fields, subdomain-specific LLMs will become increasingly feasible, enhancing the precision and utility of AI in niche domains.

Another promising area of research focuses on expanding the modalities of input data that AI models can process. While traditional LLMs primarily handle text, researchers are increasingly exploring multimodal approaches that not only integrate input data in different file formats but can also process images and small videos. Vision models, though still emerging slowly, may hold promise for applications in healthcare. In 2020, Dosovitskiy et al. demonstrated that transformer architectures, when applied directly to image patches and pre-trained on large datasets, perform exceptionally well in image classification tasks.[26]

Open AIs LLMs can already ingest and interact with images and even generate them, though the accuracy of image generation still lags behind the significant progress made in language processing. Its text-to-video AI model, Sora, is capable of generating realistic and imaginative videos from text prompts. Google's PaliGemma, a vision-text model, can process both image and text inputs to produce text-based outputs. Advanced models like these exemplify the potential for combining modalities to analyze complex data. This type of integration is particularly relevant in fields like neurosurgery, where a mix of text, image and video data is abundant and such multimodal models could help physicians and surgeons in deriving meaningful insights. It represents an exciting frontier, with the potential to significantly enhance diagnostic accuracy and support clinical decision-making. Given the accessibility of these tools to non-technical users, their adoption is likely to expand rapidly.

However, it's crucial to note that while LLMs can serve as valuable medical knowledge assistants, they should be used with caution. LLMs are well-documented to suffer from hallucinations. Since these models exhibit a strong understanding of language semantics, their responses might seem accurate, but in reality, the model is often fabricating information using words. A study by the University of Massachusetts Amherst and Mendel in August 2024 found hallucinations in nearly all medical summaries generated by GPT-4o and Llama-3.[27] It is crucial for medical professionals to verify the authenticity and accuracy of information from LLMs. Over-reliance on these models and blind acceptance of their answers can lead to serious risks.

Misinformation is another significant issue with LLMs, particularly in critical fields like healthcare and neurosurgery. Researchers have shown that medical LLMs are vulnerable to data poisoning attacks, which can produce harmful results.[28,29] Such susceptibilities highlight strong concerns regarding the reliability and truthfulness of outputs generated by LLMs in healthcare. Given the widespread use of LLMs by the general public and medical practitioners, assuming that medical advice generated by these models is accurate is dangerous. Expert physician review should always be sought to ensure the credibility of AI-generated insights.

LLMs also struggle with complex concepts like causal reasoning and the interplay of environmental and genetic factors. They cannot perceive other nuances that rely on a doctor's direct observation, such as visual cues, physical examination, patient behavior and other tangible factors that are critical for accurate medical decision-making.

Data privacy is also a critical concern, particularly in healthcare and neurosurgery, where the protection of sensitive patient information is paramount. Sharing medical data with LLMs without proper security measures and compliance with regulations risks serious breaches of confidentiality and trust. Healthcare institutes should always remember to employ robust guardrails and institutional safeguards to prevent ethical, legal and medical repercussions when integrating LLMs into clinical workflows.

REFERENCES

1. McCulloch WS, Pitts W. A logical calculus of the ideas immanent in nervous activity. *Bull Math Biophys* 1943; 5(4): 115–33.
2. LeCun Y, Boser B, Denker JS, et al. Backpropagation applied to handwritten zip code recognition. *Neural Comput* 1989; 1(4): 541–51.
3. LeCun Y, Bengio Y, Hinton G. Deep Learning. *Nature* 2015; 521(7553): 436–44.
4. Friston KJ, Holmes AP, Worsley KJ, et al. Statistical parametric maps in functional imaging: A general linear approach. *Hum Brain Mapp* 1994; 2(4): 189–210.
5. Golland P, Fischl B, Spiridon M, et al. Discriminative analysis for image-based studies. *Lect Notes Comput Sci* 2002; 2488: 508–15.
6. Lao Z, Shen D, Xue Z, et al. Morphological classification of brains via high-dimensional shape transformations and machine learning methods. *Neuroimage* 2004; 21(1): 46–57.

7. Breiman L. Random forests. *Mach Learn* 2001; 45(1): 5–32.
8. Lee J, Burkett BJ, Min HK, et al. Deep learning-based brain age prediction in normal aging and dementia. *Nat Aging* 2022; 2(5): 412–24.
9. Porwal MH, Feller C, Kumar D, et al. MedCDI: A technology-based documentation and quality improvement initiative in neurosurgery. *Surg Neurol Int* 2022; 13: 271.
10. Ali R, Syed S, Sastry R, et al. Toward more accurate documentation in neurosurgical care. *Neurosurg Focus* 2021; 51(5): E11–1.
11. Casey A, Davidson E, Poon M, et al. A systematic review of natural language processing applied to radiology reports. *BMC Med Inform Decis Mak* 2021; 21(1): 179.
12. Ghosh R, Farri O, Karn SK, et al. RadLing: Towards efficient radiology report understanding. *arXiv:2306.02492v1*, 2023.
13. Kim Y, Xu X, McDuff D, et al. Health-LLM: Large language models for health prediction via wearable sensor data. *arXiv:2401.06866v2*, 2024.
14. Mir JM, Kurland DB, Cheung ATM, et al. The evolution of pediatric spine surgery: A bibliometric analysis of publications from 1902 to 2023. *Neurosurg Open* 2024; 5(3): e00092.
15. Cheung ATM, Kurland DB, Neifert S, et al. Developing an automated registry (autoregistry) of spine surgery using natural language processing and health system scale databases. *Neurosurgery* 2023; 93(6): 1228–34.
16. Shost MD, Meade SM, Steinmetz MP, et al. Surgical classification using natural language processing of informed consent forms in spine surgery. *Neurosurg Focus* 2023; 54(6): E10–0.
17. Ortiz AV, Feldman MJ, Yengo-Kahn AM, et al. Words matter: Using natural language processing to predict neurosurgical residency match outcomes. *J Neurosurg* 2023; 138(2): 559–66.
18. Vaswani A, Shazeer N, Parmar N, et al. Attention is all you need. *arXiv:1706.03762v7*, 2017.
19. Kurland DB, Alber DA, Palla A, et al. Augmenting large language models with automated, bibliometrics-powered literature search for knowledge distillation: A pilot study for common spinal pathologies. *Neurosurgery* 2025; 97(2): 387–98.
20. Hartman VC, Bapat SS, Weiner MG, et al. A method to automate the discharge summary hospital course for neurology patients. *J Am Med Inform Assoc* 2023; 30(12): 1995–2003.
21. Jiang LY, Liu XC, Nejatian NP, et al. Health system-scale language models are all-purpose prediction engines. *Nature* 2023; 619 (7969): 357–62.
22. Guo E, Gupta M, Sinha S, et al. NeuroGPT-X: Toward a clinic-ready large language model. *J Neurosurg* 2023; 140(4): 1041–53.
23. Merritt R. Why GPUs are great for AI. NVIDIA Blog, 2023. Available from: https://blogs.nvidia.com/blog/why-gpus-are-great-for-ai/ (Accessed May 2026).
24. Singhal K, Tu T, Gottweis J, et al. Towards expert-level medical question answering with large language models. 2025; 31(3): 943–50.
25. Wu S, Irsoy O, Lu S, et al. BloombergGPT: A large language model for finance. *arXiv:2303.17564v3*, 2023.
26. Dosovitskiy A, Beyer L, Kolesnikov A, et al. An image is worth 16x16 words: Transformers for image recognition at scale. *arXiv:2010.11929v2*, 2020.
27. Rumale P, Tiwari S, Naik T, et al. Faithfulness hallucination detection in healthcare AI, 2024. Available from: https://openreview.net/pdf?id=6eMIzKFOpJ (Accessed May 2026).
28. Alber DA, Yang Z, Alyakin A, et al. Medical large language models are vulnerable to data-poisoning attacks. *Nat Med* 2025; 31(2): 618–26.
29. Han T, Nebelung S, Khader F, et al. Medical large language models are susceptible to targeted misinformation attacks. *NPJ Digit Med* 2024; 7(1): 1–9.

16

Federated Learning in Neurosurgery

AKIS LINARDOS, UJJWAL BAID, SARTHAK PATI, MATTHEW W. PEASE AND SPYRIDON BAKAS

FEDERATED LEARNING: THE NEXT FRONTIER FOR COLLABORATIVE AI SCIENCE

The road to fair and effective biomedical AI is paved in collaborative studies. While algorithms have shown remarkable potential on automated brain cancer diagnosis and risk assessment, they have mostly been restricted to data from individual institutions. This limits their capacity to perform well in a heterogeneous, real-world center that spans multiple centers and even countries. The evaluation of such performance is also constrained, as a single center, or even a few are not enough to encompass the necessary diversity in terms of ethnicity, financial status and even clinical equipment. Further, data scarcity limits the capabilities of a trained model, in particular for cases of very rare diseases such as glioblastoma (GBM). The limitations of single center training have been evidenced by neurosurgery studies that have showcased performance drops when the models are evaluated on an unseen site.[1,2]

Data scarcity, heterogeneity and fairness may only be tackled through collaborative studies, where those algorithms are informed on cases from an international, ideally global, scale. The traditional solution for such a setting is data pooling: institutions bringing their data together into a single centralized server upon which the AI model trains on. However, that is not practical either, as the privacy of subjects is compromised by allowing data transfer, a right enforced by well-placed limitations on data sharing, e.g. laws of data protection such as General Data Protection Regulation (GDPR) and Health Insurance Portability and Accountability Act (HIPAA).

Federated Learning (FL) offers a potential solution. Under this framework, the collaborating sites never share the data, but instead, host the algorithm in their servers throughout the process of training. The data analyst designs the model in a central node (CN) of their respective institution which communicates with all the local nodes (LNs) of collaborators providing the data. The data never leave their original sites. It is the algorithm itself that traverses the distribution of sites during its training process. Clones of the model are distributed to each registered LN, train locally, then return to CN and aggregate the information to one global model before splitting across LNs again. The process then repeats until the global model reaches convergence, as defined by the data analyst handling the process, often based on validation scores from each site. An overview of this process is provided in **Figure 16.1**.

FEDERATED LEARNING IN NEUROSURGERY

FL benefits neurosurgery similarly to other medical subspecialties: by extending studies beyond the restriction of a single center to multiple, increasing overall patient / data volume and diversity. Single-center studies are prone to bias from varying practice patterns, differences in surgical approaches or skill, patient populations or simply chance. In neurosurgery, as in other fields of

DOI: 10.1201/9781003471165-16

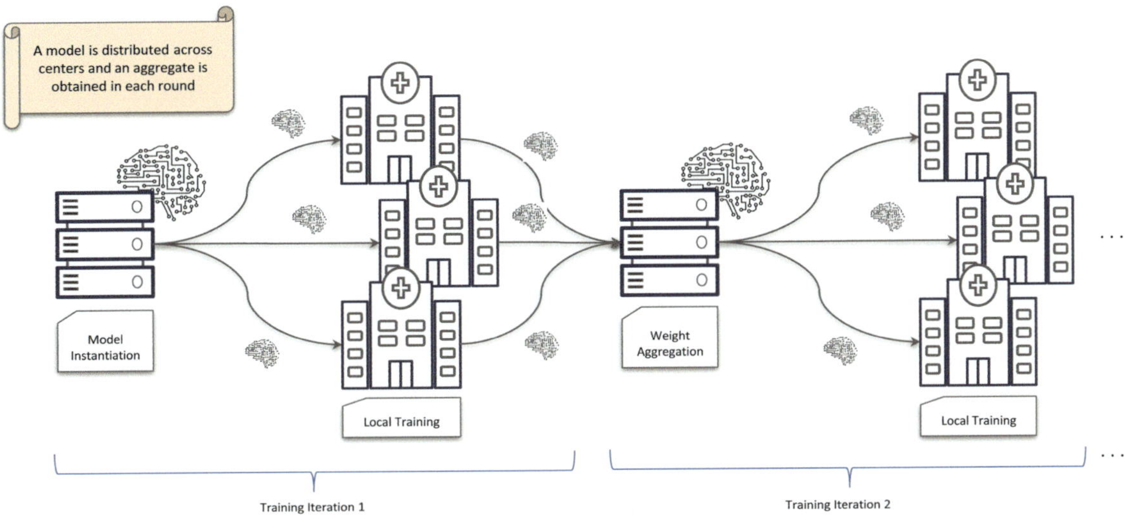

Figure 16.1 Overview of the federated learning framework. The AI models are distributed across sites then aggregated in the central server.

medicine, large, multi-institutional studies provide the highest quality of clinical evidence science and machine learning (ML) studies, external validation or incorporation of outside data sources into study design is crucial to demonstrate model reliability. Data shift, where the underlying distribution of the outcome of interest changes from one data source to another, is a common problem that negatively impacts model performance.[3] One of the first studies to demonstrate this phenomenon used chest X-rays from three different data sources with up to ten-fold difference in rates of pneumonia.[4] Model performance varied widely depending on which data source was used for training and validation. Of note, models with pooled data performed better than models trained on data from a single site. Many studies in neurosurgery, ranging from predicting surgical outcomes in GBM patients to functional outcomes after traumatic brain injury (TBI), have demonstrated the importance of data shift, with a decline in performance on external datasets.[1,2] One study reported that a DL model trained on CT scans from a single institution substantially declined in performance when validated on an external TBI dataset drawn from 18 institutions.[1] This discrepancy likely reflects heterogeneity in TBI care across centers, as well as demographic differences and subtle variations in patient populations that influence outcomes. Similar findings have been reported in GBM,[2] where models trained at a single institution demonstrate variable success when externally validated. These findings strongly suggest that reliance on single-institution datasets in neurosurgery is insufficient for developing robust models, given their limited size and the large inter-institutional variability in patient populations.

Onerous data safety regulations, while necessary to protect patient privacy, severely limit the ability to perform high-quality, multi-institutional studies. Data sharing agreements add months to study turnaround times and frequently require lawyer involvement. These challenges are best highlighted if we consider the difficulties in sharing data across published studies. Although there has been an increase in transparency with manuscripts providing data availability statements, in practice nearly 40% of researchers ignore requests to share data.[5] Using FL to ease the time and financial costs of sharing data can improve cooperation between centers.

Last, many diseases in neurosurgery are rare, and so suffer from data scarcity, whereas AI performance hinges on large datasets. For example, chordoma has only a few thousand surgical cases performed each year, which means single centers won't have enough cases for reliable AI development.[6] Even other more common diseases like GBM have typically less than 50–100 cases at

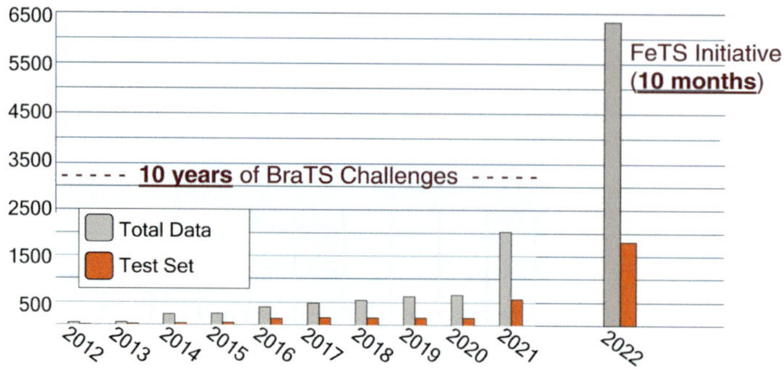

Figure 16.2 Growth of BraTS and FeTS datasets from 2012 to 2022, showing a sharp increase in total imaging data and test set size following the launch of the FeTS Initiative.

large academic medical centers each year. With an FL approach, however, this obstacle is circumvented by utilization of such rare case samples across multiple institutions.

FL research has a strong momentum, with rapidly evolving frameworks to facilitate it such as OpenFL,[7] NVFlare,[8] Flower,[9] PySyft.[10] The most significant leap was made in 2022 with the Federated Tumor Segmentation (FeTS) Initiative,[11] which introduced the largest real-world FL study to date. This study focused on automatic boundary detection on the aforementioned rare disease of GBM and enabled the analysis of the largest GBM cohort to-date (6314 cases from 71 sites across 6 continents), dwarfing the cumulative 2360 cases from a decade of Brain Tumor Segmentation (BraTS) Challenges (**Figure 16.2**). The final consensus model (FCM) developed on the entire data was compared to a public initial model (PIM), against out-of-sample data, showing significant ($p < 0.01$) performance boost for enhancing tumor (ET) (15%), tumor core (TC) (27%) and whole tumor (WT) (16%). Overall, this exemplifies how FL successfully expedited a big data analysis that resulted in a far superior model to the initial public one.

FEDERATED LEARNING ENABLES MORE TRUSTWORTHY AND ETHICAL ARTIFICIAL INTELLEGENCE

As with any powerful technology, AI ushers forward a world of increased automation, which also brings a slew of ethical concerns in all fields. The biomedical sector has formed a history of ethical studies and principles over the past century, largely as a response to cruel research ethical felonies committed, like the Tuskegee Syphilis Study,[12] among others. Follow-up resistance to these cruel methods sparked a long discussion around ethics, which eventually culminated in the four principles of biomedical ethics: non-maleficence, beneficence, autonomy, and fairness.[13] This largely overlaps with AI ethics, which also include transparency as a fifth principle.[14]

FL is relevant in affirming two of these principles: Fairness and Transparency.

Fairness

Fairness in AI means building models that are not liable to discriminating, i.e. performing selectively better on certain populations that for societal reasons have a higher presence in cleaner datasets. In single-center studies this is hard or even impossible to implement or evaluate, as these centers will be inherently limited to their own patients, or at best a more constrained pool of datasets that passed through various time-consuming agreements to be gathered in a single institution. As FL allows a model to learn locally from multiple institutions across the globe (as proven by FeTS[11]) it also makes it possible for the model to understand a much wider diversity of patients.

A limitation remains though, that these models require significant computing power to train, which again gives a disadvantage to the less wealthy participants that might not have the same level of computational infrastructure. Further, the conventional FL algorithm uses a method of voting to aggregate the information of models, which gives a higher vote to institutions that have a higher number of data (Federated Averaging). This choice stems from the original design for FL by Google[15] which was aimed at collecting data from mobile phones for the utility of saving bandwidth. As the stakes of healthcare are more obvious, however, different algorithms are already being developed to amend that.

Participants of the FeTS challenge included various methods of aggregation that aimed at alleviating the communication burden while improving the fairness of the voting system. Most prominent among the best performing methods was the usage of selective sampling in each federated round: the model trained on different subsets of the overall consortium instead of everywhere at all times. In the conventional Federated Averaging method, the model is trained on all LNs each round, and when *everyone* finishes, it's aggregated in the CN with models trained on wealthier centers gaining greater vote. By replacing that with selective sampling, each voting round includes different LNs, and by extension training is not consistently slowed down by the slowest LN, nor is the voting overwhelmed by the wealthiest one.

Besides selective sampling, there's active research on alternative methods for the algorithm of aggregation itself. It has been shown that the traditional algorithm for FL aggregation (Federated Averaging) suffers from slow and unstable convergence when dealing with heterogeneous data,[17] which further handicaps diversity studies. This effect has sparked an interest in novel methods for aggregation. We briefly mention a few of them here:

- *SCAFFOLD*:[16] This method applies "variance reduction" to balance the drift in the updates of LNs, correcting the variability responsible for the unstable training
- *FedPIDAvg*:[17] This is the winning method of the FeTS challenge 2022, building on top of the previous winner of FeTS 2021, FedCostWAvg.[18] It uses the cost reductions of LNs as an additional weighting variable during aggregation at the CN
- *FedDP*:[19] In this case, DP stands for "dual personalization." Part of each model is decoupled to be fine-tuned to each LN, adapting to the respective feature distribution of the site. It further calibrates prediction-level inconsistencies between sites, penalizing larger inconsistencies pixel-wise. As a result, the overall predictions are better tailored to each LN without sacrificing global performance

As aggregation functions govern the voting mechanism, they play a crucial role in ascertaining no discrimination regarding LN bias during FL-based studies. Selective sampling is usually coupled with such an advanced function, and both come together for a better outcome in terms of efficiency, performance and fairness.

Transparency

The principle of Transparency encompasses all fields of AI as a means to trustworthy models. It is further divided into Explainability (understanding what evidence in the data leads a model to a specific decision) and Traceability (monitoring the life cycle of a model from design to real-world application, including what type of data it has been trained on). FL studies naturally assists the Explainability aspect by introducing a higher diversity of data, and thus a more comprehensive means of explaining decisions, but shines further in its potential of affirming Traceability. Due to the structure of the FL framework, a communication network is established between the data providers (LNs) and the data analyst (CN). Compared to the data sharing approach of centralizing all the training on one institution, this enforces a level of Traceability by design as the AI developer is held accountable for the data decisions of the product by their collaborators.

More concretely, the international consensus for healthcare AI guidelines (FUTURE-AI)[21] has agreed on the following recommendation to assure Traceability:

1. Implement a risk management process throughout the AI life cycle.
2. Provide documentation (e.g. technical, clinical).
3. Define mechanisms for quality control of the AI inputs and outputs.
4. Implement a system for periodic auditing and updating.
5. Implement a logging system for usage recording.
6. Establish mechanisms for human oversight and governance.

The current form of FL as presented in large-scale studies enables most of these points:

1. FL enables a multistep risk management process, where deviations are first identified on global level at the CN then further dissected on a more focused LN.
2. As clear communication between AI experts and clinicians is a big part of the kickstarting stages of large-scale FL studies, documentation on both technical and clinical parts is in most cases a necessity for smooth implementation.
3. Quality control of the inputs and outputs is assured by clinicians having direct access to the relevant data, whereas the outputs are evaluated by the LN collaborators and the CN data analyst.
4. To be applied on a large scale, FL mandates flexible ways to introduce new centers into a consortium. As the technology matures, auditing will also be necessary to avoid malicious actors.
5. A logging system is an inherent part of an FL system, as the collaborative nature necessitates clear instructions of data used from each institution to assure compatibility with the deployed model. The training process is also logged on both local and global levels.
6. As each LN is responsible for the data they own, human oversight remains part of the loop across the FL network. The set up of an FL study further encourages data providers and AI developers to develop a governance system where AI errors are discussed and addressed.

FUTURE OUTLOOK

The initiatives we outlined have set the stage for FL by proving its feasibility and effectiveness given the right set up. The next step is bringing together what has been developed toward applications of higher clinical impact that are more widely applied.

Higher clinical impact with FL 2.0: The exemplar case of MedPerf

For AI fields to thrive, benchmarks are necessary to assure the reliability and safety of AI models. MedPerf is an open-source framework meticulously crafted to address this critical need. It brings a holistic approach to AI model assessment, with a goal to bridge the gap between cutting-edge AI technology and the intricate healthcare ecosystem. Its mission is to benchmark AI models rigorously, ensuring they not only meet clinical efficacy standards but also uphold patient privacy. This is done by utilizing the following components:

1. *Federated Evaluation*. MedPerf pioneered this through multiple large-scale pilot studies. In this decentralized approach, AI models are securely distributed across various healthcare facilities. Each facility evaluates the model's performance within its unique context, all while safeguarding patient data. This collaborative process accelerates evaluation, minimizes legal and regulatory risks and fosters knowledge sharing.
2. *Privacy First by Design*. MedPerf ensures that sensitive patient information never leaves the confines of individual facilities. By avoiding cross-facility data exchange, it balances evaluation efficiency and privacy protection.
3. *Human-Supervised Verification*. MedPerf includes a human-in-the-loop framework, pausing for healthcare organizations to assess and verify AI model performance efficiently. This affirms the previously mentioned point of traceability, ensuring accountability and alignment with clinical expertise.

Thanks to these components, MedPerf alleviates the need for data sharing, reducing the risk for privacy leakage and the substantial financial and operational cost. By including healthcare providers in the loop, it enhances the clinical relevance of the FL field, which is a necessary step to eventual adoption. MedPerf is currently the only open-source solution that adheres to the international consensus guidelines for healthcare AI[20] and achieves maximum validation potential for AI models. As the field matures, more frameworks of this nature will likely pop up to enhance the trustworthiness of FL pipelines throughout the healthcare industry.

Privacy leakage: Federated learning's private-by-design principle is insufficient at scale

In collaborative networks at scale, even exposure of model updates may pose risks for the LNs if we consider the case of "malicious" collaborators at any of the sites (a likelihood that increases with larger studies) or even the aggregator at the CN. Local model updates carry information about the respective LN's data, which an adversary may reverse-engineer to infer sensitive healthcare information.[21,22] There are two main risks of data exposure:

- *Data attribute inference*,[21,23] which involves inferring training data characteristics (e.g. scanner type) exposing information about the institutions of the cohort
- *Membership inference attacks* (MIAs),[21,24] which involve inferring whether a specific patient existed in the training cohort, severely compromising the privacy of individuals that are likely not fully aware of the dangers or the particular project taking place

While there are no known occurrences of such incidents in neurosurgery, the field is moving fast, and future studies should account for both of these and assure protection against privacy leakage. Several technical strategies have been proposed to reduce the risks of data exposure in collaborative networks. On the algorithmic side, *differential privacy*[25] can be applied to local updates to ensure that the contribution of any individual record remains statistically indistinguishable. Secure aggregation through *homomorphic encryption* allows model updates to be combined in a way that prevents the aggregator or other collaborators from inspecting them directly.[26,27] These approaches, combined with diligent clinical governance, are promising defense mechanisms to address concerns of privacy leakage.

LARGE-SCALE CHALLENGES AND STUDIES TO EXPAND BEYOND SEGMENTATION

International medical challenges enable a framework where talent is crowdsourced, and resources offered to scientists across the globe. FL training in particular involves more nuanced complexities to the traditional single-center studies, such as multiple machines of various hardware capacities, coordinating with participants for training in sync, alleviating the logistical hurdle of exposing data to involved models, and aggregating to a different server. All these make it particularly hard for budding scientists to become involved in the field, or at the very least handicaps a good chunk of their initial research stage to resolving communication with different sites and the involved logistics. Since its initial kickstart in 2021 and its yearly returns in 2022 and 2024, the aforementioned FeTS challenge has set the stage for collaborative FL studies of this nature, offering scientists across the world a lower barrier to entry in studying this field. Whereas this challenge focused on segmentation of brain tumors, future studies might encompass issues of higher clinical relevance, such as full diagnosis, risk assessment and even longitudinal data.

Further touching on other concerns raised in this chapter, future challenges and large-scale projects should focus on advancing the aspects of AI fairness and transparency or safeguarding the FL framework against privacy leakage. The future of FL is paved in collaborative studies, and its journey in bringing together healthcare research across the world is only beginning.

REFERENCES

1. Pease M, Arefan D, Barber J, et al. Outcome prediction in patients with severe traumatic brain injury using deep learning from head CT scans. *Radiology* 2022; 304(2): 385–94.
2. Pease M, Gersey ZC, Ak M, et al. Pre-operative MRI radiomics model non-invasively predicts key genomic markers and survival in glioblastoma patients. *J Neurooncol* 2022; 160(1): 253–63.
3. Li J, Arefan D, Pease M, et al. An automatic pipeline for data shift detection and mitigation to improve outcome prediction of traumatic brain injury. 2024; 12931: 66–71. Available from: https://www.spiedigitallibrary.org/conference-proceedings-of-spie/12931/129310C/An-automatic-pipeline-for-data-shift-detection-and-mitigation-to/10.1117/12.3009348.full (Accessed May 2026).
4. Zech JR, Badgeley MA, Liu M, et al. Variable generalization performance of a deep learning model to detect pneumonia in chest radiographs: A cross-sectional study. *PLoS Med* 2018; 15(11): e1002683.
5. Tedersoo L, Küngas R, Oras E, et al. Data sharing practices and data availability upon request differ across scientific disciplines. *Sci Data* 2021; 8(1): 192.
6. Barber SM, Sadrameli SS, Lee JJ, et al. Chordoma—current understanding and modern treatment paradigms. *J Clin Med* 2021; 10(5): 1–18.

7. Foley P, Sheller MJ, Edwards B, et al. OpenFL: The open federated learning library. *Phys Med Biol* 2022; 67: 214001.
8. Roth HR, Cheng Y, Wen Y, et al. NVIDIA FLARE: Federated learning from simulation to real-world. *arXiv:2210.13291v3*, 2022.
9. Beutel DJ, Topal T, Mathur A, et al. Flower: A friendly federated learning research framework. *arXiv:2007.14390v5*, 2020.
10. Ziller A, Trask A, Lopardo A, et al. PySyft: A library for easy federated learning. *Stud Comput Intell* 2021; 965: 111–39.
11. Pati S, Baid U, Edwards B, et al. Federated learning enables big data for rare cancer boundary detection. *Nat Commun* 2022; 13(1): 7346.
12. White RM. Misinformation and misbeliefs in the Tuskegee Study of Untreated Syphilis fuel mistrust in the healthcare system. *J Natl Med Assoc* 2005; 97(11): 1566–73.
13. Page K. The four principles: Can they be measured and do they predict ethical decision making? *BMC Med Ethics* 2012; 13: 10.
14. Floridi L, Cowls J. A unified framework of five principles for AI in society, 2019. Available from: https://hdsr.mitpress.mit.edu/pub/l0jsh9d1/release/8 (Accessed May 2026).
15. Brendan McMahan H, Moore E, Ramage D, et al. Communication-efficient learning of deep networks from decentralized data. *arXiv:1602.05629v4*, 2016.
16. Karimireddy SP, Kale S, Mohri M, et al. SCAFFOLD: Stochastic controlled averaging for federated learning. *arXiv:1910.06378v4*, 2019.
17. Mächler L, Ezhov I, Shit S, Paetzold JC. FedPIDAvg: A PID controller inspired aggregation method for federated learning. *arXiv:2304.12117v1*, 2023.
18. Mächler L, Ezhov I, Kofler F, et al. FedCostWAvg: A new averaging for better federated learning. *arXiv:2111.08649v1*, 2022.
19. Wang J, Jin Y, Stoyanov D, Wang L. FedDP: Dual personalization in federated medical image segmentation. *IEEE Trans Med Imaging* 2024; 43(1): 297–308.
20. Lekadir K, Feragen A, Fofanah AJ, et al. FUTURE-AI: International consensus guideline for trustworthy and deployable artificial intelligence in healthcare. *Br Med J* 2023; 388: e081554.
21. Hitaj B, Ateniese G, Perez-Cruz F. Deep models under the GAN: Information leakage from collaborative deep learning. *arXiv:1702.07464v3*, 2017.
22. Tramèr F, Zhang F, Juels A, et al. Stealing machine learning models via prediction APIs. *arXiv:1609.02943v2*, 2016.
23. Carlini N, Ippolito D, Jagielski M, et al. Quantifying memorization across neural language models. *arXiv:2202.07646v3*, 2022.
24. Nasr M, Shokri R, Houmansadr A. Comprehensive privacy analysis of deep learning: Passive and active white-box inference attacks against centralized and federated learning. *arXiv:1812.00910v2*, 2018.
25. Abadi M, Chu A, Goodfellow I, et al. Deep learning with differential privacy. *arXiv:1607.00133v2*, 2016.
26. Munjal K, Bhatia R. A systematic review of homomorphic encryption and its contributions in healthcare industry. *Complex Intell Syst* 2023; 9(4): 3759–86.
27. Xie Q, Jiang S, Jiang L, et al. Efficiency optimization techniques in privacy-preserving federated learning with homomorphic encryption: A brief survey. *IEEE Internet Things J* 2024; 11(14): 24569–80.

17

Policy Perspective on the Regulatory Landscape, Evaluation and Translation of Artificial Intelligence for Neurosurgery

SAMUEL BROWD

INTRODUCTION

The integration of artificial intelligence (AI) in neurosurgery is rapidly transforming the field by offering unprecedented advancements in diagnosis, surgical precision, patient-facing domains and commercialization potential. However, this rapid growth requires a comprehensive policy review to address the regulatory, ethical and practical challenges associated with AI adoption. This chapter examines pivotal moments in the development of AI and highlights how these technologies are reshaping neurosurgical practices. We implore the critical importance of establishing robust frameworks that promote equitable, ethical and transparent AI-driven solutions.

MILESTONES IN HEALTHCARE ARTIFICIAL INTELLIGENCE

Computer-assisted clinical decision-making has existed since the 1970s, with nascent systems such as MYCIN, which used rule-based logic to assist in diagnosing bacterial infections and recommending appropriate antibiotics.[1] This was limited by their reliance on manually coded knowledge and decision trees, which did not enable it to generalize to larger problems. A pivotal development in AI systems was the backpropagation algorithm, which allowed neural networks to effectively learn from data, enabling the training of deeper and more complex models.[2] In 2012, revolutionary techniques in deep convolutional neural networks ("AlexNet") dramatically improved image classification performance, shepherded the usage of graphic processing units for efficient training, and introduced new architectural components such as Rectified Linear Units (ReLUs), data augmentation and dropout.[3] These techniques allowed for considerable advances for radiology tasks such as mammography interpretation,[4] cardiac function assessment[5] and lung cancer screening.[6] Neurosurgical applications included brain tumor classification,[7,8] predicting risk of adjacent segment disease[9] and prediction of nonroutine hospital discharges.[10]

One of the most significant advances in AI is the development of large language models (LLMs), which now enable applications to reach beyond healthcare providers into consumer and patient-facing domains. LLMs are deep learning (DL) models based on transformers and attention mechanisms that can generate language that resembles those spoken by humans.[11] These models are able to encode medical knowledge,[12] perform exceedingly well on standardized medical exams[13] and produce

DOI: 10.1201/9781003471165-17

empathic language comparable to a human healthcare provider.[14] Applications are vast; LLMs have been used to simplify procedural consent documents,[15,16] translate inpatient discharge summaries into a patient-friendly format[17] and act as chatbots in clinical workflows.[18]

ETHICAL CONCERNS

Healthcare providers are pressured to adopt AI due to several factors involving efficiency and cost reduction, clinical outcomes and innovation and competitiveness. Industry trends, peer pressure and industry advocacy also create incentive on healthcare systems to adopt these nascent technologies.[19] However, these advancements introduce complex ethical challenges. Key issues include the risk of bias in AI training data, which, when propagated in inference, can lead to inequitable clinical decision-making.[20] Other issues include the lack of transparency in AI decision-making processes—often referred to as the "black box" problem, and concerns surrounding patient autonomy, consent and privacy.[21]

Bias in AI models

Bias in AI models typically arises from imbalances in the training data, where certain populations are overrepresented or underrepresented.[22] This lack of balance can skew the model's performance, leading to disparities in how the model interprets data and makes decisions.[23,24] For example, an algorithm trained on hospital data in one country may not perform well in another, which can be due to disparities in the racial, socioeconomic and gender makeup.[25] In the surgical realm, an AI model trained on videos of intraoperative surgical activity to assess surgeon skills exhibited under-skilling and over-skilling bias at different rates across specific surgeon sub-cohorts.[26] Within this model, the authors developed a mitigating strategy called training with explanations (TWIX) which teaches an AI system to provide a visual explanation for its skill assessment that otherwise would have been provided by human experts.

Strategies for mitigating bias include diversifying training datasets, regular audits and incorporation of human oversight. Several regulatory initiatives have been developed to assist in these endeavors. The STANDING-Together (Standards for Data Diversity, Inclusivity, and Generalizability) initiative is an international, consensus-based initiative that aims to develop recommendations for the composition and reporting of datasets that form the basis for medical AI models.[27] The FDA provides an AI/ML-Based Software as a Medical Device (SaMD) Action Plan, which outlines a regulatory framework to ensure safe, effective and unbiased AI/ML medical devices by promoting best machine learning (ML) practices and supporting real-world performance monitoring.[28]

The "black box" problem

The "black box" problem in AI refers to the difficulty in understanding how the technical underpinnings of AI algorithms—particularly those based on DL—arrive at their decisions.[29] Healthcare providers may find it challenging to trust or justify clinical decisions driven by AI if the underlying process is not transparent.

DL models are built upon layers of artificial neural networks that consist of multiple nodes ("neurons"), where each layer transforms the input data into increasingly abstract representations ("perceptrons").[2,30] Each transformation can result in an exponential increase in the number of parameters—often billions of connections between neurons—which do not follow a simple linear path that can be easily traced or explained. The final parameters of a prediction model is dependent on the weights of connections between neurons learned during the training process, which may not have any interpretable meaning in it of itself, making it challenging to understand how specific inputs are transformed into outputs, or to provide a clear rationale for the model's decision.

For example, the analysis of radiographic images is well-positioned for the adoption of AI.[31] Suppose an AI model is implemented to assist in the classification and diagnosis of brain tumors based on MRI scans. The model can identify subtle patterns in the imaging data that may not be apparent to experienced neurosurgeons or radiologists, if the model was trained on MRI scans in addition to the final neuropathological diagnosis. Even if the model outputs a classification with a high level of confidence, the physician is not provided with an explanation of why this conclusion was provided. This can raise issues with trust, accountability and informed decision-making, especially if the query involves analysis of pathologies with subtle characteristics, but with drastically different management strategies, for example, recurrent glioma versus radiation necrosis.

Mitigating the black box problem involves several strategies aimed at making AI models more interpretable and understandable, with Explainable AI (XAI) providing a framework for achieving transparency and clarity in AI decision-making processes. Techniques such as TWIX (requiring AI to generate explanations for its predictions),[26] Local Interpretable Model-Agnostic Explanations (LIME, approximating a complex model with an interpretable one),[29] and SHapley Additive ExPlanations (SHAPs, providing measures of feature importance using cooperative game theory)[32] have been developed within the XAI framework. Other strategies to consider include workflow compartmentalization using more interpretable models, attention mechanisms,[33] saliency maps and feature visualization,[34] activation maximization[35] and human-in-the-loop systems.[36] However, even with XAI frameworks in place, the user must be cognizant of potential hallucinations in AI-generated outputs or explanations of the output. Because hallucinations can sound convincingly real, it is crucial for users to apply their own domain expertise and have verification methods in place to assess the reliability of AI-generated outputs. This ensures that AI remains a tool for augmentation rather than a sole authority in decision-making.

PRIVACY CONCERNS

Whenever protected health information (PHI) is used in medical research, there is a risk of a data breach, potentially leading to loss of privacy, identity theft or discrimination based on health status.[35] Therefore, every effort to safely and securely handle PHI in healthcare-related AI applications must be undertaken. The sheer volume of data required to properly train AI models only adds to the risk of data breach.[37] Consumers are understandably hesitant to share personal data due to the risks of identity theft and data breaches, making it challenging to create unbiased, comprehensive datasets needed to train accurate AI models.[38]

By necessity, non-clinicians will be involved in data collection, processing and analysis when using EHR data for the development of AI applications. These individuals may not fully understand the consequences of data breaches or which parts of a medical record are truly sensitive.[39]

To mitigate these concerns, synthetic patient data has been offered as a potential solution to these privacy concerns. Generative adversarial networks (GANs) are a form of ML frameworks which can create synthetic patient data trained on real patient records.[40] GANs work by employing two neural networks—a generator that creates synthetic data and a discriminator that attempts to differentiate between real and synthetic data—thus refining the synthetic outputs to closely mimic actual patient data. This approach helps alleviate data privacy concerns by allowing AI models to be trained on large, realistic datasets without exposing sensitive patient information, and it can also increase the speed and efficiency of model training by expanding the available data pool.[41]

Models derived from synthetic data have been validated through several mechanisms. Differential privacy is a statistical technique that produces a quantitative value which can be used to evaluate the privacy of individuals involved in a study.[42] Other measures, such as the ϵ-identifiability value, help posit the risk that patients from a GAN may be actually identified.[43] These measures are particularly useful when studying rare diseases as the patient datasets are much smaller and have a higher risk of information breach.[41]

Regulations within AI

SaMD is deemed a "software intended to be used for one or more medical purposes that perform these purposes without being part of a hardware medical device," by the International Medical Device Regulators Forum.[44] The FDA recently released guidelines for the submission of medical software either as a novel technology or through a pre-market approval (PMA) application.[45] These pathways require that developers outline potential risks to the users and/or patients in their application prior to the public distribution of their software. Additionally, any updates to the software that may introduce a novel, harmful risk or affect a present risk to users, a change to the risk assessment controls of the device or a change that impacts the usability or functional capacity of the device, require additional clearance through one of the aforementioned pathways.

This is of particular importance when addressing AI models that learn and update the algorithm each time new information is entered into the machine. Initially, the FDA only approved algorithms that were considered "locked," meaning that the utility of the software was only approved to function based on its pre-market specifications.[45] More recently, as AI models have been designed to continuously update and improve based on the training data input, a new FDA-approved configuration to device modifications has been proposed.

The configuration is called the total product lifecycle (TPLC) approach, which provides functional protections while enabling continuous device modification. Although it is not a final regulatory proposal from the FDA, the TPLC seeks to harness the utility of AI's auto-improvement mechanisms while prioritizing patient safety. This is done through:

1. Establishing accepted beliefs about good practices in ML.
2. Completing thorough pre-market safety evaluations and specifications for any novel SaMD released.
3. Ensuring continuous monitoring of the software by industry manufacturers.
4. Disclosing performance and safety in a clear manner to both the consumers and the FDA.[46]

As of August 2024, a pilot program was initiated for the Total Product Life Cycle Advisory Program, and as of April, 2026, there are 122 devices enrolled with many more on the horizon.[47]

In 2021, the FDA, Health Canada and the United Kingdom's Medicines and Healthcare Products Regulatory Agency (MHRA) released 10 guidelines for good ML practice (GMLP).[48] These principles prioritize safety, efficacy and quality of AI/ML technologies that learn from their intended use, and, when appropriate, improve their own performance based on these data. Transparency of device performance is another priority of GMLP. A cornerstone of transparency is communicating the decisions and reasoning that led to a particular result or finding in the device. The guiding principles of transparency focus on:

1. The intended audience (users and recipients) for the device.
2. Motivation behind device development and its intended use.
3. Relevant information that is shared about the uses, users and intended goals of the device.
4. Placement of device information in a user-friendly way.
5. Appropriately timing the communication of device information in critical portions of the workflow.
6. Supporting transparency through the entire user experience.[49]

The guiding principles have been recommended primarily as considerations to software developers who intend to carry-out GMLP. The FDA recognizes that these considerations will change as the field of ML changes. Continued insights from clinicians, members of industry and patients will help develop these recommendations to ensure the highest quality of practice.

BEST PRACTICES FOR OPTIMIZING TRANSLATIONAL CAPACITY

Crigger et al. provide an excellent framework for developing trustworthy AI within healthcare.[21] The authors highlight six common themes across AI development and regulation:

1. Accountability
2. Safety and security
3. Transparency and explainability
4. Human control of technology
5. Professional responsibility
6. Promotion of human values

Ensuring appropriate data sourcing for a model is critical to produce reliable results.[50] Measurable data points are crucial to assess the validity and accuracy of a model.[51] The protocols for assessing and mitigating bias in models should be clear as they are introduced and updated. The legal implications of the algorithm and the product should be explored and explicitly defined.[52] Appropriate safeguards should be enacted to ensure that patient data and integrity is maintained.[53]

Crossnohere et al. provide a comprehensive review of the literature for studies that evaluate the framework of AI.[52] There appeared to be some deficits in the current guidelines for assessing quality within the development of AI algorithms. First, there was a lack of assessment for transparency within the training and programming. Second, there was a paucity of guidance for assessing the extent of surveillance for these algorithms. Both of these criteria are well defined for other medical solutions and innovations, however with the rapid evolution of AI, the regulatory framework seems to be lagging behind.

Within neurological surgery, Huang et al. provide a systematic review and evaluation of DL-related studies within the field.[54] Once again, the use of single institution, limited datasets provides inherent bias based on an initial narrowing of the data inputs. Further, transparency was once again highlighted as a key issue of the 35 neurological surgery DL studies included in their analysis.

Data integrity and patient transparency is essential for creating an AI algorithm that falls within an acceptable standard of practice. The extent of data, risks of breach and risk of additional information being deduced regarding a patient's health record are all information that need to be articulated to a patient when agreeing to enroll in an AI-driven solution.[52]

FUTURE DIRECTIONS

At the time of writing, the United States (US) has no comprehensive AI regulation legislation. This is almost certainly subject to change in the coming years, with continued advancements that will solve challenging problems in healthcare and beyond, but also have the potential to threaten our privacy, along with financial, psychological and physical well-being.

Unlike the United States, the European Union (EU) has officially passed a comprehensive AI legal framework. The AI Act was signed in 2024 and full implementation of the EU AI Act is expected to continue through 2030 across industries and member states.[55] This policy stratifies AI systems based on their risk and prescribes varying levels of oversight based on that risk. Additionally, it outright bans AI systems that pose unacceptable risks to individual or societal safety and rights. For example, AI systems that aid in medical decision-making are subject to intense scrutiny, regulation and quality control, whereas systems that filter junk email are not.

Individual US states like California are pushing legislation that addresses concerns surrounding topics such as digital replication of deceased individuals, labeling political ads created with generative AI, automatic rent increases and emotional manipulation, among others, modeled after the AI act.

Further, the White House has outlined AI regulation guidelines in a blueprint for an AI bill of rights.[56] This document recommends that AI systems be vigorously vetted in five separate domains before deployment, namely: safe and effective systems, algorithmic discrimination protections, data privacy, notice and explanation, human alternatives, consideration, and fallback.

Neurosurgeons must stay abreast of the constantly changing legal landscape surrounding AI applications. They must make sure that their research and entrepreneurial efforts stay within the bounds of the law. They must also critically appraise local and national legislation being reviewed by their elected representatives that has the potential to protect their patients but also has the potential to handicap research efforts.

REFERENCES

1. Van Melle W. MYCIN: A knowledge-based consultation program for infectious disease diagnosis. *Int J Man-Mach Stud* 1978; 10(3): 313–22.
2. Rumelhart DE, Hinton GE, Williams RJ. Learning representations by back-propagating errors. *Nature* 1986; 323(6088): 533–6.
3. Krizhevsky A, Sutskever I, Hinton GE. ImageNet classification with deep convolutional neural networks. *Commun ACM* 2012; 60(6): 84–90.
4. Wu N, Phang J, Park J, et al. Deep neural networks improve radiologists' performance in breast cancer screening. *IEEE Trans Med Imaging* 2020; 39(4): 1184–94.
5. Ghorbani A, Ouyang D, Abid A, et al. Deep learning interpretation of echocardiograms. *NPJ Digit Med* 2020; 3: 10.
6. Ardila D, Kiraly AP, Bharadwaj S, et al. End-to-end lung cancer screening with three-dimensional deep learning on low-dose chest computed tomography. *Nat Med* 2019; 25(6): 954–61.
7. Buchlak QD, Esmaili N, Leveque JC, et al. Machine learning applications to neuroimaging for glioma detection and classification: An artificial intelligence augmented systematic review. *J Clin Neurosci* 2021; 89: 177–98.

8. McAvoy M, Prieto PC, Kaczmarzyk JR, et al. Classification of glioblastoma versus primary central nervous system lymphoma using convolutional neural networks. *Sci Rep* 2021; 11(1): 15219.
9. Goedmakers CMW, Lak AM, Duey AH, et al. Deep learning for adjacent segment disease at preoperative MRI for cervical radiculopathy. *Radiology* 2021; 301(3): 664–71.
10. Karhade AV, Ogink PT, Thio QCBS, et al. Development of machine learning algorithms for prediction of prolonged opioid prescription after surgery for lumbar disc herniation. *Spine J* 2019; 19(11): 1764–71.
11. Clusmann J, Kolbinger FR, Muti HS, et al. The future landscape of large language models in medicine. *Commun Med (Lond)* 2023; 3(1): 141.
12. Singhal K, Azizi S, Tu T, et al. Large language models encode clinical knowledge. *Nature* 2023; 620(7972): 172–80.
13. Kung TH, Cheatham M, Medenilla A, et al. Performance of ChatGPT on USMLE: Potential for AI-assisted medical education using large language models. *PLOS Digit Health* 2023; 2(2): e0000198.
14. Ayers JW, Poliak A, Dredze M, et al. Comparing physician and artificial intelligence chatbot responses to patient questions posted to a public social media forum. *JAMA Intern Med* 2023; 183(6): 589.
15. Decker H, Trang K, Ramirez J, et al. Large language model–based chatbot vs surgeon-generated informed consent documentation for common procedures. *JAMA Netw Open* 2023; 6(10): e2336997.
16. Mirza FN, Tang OY, Connolly ID, et al. Using ChatGPT to facilitate truly informed medical consent. *NEJM AI* 2024; 1(2). doi/10.1056/AIcs2300145.
17. Zaretsky J, Kim JM, Baskharoun S, et al. Generative artificial intelligence to transform inpatient discharge summaries to patient-friendly language and format. *JAMA Netw Open* 2024; 7(3): e240357.
18. Mehandru N, Miao BY, Almaraz ER, et al. Evaluating large language models as agents in the clinic. *NPJ Digit Med* 2024; 7(1): 84.
19. Lamb J. Generative AI in healthcare: Adoption trends and what's next. Available from: https://www.mckinsey.com/industries/healthcare/our-insights/generative-ai-in-healthcare-adoption-trends-and-whats-next (Accessed May 2026).
20. Shah NH, Entwistle D, Pfeffer MA. Creation and adoption of large language models in medicine. *JAMA* 2023; 330(9): 866–9.
21. Crigger E, Reinbold K, Hanson C, et al. Trustworthy augmented intelligence in health care. *J Med Syst* 2022; 46(2): 12.
22. Mittermaier M, Raza MM, Kvedar JC. Bias in AI-based models for medical applications: challenges and mitigation strategies. *NPJ Digit Med* 2023; 6(1): 113.
23. Seyyed-Kalantari L, Zhang H, McDermott MBA, et al. Underdiagnosis bias of artificial intelligence algorithms applied to chest radiographs in under-served patient populations. *Nat Med* 2021; 27(12): 2176–82.
24. Yang J, Soltan AAS, Eyre DW, et al. An adversarial training framework for mitigating algorithmic biases in clinical machine learning. *NPJ Digit Med* 2023; 6(1): 55.
25. Obermeyer Z, Powers B, Vogeli C, Mullainathan S. Dissecting racial bias in an algorithm used to manage the health of populations. *Science* 2019; 366(6464): 447–53.
26. Kiyasseh D, Laca J, Haque TF, et al. Human visual explanations mitigate bias in AI-based assessment of surgeon skills. *NPJ Digit Med* 2023; 6(1): 54.
27. Ganapathi S, Palmer J, Alderman JE, et al. Tackling bias in AI health datasets through the STANDING Together initiative. *Nat Med* 2022; 28(11): 2232–3.
28. FDA. Artificial Intelligence/Machine Learning (AI/ML)-Based Software as a Medical Device (SaMD) Action Plan. US Food and Drug Administration, 2021. Available from: https://www.fda.gov/media/145022/download (Accessed May 2026).
29. Ribeiro MT, Singh S, Guestrin C. "Why should I trust you?": Explaining the predictions of any classifier. *arXiv:1602.04938v3*, 2016.
30. Krizhevsky A, Sutskever I, Hinton GE. ImageNet classification with deep convolutional neural networks. *Commun ACM* 2017; 60(6): 84–90.
31. Rajpurkar P, Lungren MP. The current and future state of AI interpretation of medical images. *N Engl J Med* 2023; 388(21): 1981–90.

32. Lundberg S, Lee SI. A unified approach to interpreting model predictions. *arXiv:1705.07874v2*, 2017.
33. Vaswani A, Shazeer N, Parmar N, et al. Attention is all you need. *arXiv:1706.03762v7*, 2017.
34. Zeiler MD, Fergus R. Visualizing and understanding convolutional networks. *arXiv:1311.2901v3*, 2013.
35. Yosinski J, Clune J, Nguyen A, et al. Understanding neural networks through deep visualization. *arXiv:1506.06579v1*, 2015.
36. Mosqueira-Rey E, Hernández-Pereira E, Alonso-Ríos D, et al. Human-in-the-loop machine learning: A state of the art. *Artif Intell Rev* 2023; 56(4): 3005–54.
37. Rahman MA, Victoros E, Ernest J, et al. Impact of artificial intelligence (AI) technology in healthcare sector: A critical evaluation of both sides of the coin. *Clin Pathol* 2024; 17: 2632010X241226887.
38. Azimi V, Zaydman MA. Optimizing equity: Working towards fair machine learning algorithms in laboratory medicine. *J Appl Lab Med* 2023; 8(1): 113–28.
39. Ozair FF, Jamshed N, Sharma A, Aggarwal P. Ethical issues in electronic health records: A general overview. *Perspect Clin Res* 2015; 6(2): 73–6.
40. Baowaly MK, Lin CC, Liu CL, Chen KT. Synthesizing electronic health records using improved generative adversarial networks. *J Am Med Inform Assoc* 2019; 26(3): 228–41.
41. Pezoulas VC, Zaridis DI, Mylona E, et al. Synthetic data generation methods in healthcare: A review on open-source tools and methods. *Comput Struct Biotechnol J* 2024; 23: 2892–910.
42. Appenzeller A, Leitner M, Philipp P, et al. Privacy and utility of private synthetic data for medical data analyses. *Appl Sci* 2022; 12(23): 12320.
43. Shi J, Wang D, Tesei G, Norgeot B. Generating high-fidelity privacy-conscious synthetic patient data for causal effect estimation with multiple treatments. *Front Artif Intell* 2022; 5: 918813.
44. IMDRF SaMD Working Group. Software as a Medical Device (SaMD): Key Definitions, 2013. Available from: https://www.imdrf.org/sites/default/files/docs/imdrf/final/technical/imdrf-tech-131209-samd-key-definitions-140901.pdf (Accessed May 2026).
45. FDA. US Food and Drug Administration. Developing a software precertification program: A working model, 2019. Available from: https://www.fda.gov/media/119722/download (Accessed May 2026).
46. FDA. US Food and Drug Administration. Proposed regulatory framework for modifications to artificial intelligence/machine learning (AI/ML)-based software as a medical device (SaMD). Available from: https://www.fda.gov/files/medical%20devices/published/US-FDA-Artificial-Intelligence-and-Machine-Learning-Discussion-Paper.pdf (Accessed May 2026).
47. FDA. Total Product Life Cycle Advisory Program (TAP), 2024. Available from: https://www.fda.gov/medical-devices/how-study-and-market-your-device/total-product-life-cycle-advisory-program-tap (Accessed May 2026).
48. FDA. Good machine learning practice for medical device development: Guiding principles, 2023. Available from: https://www.fda.gov/medical-devices/software-medical-device-samd/good-machine-learning-practice-medical-device-development-guiding-principles (Accessed May 2026).
49. FDA. Transparency for machine learning-enabled medical devices: Guiding principles, 2024. Available from: https://www.fda.gov/medical-devices/software-medical-device-samd/transparency-machine-learning-enabled-medical-devices-guiding-principles (Accessed May 2026).
50. Emani S, Swaminathan A, Grobman B, et al. Critically reading machine learning literature in neurosurgery: A reader's guide and checklist for appraising prediction models. *Neurosurg Focus* 2023; 54(6): E3.
51. Finlayson SG, Subbaswamy A, Singh K, et al. The clinician and dataset shift in artificial intelligence. *N Engl J Med* 2021; 385(3): 283–6.
52. Crossnohere NL, Elsaid M, Paskett J, et al. Guidelines for artificial intelligence in medicine: Literature review and content analysis of frameworks. *J Med Internet Res* 2022; 24(8): e36823.

53. Rahmani K, Thapa R, Tsou P, et al. Assessing the effects of data drift on the performance of machine learning models used in clinical sepsis prediction. *Int J Med Inform* 2023; 173: 104930.
54. Huang J, Shlobin NA, DeCuypere M, Lam SK. Deep learning for outcome prediction in neurosurgery: A systematic review of design, reporting, and reproducibility. *Neurosurgery* 2022; 90(1): 16–38.
55. Council of the European Union. Regulation (EU) 2024/1689 of the European Parliament and of the Council of 13 June 2024 laying down harmonised rules on artificial intelligence and amending Regulations (EC) No 300/2008, (EU) No 167/2013, (EU) No 168/2013, (EU) 2018/858, (EU) 2018/1139 and (EU) 2019/2144 and Directives 2014/90/EU, (EU) 2016/797 and (EU) 2020/1828 (Artificial Intelligence Act) (Text with EEA relevance), 2024. Available from: http://data.europa.eu/eli/reg/2024/1689/oj/eng (Accessed May 2026).
56. The White House. Blueprint for an AI Bill of Rights, OSTP. Available from: https://data.aclum.org/storage/2025/01/OSTP_www_whitehouse_gov_ostp_ai-bill-of-rights.pdf (Accessed May 2026).

18

Neurosurgical Data Sources and Data Needs for Artificial Intelligence

MARIA ISABEL BARROS GUINLE, DHIRAJ PANGAL,
MARIA JOSÉ CAVAGNARO, THOMAS JOHNSTONE AND JOHN K. RATLIFF

INTRODUCTION

The successful development, implementation and monitoring of artificial intelligence (AI) models in neurosurgery hinges on access to high-quality data. Models trained on data, which are not representative of that which the model will encounter in production, do not perform well in practice. Curating high-quality, well-prepared data can be particularly complex, given the heterogeneity in modality (e.g. CT, MRI), heterogeneity within a given modality (e.g. differences in quality, interpretation, etc.), lack of structure (progress notes, operative reports), and siloed data which is outside traditional electronic health records (EHRs) (e.g. operative video, real-time vitals monitoring). Privacy concerns, the need for anonymization and costs around storage and retrieval make data generation a non-trivial problem for AI applications in neurosurgery. In this chapter, we will discuss the components of data generation for AI, key challenges, possible solutions and future directions.

THE NEED FOR DATA TO TRAIN MODELS

AI models use a variety of model architectures to simulate, or model, the relationships between a variety of inputs and outputs. A deep learning (DL) model designed to identify pneumonia on a chest X-ray, for instance, may take a chest X-ray as input, and output an annotated image or body of text, describing radiological findings. These models often function as black boxes, while internally they may break down an image into its component sections, lines and color gradients. To do this, the model must first "learn" how those components look in normal radiographs and in radiographs with pneumonia. In this example, learning is made possible by annotated training data. Since models only learn information based on the data used at training time, if we wish to train a general-purpose model, our training data must generalize. In the extreme case, large language models (LLMs), popularized by models such as OpenAI's GPT[1] and Google's Gemini[2] model families, aim to generally model natural language. Thus, they have been trained on data that approaches all written text on the internet, like the Common Craw dataset.[3,4]

Training

Once a model architecture has been chosen, the model of choice can be trained to learn the pattern desired. During training, the model will process the data, make predictions on input training data, and adjust its internal parameters, known as "weights," to reduce errors in predictions. Errors are quantified by a predetermined loss function, which can also attribute errors to weights through partial differentiation, a process known as "backprop." To reduce errors, we update weights

DOI: 10.1201/9781003471165-18

according to this error attribution.[5] Training happens across several iterations of this same process, feeding training data in and updating weights based on errors, which ultimately optimizes the model's performance. As is evident by the training process, in the case of neural networks, the training data distribution determines the learned weights. Thus, any inputs outside of this distribution will have unknown outputs.

We have primarily discussed a method of training known as supervised learning. This method requires labeled datasets to train an algorithm to recognize patterns. In neurosurgery, this could mean inputting several MRI scans labeled with information such as tumor presence or absence and type of tumor, if present. Once the model learns to differentiate between scans with and without tumors with the training data, it can be fed images without these labels and categorize them appropriately.

Another method of training is unsupervised learning (UL), which does not utilize labeled data for training. UL can be used to uncover hidden patterns. For example, UL can be useful in detecting shared characteristics among MRI scans that had not been documented prior to using the algorithm. While supervised learning is more useful for classification of data, UL may be more useful in anomaly detection and data clustering.

Training relies heavily on quantity and quality of data. Thus, an important consideration for DL model training is data augmentation. Because neurosurgical datasets can be limited, techniques like data augmentation allow datasets to be artificially increased to improve the generalizability of the model.[6] For example, images may be purposefully perturbed through image processing (e.g. rotating images, adding noise or changing brightness) to better represent the full range of data that the model may encounter and to reduce predictive biases.

To reduce the amount of data required to train a performant model, we can take advantage of transfer learning (TL). With TL, we typically take a large, general purpose base model, trained on petabytes of data, and fine-tune the model for a specific use case on much less data. This method was popularized with the advent of transformer-based language models, which initially learned to predict the next-word in a body of text through token masking (an example of semi-supervised training).[7] Although these base models may only know how to predict next tokens, they can be fine-tuned to do something like diagnose patients based on clinical notes. Base models may even be more domain specific, with hopes of improving model results, as Schmidgall et al. demonstrated when training a base model for general surgery video.[8] Given a base model, fine-tuning models based on human feedback (vs optimizing a mathematical loss function), a concept known as reinforcement learning with human feedback (RLHF), is a growing and popular mechanism for improving model performance.[9]

Inference

Once DL models have been appropriately trained on certain images, they can be applied to new data, done—typically—at the point of interaction by a user. This works because weight values were determined at training time. Thus, at inference time, we reuse these existing weights and simply skip the error attribution/weight updating step. As an example of inference vs training, companies identifying stroke in-real-time on MRI may have *trained* on millions of scans to build their AI model. However, when a new scan is input to the model, the output (e.g. infarct/ no infarct) would be considered *inference.*

Although large models trained on lots of data are highly performant and can handle multiple input data modalities (e.g. Gemini 1.5 Pro can perform inference on 2 hours of video, 22 hours of video and over 1.4 million words), they are expensive. Smaller model architectures have also proven performant and are much more efficient, like the widely used U-Net architecture for medical imaging. U-Net-based models are used for image segmentation and classification.[10]

DATA TYPES IN NEUROSURGERY

Imaging

MRI, CT scans and other imaging modalities offer invaluable anatomic information that guides neurosurgical diagnoses and treatments. DL can be used to unlock the hidden potentials of medical imaging within neurosurgery. Convolutional neural networks (CNNs) such as U-Net, introduced earlier, are particularly useful at analyzing MRI,

CT and other brain images. Imaging data varies across institutions, acquisition protocols and scanners. This lack of standardization necessitates pre-processing steps such as noise reduction and normalization to create successful DL models.[10] Once pre-processed, MRI and CT scans can be fed to trained CNNs, which can perform tasks such as tumor segmentation and other pattern recognition techniques.

The Brain Tumor Segmentation (BraTS) Challenge[11] is a prime example of a robust imaging data source. This resource began as an annual challenge in 2012 with the goal of improving BraTS in MRI scans. Therefore, this publicly available dataset was constructed through multi-institutional efforts to provide high-quality, preoperative brain MRI scans for patients with gliomas. The BraTS dataset provides multi-parametric (T1, T1c, T2 and T2-FLAIR) MRI scans of patients with gliomas as well as manual annotations regarding tumor characteristics (e.g. enhancing, non-enhancing, necrotic and with edema). Crucially, each scan is paired with manual, expert-verified labels that segment the tumor into distinct sub-regions (e.g. enhancing tumor, necrotic core, edema). Research groups have used BraTS to train and validate novel segmentation models, significantly advancing the field of automated tumor delineation for surgical planning and treatment response assessment.[11]

PATHOLOGY

Pathology is an essential component of neurosurgical diagnosis and treatment planning. When a spine or brain tissue is biopsied, the pathology results help guide whether treatment will involve surgery or not, and how or to what extent surgery will be involved. DL offers exciting possibilities for automating and enhancing neuropathology. These advancements may lead to faster and more accurate diagnoses. Potential applications of DL in neuropathology include tumor grading and classification and predictive analytics.

DL models have been previously trained to identify and classify different types of tumors. This includes classification of benign versus malignant, as well as subtyping tumors. CNNs are particularly useful for tumor grading and classification, and some studies have shown that certain CNNs achieve accuracies comparable to human pathologists.[10] Once tumors have been classified and/or graded, DL models can be applied to analyze pathologic features and predict patient prognosis or therapeutic responses.[12,13]

A key example of a data source in pathology is The Cancer Genome Atlas (TCGA) program from the National Cancer Institute and Nation Human Genome Research Institute.[14] Specifically, the TCGA-GBM and TCGA-LGG databases glioblastoma multiforme (GBM) and low-grade glioma (LGG) are important datasets within neurosurgery. These TCGA datasets were constructed using tissues samples and clinical data from thousands of patients, accumulating over 2.5 petabytes of data. Cases represented in these two datasets include whole-slide pathology images of tumor tissue with their corresponding histopathologic diagnoses and genomic, transcriptomic, epigenomic and clinical outcome data.

Models trained on TCGA datasets have successfully predicted crucial molecular markers such as IDH mutation status and 1p/19q co-deletions from slide images alone, when such tasks would normally require expensive and time-consuming sequencing protocols.[13] This once again highlights the role AI neurosurgical pathology data and the importance of integrating different types of data (e.g. radiology scans and molecular data) to create multimodal models for better tumor characterization in neurosurgery.

Electronic health records

EHRs contain rich clinical data that includes objective information such as specific diagnoses, which medications patients are taking, or past procedures they have undergone. EHRs also contain subjective data including clinical assessment of the patient and each patient's individual treatment plan. EHR data can be categorized into structured, semi-structured and unstructured formats.[15] Structured data follows a predetermined format, such as dates for a procedure or numerical values of laboratory results. Semi-structured data includes test results or diagnoses written in text form. Finally, examples of unstructured data are medical notes and other free-text entries in which data is reported without a defined structure.

Karhade et al. have employed natural language processing (NLP) algorithms to identify incidental durotomies during spine surgery.[16] Their goal was to improve the process of automated detection of this complication by using NLP to filter through free-text sections of operative reports of patients who underwent spine surgery. Algorithms such as these offer a promising improvement to current protocols that use current procedural terminology (CPT) and international classification of diseases (ICD) codes to identify durotomies. As discussed in prior sections, AI applications are particularly useful for large databases. This NLP algorithm could be used to explore national registries and to improve hospital quality and safety measurements with automated tracking of complications.

One of the most robust examples of this application is the National Neurosurgery Quality and Outcomes Database (QOD, formally known as N^2QOD).[17] This prospective clinical registry was developed by the American Association of Neurological Surgeons (AANS). N^2QOD allows researchers to track the quality of neurosurgical care across thousands of patients in over 100 hospitals in the United States. The dataset includes detailed structured labels such as patient demographics, ICD codes, surgical procedures (i.e. CPT codes) and patient-reported outcomes at several time points.

The N^2QOD dataset has been used in training models to predict a wide range of outcomes such as readmission risk, mortality and quality of life after spine and cranial surgeries. However, the use of unstructured data remains limited.[18,19] The future of EHR-based data construction should aim to integrate more unstructured data such as clinical notes and operative reports as well as other data sources such as pathology and imaging repositories.

Non-traditional sources of data

Applying DL tools to medical images can aid with tumor detection, operative planning and brain mapping of functional areas. Intraoperative guidance is another area in which DL has been particularly useful. By using real-time surgical images and sensors, these models can provide live feedback to neurosurgeons.[20] Surgical videos can also be used to train AI models.[21] The Simulated Outcome for Durotomy Repair in Minimally Invasive Spine Surgery (SOSpine) is a database that exemplifies well how non-traditional sources of data may be used in AI models in neurosurgery.[22] Researchers captured videos from endoscopic spine surgeries to develop predictive AI models. These researchers used a cadaveric dual repair simulator to teach neurosurgery residents and uploaded the surgical microscope video recordings paired with outcome data to the public SOSpine database to allow for development of surgical AI models. Future data construction could aim to create larger-scale, multi-institutional datasets of real intraoperative videos (i.e. rather than simulations) and link video analytics to long-term patient outcomes.

PREPARING NEUROSURGICAL DATA FOR DEEP LEARNING: OVERCOMING CHALLENGES

Successful utilization of DL within neurosurgery relies heavily on large, well-annotated datasets for training and validation. Since data curation and preparation are crucial to developing successful algorithms, it is important to review their role.

Data quality, quantity, pre-processing and standardization

Large datasets are essential for DL models to identify complex patterns accurately and efficiently. The more data available, the more robust and generalizable a model becomes. This is particularly important for neurosurgical data, which may be used to guide clinical decision-making or surgical approaches. Acquiring medical data presents significant challenges. Patient privacy is tightly regulated through legislation and regulations such as the Health Insurance Portability and Accountability Act (HIPAA) in the United States, or the General Data Protection Regulation (GDPR) in Europe.[23] Both HIPAA and GDPR were created to ensure patient safety and anonymity. These regulations create challenges for collaboration and data sharing across institutions.

Neurosurgical data is inherently heterogeneous. Data formats, imaging protocols, surgical techniques and outcomes all vary widely across patients with the same or similar diagnoses. This variability necessitates robust data pre-processing and standardization protocols, both of which have been described in more detail in earlier parts of this chapter. Other techniques for data standardization include data normalization, use of ontologies and data schemas.

Data normalization involves scaling data to a shared range, which allows for consistent model performance. Ontologies are structured vocabularies used in DL to define concepts and relationships within data. Ontologies function similarly to our own vocabulary: allowing standardized communication about data across institutions. Data schemas define the structure of the data itself. They specify how elements of a dataset relate to each other. When implemented appropriately, these techniques allow for efficient querying, analysis and utilization of data for DL applications. However, if improperly implemented, these steps can yield inconsistent results and inaccurate algorithms that lack external validity or clinical utility.

Public and proprietary databases

Public and proprietary databases offer a plethora of opportunities to apply DL to neurosurgical data. In addition, they highlight the strengths and challenges faced when implementing AI into the neurosurgical field. Two prominent examples of large neurological databases are discussed below.

The Alzheimer's Disease Neuroimaging Initiative (ADNI) is a database that utilizes longitudinal data on Alzheimer's disease (AD) and mild cognitive impairment (MCI).[24] Data included in ADNI encompasses MRI and PET scans, cognitive assessments, genetic information, cerebrospinal fluid (CSF) biomarkers and more. ADNI data can provide information on brain structure and atrophy and can guide clinical decision-making. ADNI is a publicly available dataset that allows registered researchers to access a plethora of clinical data for their studies. This access enables researchers to develop and test algorithms with the goal of improving early detection of AD or MCI, treatment response and more. ADNI is an excellent example of how crucial data standardization is in DL and AI more broadly. Since ADNI offers public, standardized data, researchers from around the world can contribute to data collection, sharing, validation and testing, creating better algorithms.

The BraTS Challenge[11] introduced earlier in this chapter is another example of how DL can leverage large databases to improve medical care. The BraTS dataset is publicly available to be downloaded and can be used by researchers who compete annually to develop algorithms for brain tumor segmentation. It has catalyzed significant advancements in brain tumor segmentation methods, which are essential for tumor categorization and enhanced surgical planning.

Both of these large databases prioritize high-quality data that utilize standardized acquisition protocols and manual annotations for their inclusion in the dataset. They serve as valuable resources for researchers developing DL algorithms. Furthermore, they offer a pathway for successful implementation of AI in the neurosurgical field.

FUTURE DIRECTIONS IN NEUROSURGICAL DATA AND DEEP LEARNING

DL is rapidly revolutionizing neurosurgical care and research. By allowing physicians and scientists to harness the power of vast, complex datasets and utilize image guidance pre- and intraoperatively, DL algorithms can transform the neurosurgical field as we know it. However, to unlock the full potential of DL applications to this field, advancements in data collection, processing/training and application are essential.

Advancements in data collection

The progress of DL application in neurosurgery hinges on the ability to gather increasingly complex medical data. Several technological advancements are on the horizon, including wearable technologies, Internet of Things (IoT) devices, advanced neuroimaging and enhanced surgical guidance.

Wearable and IoT devices include smart watches, fitness trackers and virtual reality (VR) or augmented reality (AR) headsets, among many others. We may not be far away from a future in which wearable sensors monitor a patient's neurological state (e.g. vital signs, brain activity or even subtle movement patterns). This continuous stream of data can then be used within DL models to predict neurological events, track disease progression or provide personalized treatment plans.

Emerging neuroimaging modalities such as magnetoencephalography (MEG) and diffusion tensor imaging (DTI) offer unparalleled image resolution that can capture the brain's structure and function better than other imaging modalities. We expect neuroimaging to advance further and further. MRIs were first introduced to hospitals in the 1980s, and in 2020, the first portable

MRI was invented.[25] As neuroimaging improves, DL algorithms can leverage these advancements to create highly detailed maps of the brain and nervous system to assist in diagnosis, preoperative planning, intraoperative guidance and postoperative assessment.

Operating rooms are also becoming increasingly digitized, utilizing robotic surgical systems and real-time surgical guidance. Live data collected from these tools can be integrated with DL models to provide real-time feedback during surgery. The future of intraoperative guidance may include systems that analyze surgical maneuvers and identify potential complications, allowing for immediate adjustments, greater precision and improved surgical outcomes.

Training: The role of synthetic data and simulations

Despite the hope for emerging technologies, applications of neurosurgical data can be limited by privacy concerns, ethical considerations and the rarity of certain neurological conditions. This is when synthetic data generation becomes key for the advancement of DL in medicine.

Synthetic data and simulations allow artificial datasets generated to mimic real-world data when said data are unavailable for any of the many possible reasons listed above.[26] DL models can be trained on these synthetic datasets, allowing them to learn complex relationships and generalize to real-world scenarios when real data are scarce. For example, generative adversarial networks (GANs) are actively used in research to create realistic medical images. In neurosurgery, GANs have been trained on datasets like the BraTS to generate new, artificial, multi-parametric MRI scans of brain tumors.[27] The synthetic data that produce new images are constructed by the model itself after learning complex statistical patterns of real MRIs. A major advantage of this approach is that synthetic images can be generated with perfect, corresponding pixel-level labels for tumor sub-regions, creating an unlimited source of training data. This is particularly important for rare pathologies that are underrepresented in real datasets.

Data simulation is not the only way in which synthetic data can be useful. As surgical simulations technologies improve, through VR and AR technologies, surgeons can train complex procedures and provide DL models with a platform to learn and refine surgical strategies in a safe, virtual environment. By leveraging synthetic data and incorporating simulations in DL training, researchers can bridge the gap between the limited real-world data and the vast demand for data in DL technologies without compromising patient safety.

Integration of deep learning in neurosurgical practice

The future of DL in neurosurgical practice relies on a seamless integration of DL into surgical and clinical workflow. This involves preoperative planning, intraoperative guidance and post-surgical monitoring. To unlock the full potential of DL applications, its use in neurosurgical research cannot be overlooked. To achieve these goals, efforts for innovating data collection, sharing and analysis is paramount and predicates a multi-pronged approach.

In the future, DL implementation in neurosurgery may look something like this: a symptomatic patient presents to the hospital, where imaging is ordered. DL models are implemented to analyze the patient's medical history contained in their EHR, and the imaging data collected to assist the physician in developing a differential diagnosis. Once the diagnosis is established by the physician with the use of DL and other tools, the provider can use a DL model to help create a personalized surgical plan that minimizes complications and improves precision catered to the patient's specific neuroanatomy. Once in the operating room, DL models can be used for real-time surgical guidance and feedback to allow for adjustments that minimize tissue damage and improve overall outcomes. Finally, DL algorithms can be implemented in post-surgical imaging and through wearable monitors to track recovery, predict potential complications and aid in the development of a personalized postoperative plan.

Collaborative research efforts are necessary for developing robust data management and sharing frameworks that will make DL advancements in neurosurgery possible. Ethical considerations regarding data privacy and algorithmic bias need to be carefully addressed throughout the process to ensure equitable and responsible implementation of DL innovations in neurosurgery.

Interdisciplinary collaborations bridge the gap between neurosurgery and computer science, different institutions and across specialties. Collaborations between neurosurgeons, data scientists, ethicists, among other professionals, will facilitate the development of robust DL models that can improve patient care.

CONCLUSION

It is undeniable that DL has the potential to revolutionize neurosurgical care. However, this transformation hinges on several conditions:

1. The quality and abundance of data available.
2. The meticulous preparation of the data collected
3. An iterative process of evaluating the success of these algorithms. A poorly trained model using bad data and applied improperly will lead to bad outcomes.

Curating high-quality data for neurosurgical applications is uniquely challenging. The inherent heterogeneity of the data quality, source, collection and overarching privacy concerns of utilizing medical information present significant barriers to the advancement of DL in the field. Challenging problems require complex, well-executed solutions, which we have explored throughout this chapter.

This chapter serves as an introduction to the vast field of AI as it pertains to neurosurgical care. The growth of AI in neurosurgery is dependent on a collaborative effort to uphold high standards for algorithm development. To move the field forward, we must prioritize a commitment to innovation in data collection, standardization and ethical utilization. The future of DL in neurosurgery necessitates that data collection technologies—from MRI to wearable sensors—continue to advance. With this advancement should come increased efforts of standardization across institutions to allow for seamless collaboration. Ethical utilization of data is also essential to minimize algorithmic biases and ensure equitable and responsible implementation of AI.

By addressing these challenges through the techniques discussed throughout this chapter, we can move toward a future in which AI is seamlessly integrated within the neurosurgical workflow. In doing so, we can empower future generations of neurosurgeons to deliver more precise, personalized care to patients, and, ultimately, improve patient outcomes. This future may not be too far away if we continue to collaborate for the advancement of AI in neurosurgical care.

REFERENCES

1. OpenAI. Hello GPT-4o. Available from: https://openai.com/index/hello-gpt-4o/ (Accessed May 2026).
2. Google DeepMind. Gemini. Available from: https://deepmind.google/technologies/gemini/ (Accessed May 2026).
3. Common Crawl. Overview. Available from: https://commoncrawl.org/overview (Accessed May 2026).
4. Brown TB, Mann B, Ryder N, et al. Language models are few-shot learners. *arXiv:2005.14165v4*, 2020.
5. Goodfellow I, Bengio Y, Courville A. *Deep Learning*. Cambridge, MA: MIT Press; 2016.
6. Jin X, Li S, Fan Y, et al. A systematic review of deep learning data augmentation in medical imaging: Recent advances and future research directions. *Med Image Anal* 2024; 77:102339.
7. Vaswani A, Shazeer N, Parmar N, et al. Attention is all you need. *arXiv:1706.03762v7*, 2017.
8. Schmidgall S, Woong Kim J, Jopling J, Krieger A. General surgery vision transformer: A video pre-trained foundation model for general surgery. 2024. Available from: https://arxiv.org/pdf/2403.05949v1 (Accessed May 2026).
9. Christiano PF, Shlegeris B, Amodei D. training language models to follow instructions with human feedback. *arXiv:2203.02155v1*, 2022.
10. Yousef R, Khan S, Gupta G, et al. U-Net-based models towards optimal MR brain image segmentation. *Diagnostics (Basel)* 2023; 13(9): 1624.
11. Kazerooni AF, Khalili N, Liu X, et al. The Brain Tumor Segmentation (BraTS) Challenge 2023. *arXiv:2305.17033v7*, 2023.
12. Lessard L, Michalowski W, Chen Li W, et al. Predictive analytics to support real-time management in pathology facilities. *AMIA Annu Symp Proc* 2017; 2016: 772–8.

13. Hollon T, Jiang C, Chowdury A, et al. Artificial-intelligence-based molecular classification of diffuse gliomas using rapid, label-free optical imaging. *Nat Med* 2023; 29(4): 828–32.
14. The Cancer Genome Atlas Research Network, Weinstein JN, Collisson EA, et al. The Cancer Genome Atlas Pan-Cancer Analysis Project. *Nat Genet* 2013; 45(10): 1113–20.
15. Lee S, Kim HS. prospect of artificial intelligence based on electronic medical record. *J Lipid Atheroscler* 2021; 10(3): 282–90.
16. Karhade AV, Bongers MER, Groot OQ, et al. Natural language processing for automated detection of incidental durotomy. *Spine J* 2020; 20(5): 695–700.
17. Asher AL, McCormick PC, Selden NR, et al. The National Neurosurgery Quality and Outcomes Database and NeuroPoint Alliance: rationale, development, and implementation. *Neurosurg Focus* 2013; *34*(1): E2.
18. Wadhwa RK, Ohya J, Vogel TD, et al. Risk factors for 30-day reoperation and 3-month readmission: Analysis from the Quality and Outcomes Database Lumbar Spine Registry. *J Neurosurg Spine* 2017; 27(2): 131–6.
19. Asher AL, Speroff T, Dittus RS, et al. The National Neurosurgery Quality and Outcomes Database (N2QOD): A collaborative North American Outcomes Registry to advance value-based spine care. *Spine (Phila Pa 1976)* 2014; 39(22 Suppl 1): S106–16.
20. Park JJ, Doiphode N, Zhang X, et al. Developing the surgeon-machine interface: Using a novel instance-segmentation framework for intraoperative landmark labelling. *Front Surg* 2023; 10: 1259756.
21. Kiyasseh D, Ma R, Haque TF, et al. A vision transformer for decoding surgeon activity from surgical videos. *Nat Biomed Eng* 2023; 7(6): 780–96.
22. Balu A, Kugener G, Pangal DJ, et al. Simulated outcomes for durotomy repair in minimally invasive spine surgery. *Sci Data* 2024; 11(1): 62.
23. Price WN 2nd, Cohen IG. Privacy in the age of medical big data. *Nat Med* 2019; 25(1): 37–43.
24. Petersen RC, Aisen PS, Beckett LA, et al. Alzheimer's Disease Neuroimaging Initiative (ADNI): clinical characterization. *Neurology* 2010; 74(3): 201–9.
25. Science. MRI for all, 2023. Available from: https://www.science.org/content/article/mri-all-cheap-portable-scanners-aim-revolutionize-medical-imaging (Accessed May 2026).
26. IBM. What is synthetic data? Available from: https://www.ibm.com/topics/synthetic-data (Accessed May 2026).
27. Mukherkjee D, Saha P, Kaplun D, et al. Brain tumor image generation using an aggregation of GAN models with style transfer. *Sci Rep* 2022; 12: 9141.

19

Current Challenges for Deep Learning Neurosurgery: Clinically Applicable Metrics and Domain Shift

OLIVIER ZANIER, LARA M. HÖBNER, RAFFAELE DA MUTTEN, LUCA REGLI, CARLO SERRA AND VICTOR E. STAARTJES

INTRODUCTION

With the advent of machine learning (ML) into clinical research and clinical practice, measuring the performance of ML models, evaluating whether they work or not, and whether they offer a tangible benefit compared to human experts, has become paramount. A range of metrics have been developed over the years to gauge how well supervised learning models do compared to the "ground truth" labels. For unsupervised models, evaluation of performance is more intricate: either a clinical validation of its direct use or testing on some sort of labeled held-out data must be performed. Still, the majority of applications of ML in medicine remain based on supervised learning, which is why we will focus on conveying a basic understanding of metrics applicable to the evaluation of such algorithms in this chapter. In addition, we explore the topic of efficacy versus effectiveness in terms of "domain shifts" from training to real-world data.

CLINICALLY APPLICABLE METRICS: DIAGNOSTIC, PROGNOSTIC AND PREDICTIVE MODELS

In neurosurgical decision-making and patient care, the use of prediction ML models has become increasingly more prevalent.[1] Such models serve different purposes, ranging from diagnostic tools to estimation of prognosis and outcome prediction. Applied clinically, they have the potential to help guide neurosurgeons through the complex field of neurosurgical patient management.

The difference between diagnostic, prognostic and predictive models lies solely in their purpose. Diagnostic models aim to identify a certain disease in a patient based on input characteristics like imaging, symptoms, clinical scores or laboratory findings.[2] Predictive and prognostic models, on the other hand, focus on predicting the probability of future events based on patterns and trends learned from past data. The terms predictive and prognostic are often used inconsistently in literature.[3] The difference is subtle but important. Using a combination of patient-specific variables as input, prognostic models are trained to predict the course of a disease without considering any interventions (e.g. prediction of pituitary adenoma growth based on size, hormonal levels and patient age).[4] On the contrary, predictive models try to estimate the effectiveness of an intervention (e.g. predict the probability of gross total resection for glioma surgery based on tumor size, localization and grade) or might help to deduce other events associated with that intervention (e.g. surgical complications).[4] While ML models will allow finding out **if**

DOI: 10.1201/9781003471165-19

a patient has a disease or may experience an event, generally, no explanation will be provided for **why** this is the case.

In this chapter, the diverse array of metrics that are employed to evaluate the performance and clinical applicability of prediction models is explored. Binary and multiclass classification models utilized for determining categorical outcomes, regression models used to predict continuous targets, and survival models for time-to-event assessments: each offers unique insights but necessitates the use of specific metrics for performance evaluation.

CLASSIFICATION MODELS

Classification models learn patterns from labeled data (supervised) and are used to determine a categorical outcome.[5] While binary prediction models are applied to data with a question for which only two outcomes (e.g. yes/no, true/false) are possible, multiclass models are used when instances need to be categorized into more than two categories (e.g. full vs partial vs no postoperative improvement).[6,7] It is important to assess both the discrimination and the calibration performance of prediction models. Both will be discussed in more detail in the following, focusing on binary classification models.

Discrimination

The discrimination performance describes how well a prediction model can distinguish between different outcomes or classes. It assesses the model's capacity to accurately categorize both positive and negative cases while keeping misclassifications to a minimum.

Table 19.1 Confusion matrix

		Model prediction	
		Prediction positive (PP)	Prediction negative (PN)
Real condition	Positive (P)	*True positive (TP)*	*False negative (FN)*
	Negative (N)	*False positive (FP)*	*True negative (TN)*

For understanding the calculations of discrimination metrics, the confusion matrix in Table 19.1 can be helpful.

Accuracy

In ML, accuracy refers to the fraction of a model's correct predictions or classifications in relation to all cases the model was applied to:

$$Accuracy = \frac{Correct\ predictions}{All\ predictions} = \frac{(TP+TN)}{(P+N)}$$

The perfect accuracy is 100% or 1 (i.e. the model correctly predicts all data correctly), whereas a 50% or 0.5 accuracy rate denotes a performance on par with random guessing on balanced dataset.

Applications and Limitations: Accuracy is a popular and simple metric to assess a model's discrimination performance and works particularly well on balanced datasets with evenly distributed classes. However, when working with imbalanced datasets, where one class is significantly more frequent than the other, accuracy may not be the ideal metric to use, as severe class imbalance can lead to high scores despite producing useless predictions.

A neurosurgical illustration: A model aiming to predict gross total resection for meningiomas might achieve an 80–90% accuracy by solely predicting that total resection will be achieved for every patient. This model will be useless, despite its respectable accuracy, as it fails to capture the more relevant subgroup of cases where full resection may not be achieved.

In such cases, other metrics might provide a better understanding of the model's performance and will be described in the following. In general, no clinical classification model should be assessed solely on the basis of accuracy, and readers should be cautious about suspiciously high accuracy scores.

Recall (sensitivity, true positive rate)

In data science and ML, sensitivity is often named recall. It assesses a model's capacity to accurately identify all relevant (i.e. positive) instances from a dataset:

$$Recall\ (Sensitivity) = \frac{TP}{(TP+FN)} = \frac{TP}{P}$$

The percentage of subjects who are positive cases and who were accurately classified to be positive is therefore known as recall. A high recall indicates that the model is good at identifying positive instances and produces only a few false negatives.

Specificity

Specificity, on the other hand, is a metric that is especially useful when the negative class is of interest. Specificity measures a model's ability to accurately identify the true negatives:

$$Specificity = \frac{TN}{(TN + FP)} = \frac{TN}{N}$$

A high specificity indicates that the model is good at recognizing the negative class, therefore, minimizing the number of false positives.

Precision (positive predictive value)

The positive predictive value (PPV) is commonly referred to as precision in the realm of ML. It assesses the proportion of true positive predictions among all instances that are predicted positive:

$$PPV = \frac{TP}{(TP + FP)} = \frac{TP}{PP}$$

A high precision indicates that the model is good at avoiding false positives, and cases that were classified as positive by a model with a high PPV are very likely true positives.

Negative predictive value

In contrast, the negative predictive value (NPV) measures the probability that instances predicted as negative are truly negative:

$$NPV = \frac{TN}{(TN + FN)} = \frac{TN}{PN}$$

With a high NPV, a model minimizes the number of false negatives, and the likelihood of negative cases to be truly negative is high.

F1 score

The F1 score combines both the abovementioned precision and recall into a single metric, providing a comprehensive assessment of a model's performance:

$$F1 = 2 \times \frac{Precision \times Recall}{Precision + Recall}$$

Better model discrimination performance is indicated by a higher value for the F1 score. It ranges from 0 to 1, with 1 indicating the highest score. The F1 score is commonly applied in situations where both precision and recall are important.

Applications and Limitations: Depending on the goal of a classification model, the confidence threshold can either be optimized for the model to rule out (high sensitivity and NPV) or rule in (high specificity and PPV). Alternatively, a more balanced threshold can be selected to get the best of both worlds. At a minimum, clinically intended classification models should report both sensitivity and specificity, as neither metric alone captures the balance between false positives and false negatives.

Furthermore, for prediction models where one of the two predicted outcomes occurs much less frequently, PPV and NPV should be reported, as Sensitivity and Specificity on their own do not sufficiently reflect the impact of outcome prevalence on the predictions.

A simplistic neurosurgical example of the metrics' threshold dependency could be two models aimed at detecting an increase in ICP, or the absence of it. One model might do so based on the input variables hypertension, bradycardia and irregular respiration (Cushing's triad). Such a model, if trained properly, will have a high specificity but low sensitivity (i.e. "rule-in" model) by construction. The used variables are strong predictors of an increased ICP, and selecting an overly high confidence threshold can render this model useless, as it will miss cases with elevated ICP where, for example, only two of the three findings are present or only mild ICP increase is present. This will consequently negatively affect Sensitivity and NPV, even though the model might have worked well using an appropriate cutoff.

In contrast, a second model aiming to rule out an increased ICP based on the absence of a headache, vomiting, papilledema and alterations in mental status will have a much higher sensitivity but lower specificity. For this second model, applying a too low confidence threshold can be detrimental, as it would lead to an overwhelming number of patients being wrongly flagged as positive (a positive prediction having no value in a rule-out model). It has to be noted, though, that a model which is primarily aimed at ruling out (high sensitivity, negative prediction -> allows a safe rule-out) also is hampered by a too high threshold, as then the entire rule-out goal of this model is neutered because the rule-out accuracy is not near-perfect anymore. A threshold-independent measure will help identify in which scenarios a model performs well and which it does not. The receiver operating characteristic (ROC) curve and area under the ROC (AUROC) curve are such measures.

Receiver operating characteristic curve

The ROC curve is a graphical representation of the Sensitivity (true positive rate) plotted against the false positive rate (1-Specificity) at different confidence thresholds for a binary classification model.

Area under the ROC curve

The AUROC curve is used to assess a binary classification model's overall performance. In theory, perfect discrimination is represented by an area under the curve (AUC) of 1.0, whilst a discriminative performance that is not better than a random guess results in an AUC of 0.5.

In general, AUC values above 0.7 or 0.8 are indicative of a well-performing prediction model, however, this is heavily dependent on the characteristics of the dataset and the intended application of the model.

Applications and Limitations: The ROC and AUROC are good measures for obtaining a comprehensive, threshold-independent overview of a binary classification model's discrimination performance. The main drawbacks are that, since they are reliant on sensitivity and specificity, they do not capture the impact of outcome prevalence on the predictions. As a result, in datasets with severe class imbalance, models can achieve high AUC and ROC scores, yet fail to detect rare but clinically important events.

Calibration

Classification models assign a specific class to all instances with a certain confidence (0–1 or 0–100%). The binarization threshold is often set to 0.5 or selected according to the *closest-to-1.0 criterion* (displayed in **Figure 19.1**), but can also be adjusted depending on the goal of the model (rule in vs rule out).[8] This confidence of the model can also be interpreted as the absolute predicted probability of the event occurring, and, in a clinical setting, it is usually of equal or higher importance than the binary classification itself.[9]

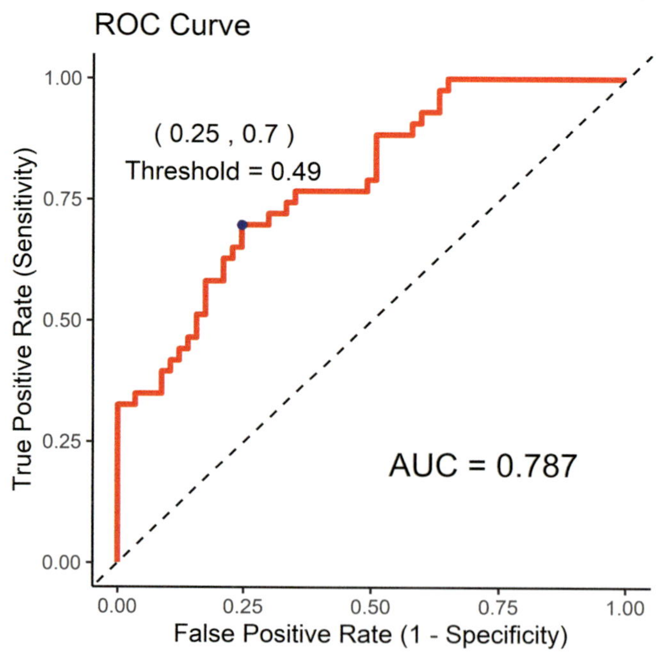

Figure 19.1 Example of a receiver operating characteristic curve.

Model calibration evaluates the alignment between the predicted probabilities and the actual occurrence of the binary outcome in the dataset.[9] It is an essential metric that should always be analyzed for clinical classification models, which, unfortunately, is still commonly neglected in practice. Calibration is generally portrayed as a plot, with the y-intercept (mostly just referred to as "intercept") and the slope reported as numerical metrics for calibration performance. A well-calibrated model, with an intercept close to 0 and a slope close to 1, produces probability estimates that are closely aligned with the actual occurrences across the entire probability spectrum.[10] In other words, such a model is capable of accurately predicting absolute probabilities of an outcome for patients with very high, medium and low actual likelihoods (and everything in-between).

Brier Score

The Brier Score includes components of both discrimination and calibration. It is the mean squared error (MSE) calculated between the predicted probabilities and the observed outcomes:[10]

$$Brier\ Score = \frac{\sum_{i=1}^{n}(P_i - O_i)^2}{n}$$

with n being the number of patients, P_i the predicted and O_i the observed outcome.

Resulting values range from 0 to 1, with 0 indicating best performance or, in other words, the smallest error.[10]

Applications and Limitations: Calibration should be assessed for all classification models where the absolute probability of the outcome occurring is clinically relevant. For example, it will be more helpful to know that a surgical complication will occur with a 60% likelihood rather than just knowing that a complication is likely to occur. Calibration alone does not allow for the assessment of discrimination and should always be reported as an adjunct to discrimination analysis.

REGRESSION MODELS

Regression models are the second main category of supervised learning techniques. They essentially learn how to accurately convert input data points into a continuous range of real numbers as an outcome (e.g. prediction of glioblastoma survival in months based on surgery, localization, methylation status, etc.).[5] They are less in use compared to classification models, one reason being that many continuous outcomes can be simplified into binary categories.[11]

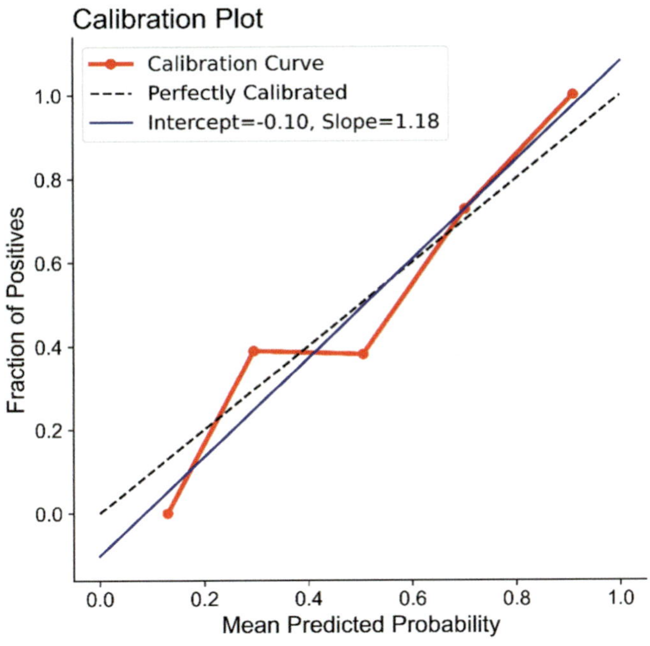

Figure 19.2 Example of a calibration plot.

The only way to assess performance for regression models is to directly compare the predicted and true values and the following metrics are commonly used to do so.

Mean absolute error

The mean absolute error (MAE) measures the average of the absolute differences between predicted and actual values. Therefore, an MAE of 0.00 would mean that there is no error at all, and any variations from 0 indicate that values are generally overestimated or underestimated:

$$MAE = \frac{\sum_{i=1}^{n} | y_i - \breve{y}_i |}{n}$$

where n is the number of samples, y_i is the actual value and $\breve{y}_i$ is the predicted value for the outcome.

Mean squared error and root mean squared error

The MSE calculates the average of the squares of the errors between the expected and actual values over a dataset:

$$MSE = \frac{\sum_{i=1}^{n} (y_i - \breve{y}_i)^2}{n}$$

where n is the number of samples, y_i is the actual value and $\breve{y}_i$ is the predicted value for the outcome.

Larger errors are penalized more severely than smaller ones because the errors are squared.

One disadvantage of MSE is that it does not have the same unit as the outcome, thus, it can be difficult to interpret. To address this issue the Root Mean Squared Error (RMSE) is used:

$$RMSE = \sqrt{MSE}$$

Better model performances are indicated by lower values for *MSE* or *RMSE*.

R-squared

R-squared (R^2) is a measure of how well the independent variables (i.e. input features) explain the variability in the dependent variable (i.e. actual outcome). The idea is that changes in the values of the independent variables directly influence the predictions made by the model. Now, if the independent variables are effective to capturing relevant patterns present in the data, the model's predictions (dependent variable) will be more accurate (i.e. closer to the actual outcomes). Accordingly, a perfect explanatory power would be shown by an R^2 value of 1.0.

Applications and Limitations: Regression models are less common compared to classification models, primarily due to the fact that most regression problems can be converted into classification tasks, which however has the drawback of losing information by a relevant margin. A neurosurgical example of this would be predicting the length of hospital stay (in days) after intracranial surgery. This can easily be converted into predicting a short versus a long stay (e.g. less than 7 days vs more than 7 days). Of course this is much less granular than trying to predict the actual number of days in hospital. However, this makes the model training process less complicated, and also allows for the use of classification metrics, which are more clinically impactful and interpretable than regression metrics.

SURVIVAL MODELS

Survival models, a sub-type of prognostic models, are devised to analyze time-to-event data for the estimation of survival probabilities, or any other event with a time component, over a specified period.[12] Two different types of survival models need to be distinguished: time-dependent and time-independent models. While time-dependent prediction models allow for individual predictions of an outcome at specific time points, time-independent models only provide a single output for each patient or instance.[13] In other words, time-independent survival models produce a summary risk for each individual at the end of one specified time period, while time-dependent models can predict the risk at more than one specified point in time. Each of them requires evaluation using separate metrics.

Censoring is a frequent obstacle when working with time to event data. Subjects lost to follow-up need to be included in the analysis as they provide valuable information up to the date of last follow-up, but must be censored thereafter.[14]

DISCRIMINATION

Time-independent models

Concordance Index, Harrell's C-Index

The Concordance Index (C-index) compares the predicted probability of event occurrence with the observed (ground-truth) time-to-event and assesses whether they are concordant. In other words, it evaluates the proportion of all possible patient pairs that have been correctly ordered by the model based on their predicted time-to-event.[15] There are different ways of how to account for censored subjects, one of the more common being the Harrell's C-index.[13,16]

Time-dependent models

Time-dependent area under the ROC curve

A time-dependent model's discrimination performance can be assessed using the time-dependent AUROC curve. This involves generating a separate ROC at specific time points and calculating the AUC for each. In contrast to conventional ROC curve analysis, calculation of time dependent ROC curves need to account for the fact that the state of outcome may change for certain subjects at specific time points.[13,17] Further, censored subjects need to be considered appropriately. There are various established methods available to do so.[17]

The time-dependent AUROC provides insight in how well a survival model performs at each specific time point when the ROC is calculated. Models achieving higher AUCs generally indicate better performance.

Integrated AUROC

The integrated AUC (iAUC) takes the time dependent AUCs one step further by applying a mathematical integration to derive a single AUC.[13,18] This iAUC is representative of all time-dependent AUROCs.

Applications and Limitations: In a neurosurgical context, a time-independent model could estimate the probability of death within 30 days after subarachnoid hemorrhage, while a time-dependent model could do much more dynamically at any day from the time of hospital admission to 30 days after the bleeding incident. Therein also lie the drawbacks of time-independent models: they do not allow for reliable predictions before or after a 30-day window, while time-dependent models generally will only become unreliable for predictions beyond the observed follow-up period. Correspondingly, single 30-day AUC overall C-index are simpler and allow for easier clinical interpretation. On the other hand, the time-dependent AUC or iAUC are much more complex, and data might be scarce for certain points within the observed timeframe, with the advantage being the ability to assess discrimination for any point within the follow-up period.

Calibration and Brier score

As previously described for classification models, Calibration and Brier score can also be used to assess the performance of survival models. However, just like the time-dependent AUROC, the calibration plots and Brier scores need to be calculated separately for each of the follow-up times.[13]

The mathematical definitions of the Harrell's C-index, time-dependent AUROC/calibration plots and integrated AUROC are considered out of scope and will not be discussed in this section. In any case, having a general idea of the purpose as well as when and how to apply these metrics already allows for the utilization of pre-coded packages to handle the calculations. This should suffice for most clinical research projects.

Other important considerations

Variable importance

Variable importance allows for an insight into the model's decision-making process. It describes the impact each variable has on the final predictions of an ML model.[19,20] In clinical scenarios, it needs to be ensured that the most impactful input variables are truly representative of the predicted outcome. A model basing its predictions solely on variables like gender or age provides only very little benefits.

External validation

Evaluation of model performance on an independent dataset from one or more separate centers is crucial to ensure generalizability of any ML model and is, therefore, mandatory for any model intended for clinical application.

CLINICALLY APPLICABLE METRICS: IMAGING

The birth of convolutional neural networks (CNNs) is often attributed to LeCun et al., who in 1998 demonstrated the capability of their LeNet-5 to recognize handwritten characters in images.[21,22]

Many improvements to the original architecture ensued over the next decade, making training more efficient and models more effective.[23,24] The breakthrough classification performance achieved by Krizhevsky et al. in 2012 on the ImageNet dataset is commonly regarded as the first application of a modern deep CNN architecture and also broadly introduced the utilization of graphical processing units (GPUs) into model training.[25,26]

The Brain Tumor Segmentation (BraTS) challenge,[27,28] which started in 2012, has been a main driving force behind the implementation of DL in the fields of Neurosurgery, Neuro-oncology and Neuroimaging. Image classification and segmentation are among the most common applications of medical image analysis in the field of computational neuroscience.[27,29,30] Newer, more preliminary approaches to the field include object detection (e.g. for anatomic structures), synthetic image generation or disease progression modeling.[28,31–34]

The performance evaluation method is heavily dependent on the task intended for imaging DL models. As a result, a wide variety of metrics have been employed. In this section, a comprehensive overview of the relevant metrics is provided for each task.

Classification

In image classification, the same metrics are used as for all classification tasks. The most important ones include Accuracy, Precision, Recall, F1 Score and AUROC or AUC. These metrics have been covered in the preceding pages.

Segmentation

Two widely applied techniques for image segmentation using DL are semantic segmentation and instance segmentation, in which each pixel in the image is classified into a certain class. However, semantic segmentation does not distinguish between multiple instances of the same object, whereas instance segmentation treats each occurrence of the same object as an individual, separate class.[35] Panoptic segmentation is a newer method that combines the advantages of both techniques by using instance identifiers.[36] Only semantic segmentation has been extensively applied in the field of computational neuroscience so far, therefore, it will be the focus for the discussion of evaluation metrics in this section.

Semantic segmentation

Accuracy (pixel accuracy)

The most rudimentary metric used to evaluate semantic segmentation performance is Accuracy, which is defined as the percentage of accurately classified pixels in an image:[37]

$$Accuracy = \frac{correct\ classifications}{all\ classifications} = \frac{nr.\ of\ correctly\ classified\ pixels}{nr.\ of\ all\ pixels}$$

The resulting values fall within the range of 0 to 1, where an Accuracy of 1 signifies flawless performance.

Despite being easy to implement, Accuracy has some disadvantages when applied to assess semantic segmentation models. First, it is heavily influenced by class imbalance, which is an extremely common issue when working with medical imaging. When the images are dominated by background, the resulting values are high, even if the model does not recognize the objects of interest at all. Second, accuracy cannot determine the spatial relation between the pixels, which is essential for understanding the quality of segmentations.

Dice similarity coefficient and intersection over union

Overlap-based metrics such as Intersection-over-Union Score (IoU, Jaccard Index) and Dice Similarity Score (DSC, Sørensen–Dice coefficient, F1 Score) are also commonly used to evaluate segmentation results:[38–40]

$$IoU = \frac{area\ of\ overlap}{area\ of\ union} = \frac{|A \cap B|}{|A \cup B|}$$

$$DSC = \frac{2 * area\ of\ overlap}{total\ area} = \frac{2|A \cap B|}{|A| + |B|}$$

where *A* and *B* correspond to ground truth and model generated mask, respectively.

IoU and DSC are similar metrics, positively correlated and ranging from 0 to 1, meaning, respectively, no overlap and perfect congruence.

Applications and Limitations: Several factors need to be considered when utilizing these two metrics. First, they are affected by the scale of the object requiring segmentation.[40,42,43] If the regions of interest are small, false positives and negatives have a greater impact on the score. Second, when working with 3D imaging, e.g. segmentation of brain tumors in MRI, there are different ways to calculate these scores: over the whole volume (in 3D) or slice-wise (in 2D). Calculating the scores in 3D is straightforward but neglects spatial information in the segmentations to some degree. When using a 2D implementation, on the other hand, some image slices will neither contain model segmentation nor ground-truth segmentation, which leads to undefined values. There are several methods to handle such undefined values (e.g. setting them to 1) that can have a considerable impact on the final scores.[42] Three, like accuracy, DSC and IoU are insensitive to the boundaries of a structure of interest.[43,44] This can be problematic as these regions are of especially high interest in neurosurgical imaging. For example, accurately detecting the boundaries of a brain tumor in an MRI is much more relevant than segmenting 95% of the tumor volume with incorrect boundaries. This is the reason why the Hausdorff Distance is commonly reported together with DSC and IOU.

Besides, for model performance evaluation, DSC and IoU are also commonly used as loss functions, and several adaptations have been explored (Focal Dice loss, Tversky loss).[45,46] This often results in higher DSC and IoU scores, but, due to the reasons outlined before, not necessarily more clinically relevant segmentations.

Hausdorff distance

In contrast to Accuracy, DSC and IoU, the Hausdorff Distance (HD) considers spatial relations as well as boundaries of the segmentations. It is defined as "the greatest of all distances from all points in one set to their closest points in the other set," and vice versa (bidirectional).[47] The two point sets are derived from the boundaries of the ground truth and algorithm segmentation.

The HD calculation can be illustrated in simple terms as follows:

For two finite point sets:

1. For each point in the first set, find the nearest point in the second set and measure the distance between them.
2. Repeat this procedure for the second set: For each point in the second set, find the nearest point in the first set and measure the distance between them.
3. The longest distance found is the HD.

A variation of the classic HD, that is widely applied as a metric for analyzing the performance of segmentation models, is the 95th percentile Hausdorff distance (HD95).[48,49] Compared to the HD, the HD95 is much less sensitive to outliers, thus providing an overall more representative measure for the performance in segmentation tasks.[48]

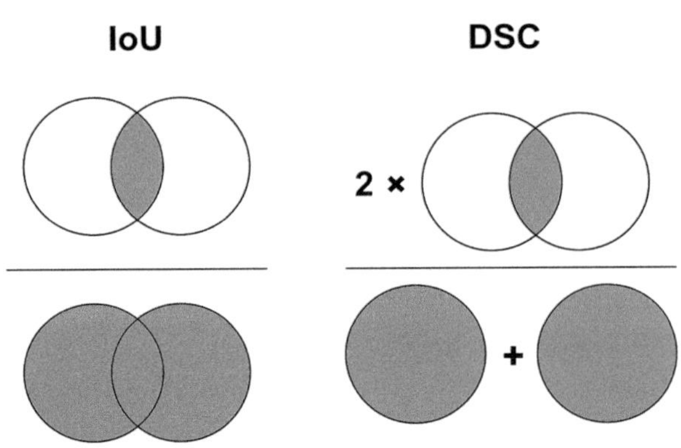

Figure 19.3 Visual representation of intersection over union score and Dice similarity coefficient. (Based on Nguyen et al.[41])

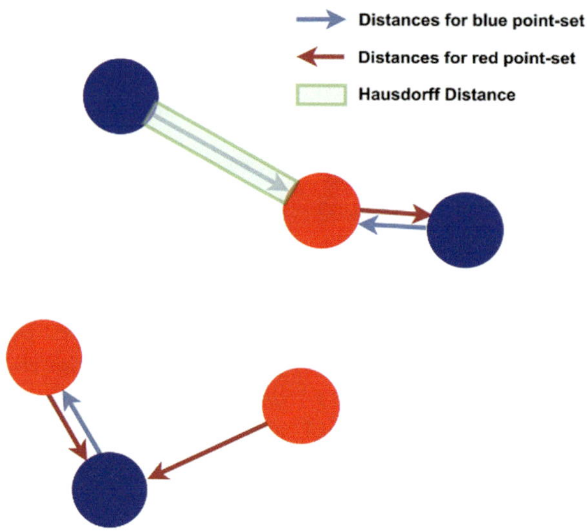

Figure 19.4 Visual representation of Hausdorff distance calculation.

When evaluating 3D segmentations, the HD can be calculated for each 2D slice (slice-wise) or once for the whole volume. When calculating its 2D implementation, handling of undefined values can pose a significant issue. There may be slices that have either algorithm or ground-truth segmentation, but not both. Further, slices without any segmentations at all may also be present. In both cases, the HD is not defined. Depending on how these undefined regions are handled, scores can differ significantly.

If correctly used, the HD (or HD95) are more relevant compared to the overlap-based metrics such as the Dice or IoU in a clinical setting. It considers spatial information and gives special attention to the perimeters of target structures.

Instance segmentation

Dice and IoU scores are not only applicable to semantic segmentation but can also be extended to instance segmentation tasks. Another crucial metric in this context is Average Precision (AP), which quantifies the accuracy of detecting various objects.[50] It is also commonly used for object detection tasks, and a more detailed exploration of AP is provided under "Object Detection".

Panoptic segmentation

For panoptic segmentation both the quality of the segmentation and recognition need to be assessed. The metric proposed is Panoptic Quality (PQ) which uses the average IoU for true positive matches (segmentation quality) together with the F1 score (recognition quality).[51] The application of panoptic segmentation in the field of neurosurgery remains to be explored.

OBJECT DETECTION

In object detection, DL is applied to videos or pictures with the aim of identifying and marking one or more objects of interest.[52] This is achieved by identifying the object's class and determining the bounding box coordinates (i.e. its location).[52] Object detection has been applied to a variety of tasks, far beyond medical imaging. Examples include self-driving cars,[53] agriculture,[54] or industrial process monitoring.[55] Benchmark datasets and challenges such as the Pattern Analysis, Statistical Modeling and Computational Learning Visual Object Classes (PASCAL-VOC) challenge[56] or the Common Objects in Context (COCO) dataset[57] influenced and introduced the following widely used metrics.

Intersection over union

The IoU score, as described in the previous section on segmentation, can also be used to evaluate the performance of object detection algorithms. It is calculated by comparing the ground truth and algorithm bounding boxes for the object of interest and calculating the mean over the whole dataset.[58]

Precision-recall curve and average precision

Calculation of the precision-recall curve (PR curve) in the context of object detection necessitates the differentiation between correct and incorrect detections of a class.[59] This differentiation is more complex than image classification. If the IoU calculated between the ground truth and algorithm bounding boxes exceeds a certain threshold, commonly 0.5, the detection is considered to be correct.[56]

By plotting precision against recall at different model confidence levels, the PR curve can then be generated.[59] AP represents the area under this PR curve and is an established metric for assessing the performance of an object-detection algorithm.[59] It is distinct from the AUROC, which represents the area under the recall (sensitivity) and fallout (1-specificity) curve.

Mean average precision

The mean average precision (mAP) extends AP and is used to evaluate the performance object detection models across multiple classes by simply taking the mean AP over all classes.[60] Normally, the same 0.5 IoU threshold is used (i.e. mAP50).

A variation of the mAP50 is mAP50–95. Instead of just using a single IoU threshold, mAP50–95 is classically calculated by averaging all mAPs obtained at IoU thresholds ranging from 0.5 to 0.95 with steps of 0.05.[61] This allows for a more comprehensive assessment of the model's detection performance not just at loose (0.5 IoU) but also at tighter matching thresholds.

Applications and Limitations: Object detection in a neurosurgical context is explored less commonly than segmentation. An example of a neurosurgical application is the detection and labeling of anatomic structures within the field of view during an endoscopic procedure. The advantage of object detection compared to segmentation is that it is much more efficient, as only the computation of four values defining the bounding box (x and y coordinates of corners or center together with width and height) is needed, whereas for segmentation tasks, each pixel needs to be classified. This is one reason why it is used more readily for real-time applications.

Regarding evaluation metrics, AP and mAP are heavily reliant on the chosen IoU threshold. If the cutoff is selected too strictly (e.g. >0.8), this can lead to missing the anatomic structures altogether. Conversely, if the cutoff is too low, it will result in inaccurate detections and false positives being included in the analysis. Furthermore, while mAP provides an overall measure across multiple classes, in contrast to AP, it can mask class-specific weaknesses. If nine out of ten structures are perfectly detected, but one is missed every time, mAP will remain high. Finally, mAP50–95 provides a threshold-independent assessment of object detection performance but, in clinical practice, performance at a specific predetermined threshold is usually more relevant than across multiple thresholds.

Further metrics

Besides IoU, AP and mAP, Precision, Recall and F1-Score are also commonly reported.

Image and text generation

Synthetic image generation is a broadly defined field wherein DL is applied to create artificial imaging using text or imaging as input. In certain scenarios, trained models can even generate such synthetic images from scratch. Current applications include image domain transfer (e.g. from MRI to CT), image style transformation, image quality enhancement or generation of enlarged training datasets to facilitate the training of independent ML models.[33,34,62–64]

In computational neuroscience, generation of synthetic CT from MRI has been broadly explored, primarily with the goal of enabling MRI-only radiotherapy.[65–67] Outside the field of MRI-only radiotherapy, generation of synthetic imaging in neurosurgery has not been extensively studied yet. Among others, investigations encompass the generation of synthetic spine X-rays to create a more extensive and diverse imaging dataset[34] or the reconstruction of a synthetic CTs from spinal radiographs.[68]

For medical text generation, structured, unstructured, text or multimodal (e.g. clinical and imaging) medical data are used by language models to produce a specific output text. This could be an operative report, patient progress notes or decision-making support.[69–71]

Due to the diverse nature of the field, the evaluation metrics used are not standardized and sometimes serve very different purposes. Further, most metrics only capture a small aspect of the essential image/text features, which further complicates evaluations of the produced generative data.

MRI-to-CT conversion

For MRI-to-CT conversion commonly employed metrics include dosimetric agreement, MAE of Hounsfield units at the voxel level or the Dice similarity coefficient for specific regions of the image (e.g. bone or brain).[72] Dosimetric agreement refers to the disparities in radiation dose when calculated on the synthetic CT compared to original CT.[65,72]

Other important metrics in a broader realm include the Fréchet Inception Distance (FID), Peak Signal-to-Noise Ratio (PSNR) or Structural Similarity Index (SSIM).

Peak signal-to-noise ratio and structural similarity index

PSNR and SSIM are used to assess the similarity of reconstructed signals, including images, to a ground truth.[73] Therefore, these two metrics are particularly useful when an artificial image is intended to resemble the original as closely as possible.[74]

When applied to imaging, PSNR can be defined as:[75]

$$PSNR = 20 * log_{10} \frac{2^n - 1}{\sqrt{MSE}}$$

where n refers to the bit depth of the image, $2^n - 1$ corresponds to the maximum image intensity for a specified bit depth image and *MSE* denotes the mean squared error.

Unlike PSNR, SSIM not only takes into account the absolute errors, but also incorporates perceptual aspects such as luminance, contrast and structural information.[76]

The two metrics have been shown to have significant limitations in terms of performance on medical imaging and correlation with human raters.[77] There are many variations to both PSNR and SSIM that aim to improve their reliability.[78,79]

The FID is determined by comparing the feature distributions of generated images with those of genuine images and serves a different purpose to PSNR and SSIM.[80] It is a measure of how well a generative model can produce images that exhibit certain characteristics or features, rather than just replicating similar patterns. Therefore, it is commonly applied to assess models meant for producing larger and more varied image datasets and is not suitable for comparison of image similarity.

For generative text quality assessment BLEU (Bilingual Evaluation Understudy) or ROUGE (Recall-Oriented Understudy for Gisting Evaluation) scores are used to assess the text overlap, and more advanced metrics like METEOR and BERTScore can capture semantic similarity.[81–84]

Applications and Limitations: As with the metrics used for the generation of synthetic imaging, these metrics capture similarities with reference texts, but do not necessarily correspond to the ones relevant in a neurosurgical or even general medical context. In other words, these metrics are "domain agnostic." To illustrate, consider the following example from a model-generated report:

> A left frontotemporal craniotomy was performed to resect a fronto-temporal tumor.

The corresponding ground truth reads:

> A left pterional craniotomy was performed to resect an insular glioma.

Although these sentences share substantial word overlap (yielding acceptable BLEU and ROUGE scores), the model entirely misses the most critical neurosurgical details, including the precise location and specific pathology. The same issue occurs with synthetic imaging, where visually plausible outputs may still fail to capture clinically relevant features. Therefore, reporting high scores for generative imaging or text alone is insufficient. A domain-specific evaluation by neurosurgeons remains essential.

THE ISSUE OF DOMAIN SHIFT

An ML algorithm that performs admirably "*in silico*" on held-out testing data may be all well and good. As discussed above, external validation is a next important step toward ensuring that the model really works in the sense that it has truly extracted generalizable relationships among the inputs and the output. Still, even if the hurdle of external validation is surpassed, an algorithm may still fail when actually applying it in clinical practice.

The reason is the same as with medications or surgical interventions, which have been tested in large randomized controlled trials (RCTs): Usually, these trials have a large amount of exclusions (when looking at their study cohort flow charts) and have quite strict inclusion and exclusion criteria. Of course, ideally, the findings of such studies should only be applied strictly to patients seen in clinical practice that fit these exact same inclusion and exclusion criteria. In reality, however, the situation is often more complex, as the RCTs' criteria may have been so very specifically selective that the clinical applicability is hampered because only a fraction of real-world patients fit the description; or, because in a clinical scenario, not all inclusion and exclusion criteria can always be screened for (due to time constraints in trauma or emergencies, for example, or for economic reasons, or because measurements are taken differently at various institutions). Off-label use in this sense is not always pernicious but requires extreme caution and Phase IV vigilance studies to make sure that treatments do remain useful rather than harmful.

The terminology applying to this phenomenon is the difference between "efficacy" and "effectiveness."[85] Whereas efficacy denotes a certain intervention's performance under ideal conditions (study with strict inclusion and exclusion criteria plus all the placebo effects), the term effectiveness denotes real-world performance in clinical practice. This is why initial RCTs are often positive with novel treatments, but real-world studies following up patients and looking at effectiveness may then sometimes show more disappointing results.

How does this apply to ML? Domain shift or domain adaptation in ML denotes the phenomenon where an algorithm is applied to slightly different novel data than it was originally trained to handle. Of course, the data that it is applied to cannot be completely different: For example, we cannot take a prediction model made to predict the 12-month outcomes after lumbar fusion in degenerative disease and then apply it to the outcome of spinal cord injury patients. That would be total extrapolation. But, possibly, the same degenerative model could be used to predict 6-month instead of 12-month outcomes, or it could potentially be applied to patients treated with a different interbody fusion technique than in the training cohort (for example, posterolateral vs lateral). Sometimes, models can handle such domain shifts. Even more often, this is not the case!

The key to domain shift, which is sometimes inevitable, is real-world validation. As always, validation is the only way to truly ensure that a medical application of ML is safe and effective. This would mean that, before actually applying such a domain-shifted model, it would need to be validated again, but this time for the new domain. Often, as stated above, the model will perform poorly after domain shift. In this case, domain adaptation (commonly "transfer learning") is then necessary. This is very common in imaging interpretation using DL algorithms. Such algorithms require massive amounts of training data and computational power to even start recognizing edges, corners, colors, patterns, etc. So, training a DL algorithm for medical image interpretation from scratch is often not feasible in practice. Instead, we have to resort to pre-trained models, which already have some ability to recognize objects (such as models having been trained to distinguish cats and dogs), and use these models in a "transfer learning" approach by continuing their training on a different domain (for example, distinguishing glioblastoma from lymphoma of the brain). Of course, as always, proper validation is also key here.

The problem of domain shifts when applying published models is often that reporting standards are not well-defined for ML in medicine.[86] For example, the exact inclusion and exclusion criteria of a prediction model are not always stated within the web-app for the model itself, which can then easily lead to extrapolation by the end user. Reporting the exact inclusion and exclusion criteria for the training cohort is thus key, as is proper external validation after models are shifted from one domain to another. There is never a way around external validation.

Another potential source of bias during domain shift are confounding variables. Imagine an ML model trained to predict outcome after spinal surgery based on patient multiparametric MRI imaging from multiple centers. Some of these centers will be advanced tertiary care centers to which complex patients were referred. However, simpler surgeries will be conducted regularly at smaller neurosurgical departments. Department expertise might be a valid variable among many for predicting patient outcome, and because of the more complex cases, outcomes at the tertiary centers might be worse than in smaller centers despite great expertise.

If now, however, most of the advanced care centers use the latest type of MRI scanner from a specific manufacturer, while the few smaller centers use older types of scanners from a different manufacturer, the specific type of MRI machine, or rather the way this affects the MRI images themselves, will influence the predictions. If this model is now applied to an independent cohort, it might start associating any images taken with such an older scanner model with a better prognosis, rather than true prognostic markers such as neural compression or degenerative changes.

There are strategies to mitigate the risk of confounders affecting the ML model's predictions, the easiest of which is ensuring an even distribution of scanners. However, especially for models trained on images, it can be difficult to detect such issues unless you specifically look for them.

CONCLUSION

This chapter conveys to the reader the intuitions behind clinically applicable evaluation metrics, and the mathematical basics to conduct these analyses independently. We focus on predictive, diagnostic and prognostic models, as well as applications in imaging. We also discuss the issue of the "domain shift," which is critical when applying trained models to clinical practice. A solid understanding of these issues is paramount for the safe and effective introduction of ML into clinical practice.

REFERENCES

1. Schilling AT, Shah PP, Feghali J, et al. A brief history of machine learning in neurosurgery. In: Staartjes VE, Regli L, Serra C (eds). *Machine Learning in Clinical Neuroscience*. Cham: Springer International Publishing; 2022, pp. 245–50.
2. Hendriksen JMT, Geersing GJ, Moons KGM, de Groot JAH. Diagnostic and prognostic prediction models. *J Thromb Haemost* 2013; 11(s1): 129–41.
3. Clark GM, Zborowski DM, Culbertson JL, et al. Clinical utility of epidermal growth factor receptor expression for selecting patients with advanced non-small cell lung cancer for treatment with erlotinib. *J Thorac Oncol* 2006; 1(8): 837–46.
4. Craddock M, Crockett C, McWilliam A, et al. Evaluation of prognostic and predictive models in the oncology clinic. *Clin Oncol* 2022; 34(2): 102–13.
5. Nasteski V. An overview of the supervised machine learning methods. *HORIZONSB* 2017; 4: 51–62.
6. Tunthanathip T, Sae-heng S, Oearsakul T, et al. Machine learning applications for the prediction of surgical site infection in neurological operations. *Neurosurg Focus* 2019; 47(2): E7.
7. Shimizu T, Suda K, Maki S, et al. Efficacy of a machine learning-based approach in predicting neurological prognosis of cervical spinal cord injury patients following urgent surgery within 24 h after injury. *J Clin Neurosci* 2023; 107: 150–6.
8. Perkins NJ, Schisterman EF. The inconsistency of "optimal" cutpoints obtained using two criteria based on the receiver operating characteristic curve. *Am J Epidemiol* 2006; 163(7): 670–5.
9. Staartjes VE, Kernbach JM. Foundations of machine learning-based clinical prediction modeling: Part III—Model evaluation and other points of significance. In: Staartjes VE, Regli L, Serra C (eds). *Machine Learning in Clinical Neuroscience*. Cham: Springer International Publishing; 2022, pp. 23–31.
10. Huang Y, Li W, Macheret F, et al. A tutorial on calibration measurements and calibration models for clinical prediction models. *J Am Med Inform Assoc* 2020; 27(4): 621–33.
11. Staartjes VE, Stumpo V, Ricciardi L, et al. FUSE-ML: Development and external validation of a clinical prediction model for mid-term outcomes after lumbar spinal fusion for degenerative disease. *Eur Spine J* 2022; 31(10): 2629–38.
12. Hajianfar G, Haddadi Avval A, Hosseini SA, et al. Time-to-event overall survival prediction in glioblastoma multiforme patients using magnetic resonance imaging radiomics. *Radiol Med (Torino)* 2023; 128(12): 1521–34.
13. Park SY, Park JE, Kim H, Park SH. Review of statistical methods for evaluating the performance of survival or other time-to-event prediction models (from conventional to deep learning approaches). *Korean J Radiol* 2021; 22(10): 1697–707.

14. Clark TG, Bradburn MJ, Love SB, Altman DG. Survival analysis part I: Basic concepts and first analyses. *Br J Cancer* 2003; 89(2): 232–8.
15. Steck H, Krishnapuram B, Dehing-oberije C, et al. On ranking in survival analysis: Bounds on the concordance index. Advances in Neural Information Processing Systems, 2007. Available from: https://proceedings.neurips.cc/paper_files/paper/2007/hash/33e8075e9970de0cfea955afd4644bb2-Abstract.html (Accessed May 2026).
16. Harrell FE Jr, Califf RM, Pryor DB, et al. Evaluating the yield of medical tests. *JAMA* 1982; 247(18): 2543–6.
17. Kamarudin AN, Cox T, Kolamunnage-Dona R. Time-dependent ROC curve analysis in medical research: Current methods and applications. *BMC Med Res Methodol* 2017; 17(1): 53.
18. Heagerty PJ, Zheng Y. Survival model predictive accuracy and ROC curves. *Biometrics* 2005; 61(1): 92–105.
19. RDocumentation. varImp: Calculation of variable importance for regression and classification models. Available from: https://www.rdocumentation.org/packages/caret/versions/6.0-92/topics/varImp (Accessed May 2026).
20. Gevrey M, Dimopoulos I, Lek S. Review and comparison of methods to study the contribution of variables in artificial neural network models. *Ecol Model* 2003; 160(3): 249–64.
21. LeCun Y, Jackel L, Bottou L, et al. Comparison of learning algorithms for handwritten digit recognition. In: *International Conference on Artificial Neural Networks*. Perth, Australia; 1995, pp. 53–60.
22. Lecun Y, Bottou L, Bengio Y, Haffner P. Gradient-based learning applied to document recognition. *Proc IEEE* 1998; 86(11): 2278–324.
23. Hinton GE, Osindero S, Teh YW. A fast learning algorithm for deep belief nets. *Neural Comput* 2006; 18(7): 1527–54.
24. Nair V, Hinton GE. Rectified linear units improve restricted boltzmann machines. In: *Proceedings of the 27th International Conference on Machine Learning* (ICML-10). 2010; pp. 807–14.
25. Krizhevsky A, Sutskever I, Hinton GE. ImageNet classification with deep convolutional neural networks. In: Advances in Neural Information Processing Systems, 2012. Available from: https://proceedings.neurips.cc/paper/2012/hash/c399862d3b9d6b76c8436e924a68c45b-Abstract.html (Accessed May 2026).
26. Chan HP, Samala RK, Hadjiiski LM, Zhou C. Deep learning in medical image analysis. In: Lee G, Fujita H (eds). *Deep Learning in Medical Image Analysis: Challenges and Applications*. Cham: Springer International Publishing; 2020, pp. 3–21.
27. Baid U, Ghodasara S, Mohan S, et al. The RSNA-ASNR-MICCAI BraTS 2021 benchmark on brain tumor segmentation and radiogenomic classification. *arXiv:2107.02314v2*, 2021.
28. Menze B, Jakab A, Bauer S, et al. Proceedings of the MICCAI Challenge on Multimodal Brain Tumor Image Segmentation (BraTS) 2012. In: MICCAI challenge on multimodal brain tumor image segmentation (BraTS). MICCAI; 2012, p. 77.
29. Mohsen H, El-Dahshan ESA, El-Horbaty ESM, Salem ABM. Classification using deep learning neural networks for brain tumors. *Future Comput Inform J* 2018; 3(1): 68–71.
30. Isensee F, Jäger PF, Full PM, et al. nnU-Net for brain tumor segmentation. In: Crimi A, Bakas S (eds). *Brainlesion: Glioma, Multiple Sclerosis, Stroke and Traumatic Brain Injuries*. Cham: Springer International Publishing; 2021, pp. 118–32.
31. Abramson HG, Curry EJ, Mess G, et al. Automatic detection of foreign body objects in neurosurgery using a deep learning approach on intraoperative ultrasound images: From animal models to first in-human testing. *Front Surg* 2022; 9: 1040066.
32. Staartjes VE, Volokitin A, Regli L, et al. Machine vision for real-time intraoperative anatomic guidance: A proof-of-concept study in endoscopic pituitary surgery. *Oper Neurosurg* 2021; 21(4): 242.
33. Zanier O, Theiler S, Da Mutten R, et al. TomoRay: Generating synthetic computed tomography of the spine from biplanar radiographs. *Neurospine* 2024; 21(1): 68–75.

34. Schonfeld E, Veeravagu A. Demonstrating the successful application of synthetic learning in spine surgery for training multi–center models with increased patient privacy. *Sci Rep* 2023; 13: 12481.
35. Hafiz AM, Bhat GM. A Survey on instance segmentation: State of the art. *Int J Multimed Inf Retr* 2020; 9(3): 171–89.
36. Kirillov A, He K, Girshick R, et al. Panoptic segmentation. *arXiv:1801.00868v3*, 2019.
37. scikit-learn. 3.3. Metrics and scoring: quantifying the quality of predictions. Available from: https://scikit-learn/stable/modules/model_evaluation.html (Accessed May 2026).
38. Jaccard P. The distribution of the flora in the alpine zone. *New Phytol* 1912; 11(2): 37–50.
39. Sorensen T. A method of establishing groups of equal amplitude in plant sociology based on similarity of species content and its application to analyses of the vegetation on Danish commons. *Biol Skr* 1948; 5: 1–34.
40. Zanier O, Da Mutten R, Vieli M, et al. DeepEOR: Automated perioperative volumetric assessment of variable grade gliomas using deep learning. *Acta Neurochir (Wien)* 2023; 165(2): 555–66.
41. Nguyen HT, Tran TB, Luong HH, Huynh TKN. Decoders configurations based on U-Net family and feature pyramid network for COVID-19 segmentation on CT images. *PeerJ Comput Sci* 2021; 7: e719.
42. Reinke A, Maier-Hein L, Müller H (eds). Common limitations of performance metrics in biomedical image analysis. *Proceedings of Medical Imaging with Deep Learning* (MIDL), 2021.
43. Zhang Y, Liu S, Li C, Wang J. Rethinking the dice loss for deep learning lesion segmentation in medical images. *J Shanghai Jiaotong Univ Sci* 2021; 26(1): 93–102.
44. Dolz J, Desrosiers C, Ben Ayed I. 3D Fully convolutional networks for subcortical segmentation in MRI: A large-scale study. *NeuroImage* 2018; 170: 456–70.
45. Wang P, Chung ACS. Focal dice loss and image dilation for brain tumor segmentation. In: Stoyanov D, Taylor Z, Carneiro G, et al. (eds). *Deep Learning in Medical Image Analysis and Multimodal Learning for Clinical Decision Support*. Cham: Springer International Publishing; 2018, pp. 119–27.
46. Salehi SSM, Erdogmus D, Gholipour A. Tversky loss function for image segmentation using 3D fully convolutional deep networks. In: Wang Q, Shi Y, Suk HI, Suzuki K (eds). *Machine Learning in Medical Imaging*. Cham: Springer International Publishing; 2017, pp. 379–87.
47. Huttenlocher DP, Klanderman GA, Rucklidge WJ. Comparing images using the Hausdorff distance. *IEEE Trans Pattern Anal Mach Intell* 1993; 15(9): 850–63.
48. Menze BH, Jakab A, Bauer S, et al. The multimodal brain tumor image segmentation benchmark (BRATS). *IEEE Trans Med Imaging* 2015; 34(10): 1993–2024.
49. Karimi D, Salcudean SE. Reducing the Hausdorff distance in medical image segmentation with convolutional neural networks. *IEEE Trans Med Imaging* 2020; 39(2): 499–513.
50. Jena R, Zhornyak L, Doiphode N, et al. Beyond mAP: Towards better evaluation of instance segmentation. In: *2023 IEEE/CVF Conference on Computer Vision and Pattern Recognition* (CVPR). Vancouver, Canada: IEEE; 2023, pp. 11309–18.
51. Kirillov A, He K, Girshick R, et al. Panoptic segmentation. In: *Proceedings of the IEEE/CVF Conference on Computer Vision and Pattern Recognition* (CVPR), 2019. Available from: https://openaccess.thecvf.com/content_CVPR_2019/html/Kirillov_Panoptic_Segmentation_CVPR_2019_paper.html (Accessed May 2026).
52. Wu X, Sahoo D, Hoi SCH. Recent advances in deep learning for object detection. *Neurocomputing* 2020; 396: 39–64.
53. Sarda A, Dixit S, Bhan A. Object detection for autonomous driving using YOLO [You Only Look Once] algorithm. In: *2021 Third International Conference on Intelligent Communication Technologies and Virtual Mobile Networks* (ICICV), 2021. Available from: https://ieeexplore.ieee.org/document/9388577 (Accessed May 2026).
54. Wosner O, Farjon G, Bar-Hillel A. Object detection in agricultural contexts: A multiple resolution benchmark and comparison to human. *Comput Electron Agric* 2021; 189: 106404.
55. Usamentiaga R, Lema DG, Pedrayes OD, Garcia DF. Automated surface defect

detection in metals: A comparative review of object detection and semantic segmentation using deep learning. *IEEE Trans Ind Appl* 2022; 58(3): 4203–13.

56. Everingham M, Van Gool L, Williams CKI, et al. The Pascal Visual Object Classes (VOC) Challenge. *Int J Comput Vis* 2010; 88(2): 303–38.
57. Lin TY, Maire M, Belongie S, et al. Microsoft COCO: Common objects in context. In: Fleet D, Pajdla T, Schiele B (eds). *Computer Vision—ECCV 2014*. Cham: Springer International Publishing; 2014, pp. 740–55.
58. Han J, Zhang D, Cheng G, et al. Advanced deep-learning techniques for salient and category-specific object detection: A survey. *IEEE Signal Process Mag* 2018; 35(1): 84–100.
59. Padilla R, Netto SL, da Silva EAB. A survey on performance metrics for object-detection algorithms. In: *2020 International Conference on Systems, Signals and Image Processing* (IWSSIP), 2020. Available from: https://ieeexplore.ieee.org/abstract/document/9145130 (Accessed May 2026).
60. Henderson P, Ferrari V. End-to-end training of object class detectors for mean average precision. In: Lai SH, Lepetit V, Nishino K (eds). *Computer Vision—ACCV 2016*. Cham: Springer International Publishing; 2017, pp. 198–213.
61. Ultralytics. YOLO Leistungsmetriken. Available from: https://docs.ultralytics.com/de/guides/yolo-performance-metrics (Accessed May 2026).
62. Liu Y, Lei Y, Wang T, et al. CBCT-based synthetic CT generation using deep-attention cycleGAN for pancreatic adaptive radiotherapy. *Med Phys* 2020; 47(6): 2472–83.
63. Liao H, Huo Z, Sehnert WJ, et al. Adversarial sparse-view CBCT artifact reduction. In: Frangi AF, Schnabel JA, Davatzikos C et al. (eds). *Medical Image Computing and Computer Assisted Intervention—MICCAI 2018*. Cham: Springer International Publishing; 2018, pp. 154–62.
64. Jing Y, Yang Y, Feng Z, et al. Neural style transfer: A review. *IEEE Trans Vis Comput Graph* 2020; 26(11): 3365–85.
65. Bourbonne V, Jaouen V, Hognon C, et al. Dosimetric validation of a GAN-based pseudo-CT generation for MRI-only stereotactic brain radiotherapy. *Cancers* 2021; 13(5): 1082.
66. Kazemifar S, Barragán Montero AM, Souris K, et al. Dosimetric evaluation of synthetic CT generated with GANs for MRI-only proton therapy treatment planning of brain tumors. *J Appl Clin Med Phys* 2020; 21(5): 76–86.
67. Maspero M, Bentvelzen LG, Savenije MHF, et al. Deep learning-based synthetic CT generation for paediatric brain MR-only photon and proton radiotherapy. *Radiother Oncol* 2020; 153: 197–204.
68. Saravi B, Guzel HE, Zink A, et al. Synthetic 3D spinal vertebrae reconstruction from biplanar x-rays utilizing generative adversarial networks. *J Pers Med* 2023; 13(12): 1642.
69. Patil A, Serrato P, Chisvo N, et al. Large language models in neurosurgery: A systematic review and meta-analysis. *Acta Neurochir (Wien)* 2024; 166(1): 475.
70. Dubinski D, Won SY, Trnovec S, et al. Leveraging artificial intelligence in neurosurgery—unveiling ChatGPT for neurosurgical discharge summaries and operative reports. *Acta Neurochir (Wien)* 2024; 166(1): 38.
71. Zhai Y, Chen Z, Luo X, et al. Generation of surgical reports for lymph node dissection during laparoscopic gastric cancer surgery based on artificial intelligence. *Int J Comput Assist Radiol Surg* 2025; 20(5): 1025–33.
72. Edmund JM, Nyholm T. A review of substitute CT generation for MRI-only radiation therapy. *Radiat Oncol* 2017; 12(1): 1–15.
73. Sara U, Akter M, Uddin MS. Image quality assessment through FSIM, SSIM, MSE and PSNR—A comparative study. *J Comput Commun* 2019; 7(3): 8–18.
74. Horé A, Ziou D. Image quality metrics: PSNR vs. SSIM. In: *2010 20th International Conference on Pattern Recognition*, 2010. Available from: https://ieeexplore.ieee.org/abstract/document/5596999 (Accessed May 2026).
75. Huynh-Thu Q, Ghanbari M. The accuracy of PSNR in predicting video quality for different video scenes and frame rates. *Telecommun Syst* 2012; 49(1): 35–48.
76. Wang Z, Bovik AC, Sheikh HR, Simoncelli EP. Image quality assessment: From error visibility to structural similarity. *IEEE Trans Image Process* 2004; 13(4): 600–12.

77. Renieblas GP, Nogués AT, González AM, et al. Structural similarity index family for image quality assessment in radiological images. *J Med Imaging* 2017; 4(3): 035501.
78. Egiazarian K, Astola J, Ponomarenko N, et al. New full-reference quality metrics based on HVS. In: *Proceedings of the Second International Workshop on Video Processing and Quality Metrics*, 2006. Available from: https://www.semanticscholar.org/paper/A-NEW-FULL-REFERENCE-QUALITY-METRICS-BASED-ON-HVS-Egiazarian-Astola/cf7dee64f8a0bcd31aa82ba7fda80463743ffd90 (Accessed May 2026).
79. Wang Z, Simoncelli EP, Bovik AC. Multiscale structural similarity for image quality assessment. In: *The 37th Asilomar Conference on Signals, Systems & Computers*, 2003. Available from: https://ieeexplore.ieee.org/document/1292216 (Accessed May 2026).
80. Heusel M, Ramsauer H, Unterthiner T, et al. GANs trained by a two time-scale update rule converge to a local Nash equilibrium. In: *Advances in Neural Information Processing Systems*, 2017. Available from: https://proceedings.neurips.cc/paper_files/paper/2017/hash/8a1d694707eb0fefe65871369074926d-Abstract.html (Accessed May 2026).
81. Papineni K, Roukos S, Ward T, Zhu WJ. Bleu: A method for automatic evaluation of machine translation. In: Isabelle P, Charniak E, Lin D (eds). *Proceedings of the 40th Annual Meeting of the Association for Computational Linguistics*. Philadelphia: Association for Computational Linguistics; 2002, pp. 311–18.
82. Lin CY. ROUGE: A package for automatic evaluation of summaries. In: Text Summarization Branches Out, 2004. Available from: https://aclanthology.org/W04-1013/ (Accessed May 2026).
83. Banerjee S, Lavie A. METEOR: An automatic metric for MT evaluation with improved correlation with human judgments. In: Goldstein J, Lavie A, Lin CY, Voss C (eds). *Proceedings of the ACL Workshop on Intrinsic and Extrinsic Evaluation Measures for Machine Translation and/or Summarization*. Ann Arbor: Association for Computational Linguistics; 2005, pp. 65–72.
84. Zhang T, Kishore V, Wu F, et al. BERTScore: Evaluating text generation with BERT. *arXiv: 1904.09675v3*, 2020.
85. Singal AG, Higgins PDR, Waljee AK. A primer on effectiveness and efficacy trials. *Clin Transl Gastroenterol* 2014; 5(1): e45.
86. Ciobanu-Caraus O, Aicher A, Kernbach JM, et al. A critical moment in machine learning in medicine: On reproducible and interpretable learning. *Acta Neurochir (Wien)* 2024; 166(1): 14.

20

Using Operating Room Audio and Video for Predictive Analytics

RECAI YILMAZ, DHIRAJ PANGAL AND DANIEL DONOHO

INTRODUCTION

Predictive analytics derived from the neurosurgical operating room (OR) hold the promise of forecasting future events and outcomes, guiding interventions and improving safety and efficiency. Intraprocedural data include a vast array of video, audio, waveform, tabular and time series data collected by a plethora of sensors during surgery. These data—including audio from team communications and video from surgical cameras—provide a rich source of information that can be harnessed to develop predictive models. These models can analyze patterns and trends, offering predictions about surgical complications, workflow inefficiencies, or equipment usage, among other factors.[1,2]

This chapter focuses on the specific application of audio and video data for predictive analytics in the OR. While traditional clinical data sources, such as electronic health records (EHRs) and physiological monitors, have been extensively studied, the potential of intraprocedural audio and video data remains relatively untapped. By exploring the integration of these multimodal data sources, we aim to shed light on their unique contributions to predictive analytics in surgery. We will also discuss how data sources specific to neurosurgery can be built into the flow of a real-time data pipeline.

DATA SOURCES IN THE OPERATING ROOM

In the OR, a diverse array of data sources contributes to a comprehensive understanding of the surgical environment (**Figure 20.1**). Among these, audio and video data stand out for their potential to provide detailed insights into surgical procedures and team dynamics.[3] This section explores the types and sources of audio and video data commonly encountered in the OR, as well as the integration of these modalities to create a cohesive data environment.

VIDEO DATA

Surgical video

There is a growing percentage of video performed with intraoperative visualization tools (e.g. laparoscope, microscope). In conjunction with improved artificial intelligence (AI) methods to "view" and analyze that video, surgical video is a rich source of data for predictive analytics. Within neurosurgery, data from the endoscope, microscope or exoscope demonstrates the interaction between anatomy, pathology and instrumentation. Analyzing these interactions, using methodologies such as computer vision (CV), and developing predictive models is a growing field of interest.[4]

DOI: 10.1201/9781003471165-20

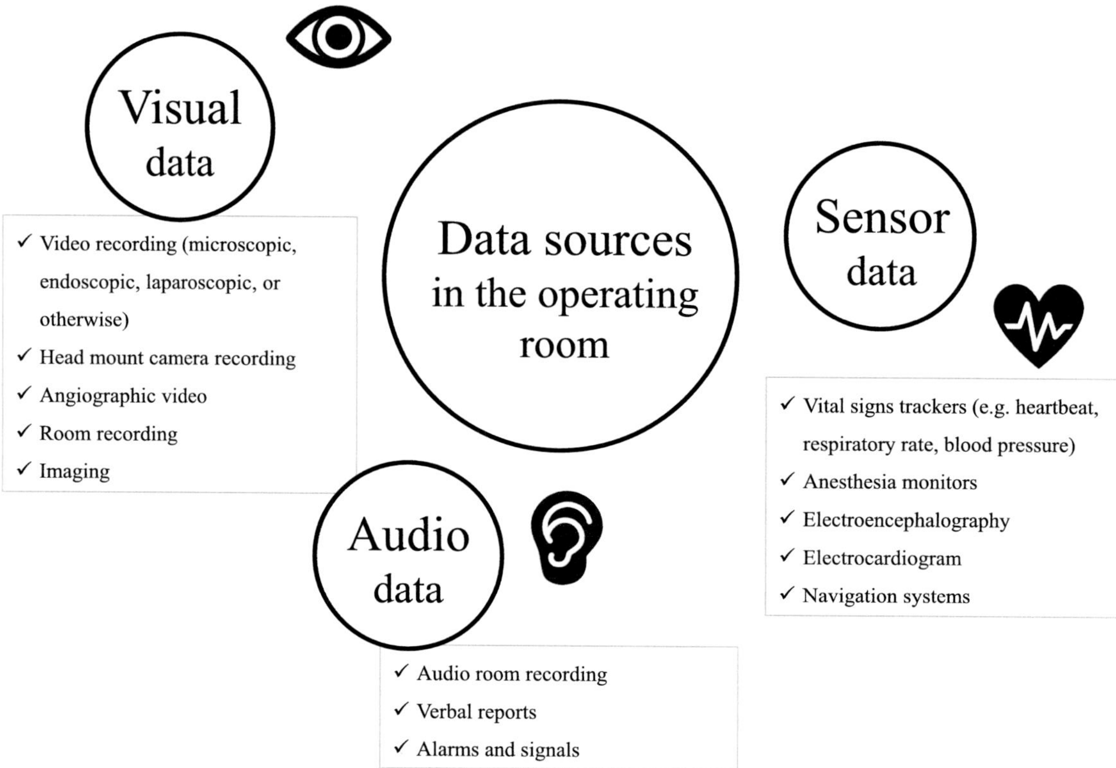

Figure 20.1 Data sources in the operating room. Intraoperative environment is a data-rich setting, encompassing visual, auditory and sensory data.

Angiographic video

While not necessarily "video" in the traditional sense, visual data from angiography suites contain critical information on the deployment of catheters, stents, coils and other endovascular devices. The real-time fluoroscopy data is often not saved unless specifically designated, but the combination of real-time fluoroscopy and the angiographic "runs" which comprise an interventional radiology case (sequences of images or a clip) can be classified as a type of procedural data.[5]

Ambient video

In the OR, ambient video refers to recordings that capture the overall environment, providing a broader context to the surgical procedure. Unlike focused procedural videos, ambient videos are often captured by cameras placed at strategic points within the OR—sometimes on overhead OR lights, in room corners (e.g. "security" camera footage), etc. These recordings include wide-angle views that encompass the surgical team, equipment and the patient. This type of video is particularly valuable for understanding the dynamics of team interactions, workflow patterns and the movement of equipment and personnel.[6]

Point-of-view video

Point-of-view (POV) video, often captured through wearable devices such as surgical loupes equipped with cameras or egocentric cameras, provides a unique and highly detailed perspective of the surgical field from the surgeon's viewpoint.[7] POV videos are particularly valuable for analyzing surgical techniques and decision-making processes at a granular level for open procedures that do not utilize surgical visualization devices such as microscopes, exoscopes or endoscopes. Predictive analytics for actions in open spine surgery, for instance, could be derived from the rich data provided from egocentric, surgeon-mounted cameras.

AUDIO DATA

Speech

Speech data can be captured through a variety of sources via a microphone. The OR in general has fewer opportunities for the natural detection of speech than video, however, with the increasing use of broadcasted surgeries, telemedicine and robotics, speech is a growing medium of capturing a surgical team's interactions and communications.[8]

Alarms and signals

The OR is filled with alarms and bells from various sensors. These could be routine vitals monitoring, distress signals or signals that an instrument is on (e.g. bipolar cautery, drills, etc.). Similarly, these are not routinely captured, but if coupled with intraoperative actions could be a rich source of intraoperative action data.

TECHNOLOGICAL INFRASTRUCTURE

The successful implementation of audio and video-based predictive analytics in the OR depends heavily on a robust technological infrastructure for data collection and analysis. This infrastructure encompasses the hardware for data capture and analysis, the software for data processing and analysis and the systems for secure storage and management of sensitive information (**Figure 20.2**). In this section, we discuss the key components of this infrastructure and the challenges associated with its deployment in a clinical setting.

Recording devices and storage

The recording of audio and video comes from cameras and microphones either embedded within the operating theater, within individual operative tools (e.g.

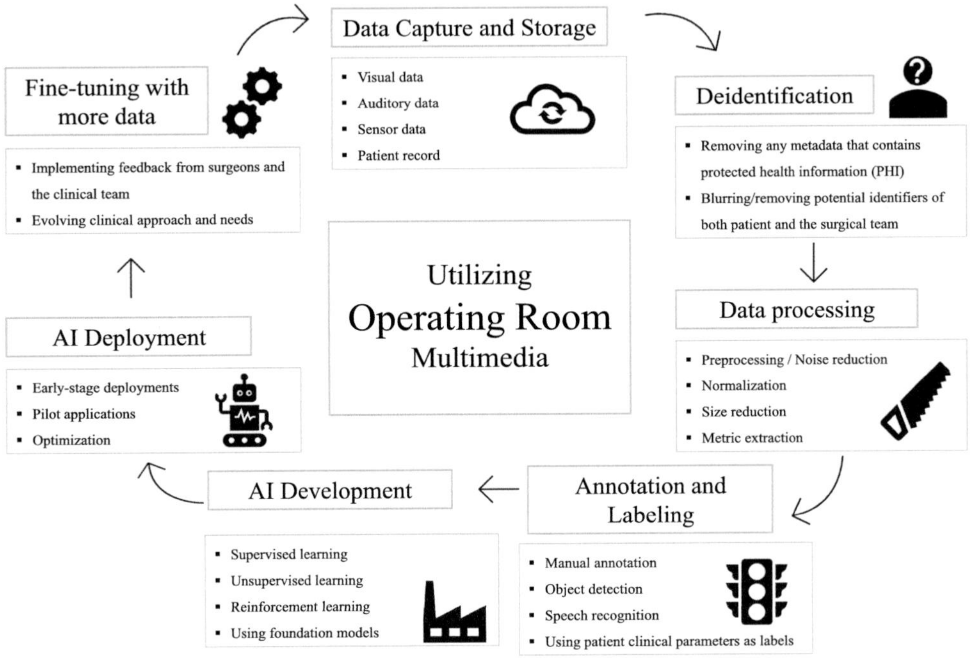

Figure 20.2 A general framework for leveraging operating room multimedia. An intraoperative AI application may incorporate strategies for collecting high-yield intraoperative data, protecting patient information, developing AI models with reliable performance, conducting early pilot deployments to ensure safety and facilitate improvement and fine-tuning the system to remain aligned with evolving needs and expectations.

microscope), or worn by surgeons or staff members on their person. Particularly in neurosurgery where cases routinely run for 8–10 hours, the storage of gigabytes of data per case, and petabytes of data per OR per year, becomes a central logistical and technical challenge.

Many OR camera towers have local storage with ~2 terabytes of video. However, with modern 4K cameras, any individual case may routinely take up ~20 GB worth of storage, rendering the entire tower capable of holding only ~50 cases before running out of room.

The systematic retrieval and storage of OR video is a challenge. While device providers often offer the ability to upload video directly to a cloud storage platform, most hospital infrastructures do not have the bandwidth in the OR to securely transmit such high volumes of data and the costs of commercial cloud storage are high. This is an unmet need and a necessity for developing predictive analytics for the OR.

Security and safety infrastructure

Following data upload, the security and safety of this data are paramount. First, de-identification steps must be taken to remove any metadata (e.g. filenames, textual tags) that contains protected health information (PHI). Second, for audio and video data, an automated process must be employed to "scrub" any sensitive data since manual obscuration of PHI is impractical at scale. These systems should be capable of removing names or identifiers in audio recordings, depictions of whole faces and other identifying data.[9]

Data processing

Effective data pre-processing and annotation are critical steps in preparing OR audio and video data for predictive analytics. These processes ensure that the data are clean, consistent, and appropriately labeled, facilitating accurate model training and analysis. This section outlines the key techniques used for pre-processing audio and video data, the methods for annotating these data, and the challenges related to data privacy and security.

Pre-processing tools and techniques

Before analysis, audio and video data often require pre-processing, such as noise reduction, normalization and segmentation. Specialized software can automate these processes, preparing the data for further analysis.

Audio data pre-processing

- *Noise Reduction*: ORs are noisy environments, with a mix of machine sounds, alarms and human speech. Noise reduction techniques, such as spectral subtraction and adaptive filtering, are used to isolate relevant audio signals from background noise.
- *Segmentation*: Audio data are segmented into meaningful units, such as individual words or sentences, which can be critical for speech recognition and analysis. This segmentation can be time-based or event-based, depending on the application.
- *Normalization*: Audio normalization adjusts the volume levels across different recordings to ensure consistency. This process helps in comparing data from different sessions or sources on a common scale.

Video data pre-processing

- *Frame Extraction and Selection*: Video data consists of numerous frames, many of which may be redundant. Frame extraction techniques select keyframes that capture critical moments or actions, reducing the data volume while preserving important information.
- *Image Enhancement*: Techniques such as contrast adjustment, deblurring and color correction are applied to enhance the quality of video frames. This step is particularly important in improving the visibility of anatomic details and surgical actions.
- *Motion Tracking*: Motion tracking algorithms are used to follow the movement of surgical instruments, team members or anatomic structures. These data are valuable for analyzing procedural dynamics and interactions.

Manual annotation

- *Labeling*: Manual annotation involves human experts reviewing audio and video data to label specific events, actions or features. This process can include labeling speech segments with the speaker's identity, tagging specific surgical instruments or noting critical procedural steps.
- *Transcription*: For audio data, transcription converts spoken words into written text, providing a searchable and analyzable text dataset. This is

particularly useful for speech recognition and natural language processing applications.

Automated annotation

- *Object Detection and Recognition*: Automated annotation tools use machine learning (ML) models to detect and recognize objects or actions in video data. For example, these tools can identify surgical instruments, monitor usage patterns or recognize specific surgical techniques.
- *Speech Recognition*: Automated speech recognition (ASR) systems transcribe spoken language in real time, offering a quick and scalable way to annotate large datasets. These systems can be trained to recognize medical terminology and context-specific vocabulary.

BUILDING AND IMPLEMENTING PREDICTIVE ANALYTICS MODELS

Predictive analytics in the OR leverage advanced ML and deep learning (DL) techniques to analyze audio and video data, offering valuable insights and forecasts that can improve surgical outcomes and operational efficiency. This section provides an overview of the key predictive models used in this context, highlighting their methodologies, applications and some case studies of successful implementations.

PAIRING ARTIFICIAL INTELLIGENCE TECHNIQUES WITH MULTIMEDIA DATA

Kinematic data from instrument movement

AI, more specifically CV models, can identify and track surgical instruments.[10] This capability enables the assessment of instrument motion over time, known as kinematics, which may help to identify patterns or surgical techniques that reveal the expertise level of the surgeon or the trainee or are influential on procedural outcome.[11] Few systems exist that can reliably identify surgical expertise or optimal performance across domains and tasks. Developing AI systems may help to assess and benchmark the expertise level of the surgeon, identify critical instrument movements and risks, and explore correlations between performance metrics and clinical outcomes. Such systems receive the same visual info that the surgeon sees (such as an endoscopic camera view), and in the future, may become able to provide feedback for risk mitigation and improved outcomes similar to feedback systems in simulation systems.[12]

For instance, kinematic data on how often and where hemostatic agents are used could be tracked with subjective surgeon assessments of "bloodiness" and correlated with postoperative blood loss or need for transfusions. This provides a granular and segmented way to analyze blood loss. This is one example of the ways in which clinical data and kinematic data are paired together to answer new research questions.

Predictive modeling with critical anatomy

Besides detecting surgical instruments, CV models are also used to identify anatomic structures, which may help the surgeon navigate the surgery and avoid the risk of injuring critical structures.[13] Each surgery is unique and different anatomic landmarks may be of importance. Proper identification and assessment (pathologic vs normal) of these structures may lead to variations in the surgical approach, the outcome and the risks associated with surgery. In the future, AI systems may provide real-time feedback to the surgeon and provide warnings about the surrounding tissues to increase the surgeon's awareness and help mitigate technical errors.

These models can be used as critical intraoperative safety stops. For instance, high-fidelity detection of standard anatomy at risk during surgery (e.g. carotid artery during endoscopic endonasal surgeries), could allow for a "safety stop" if high-risk instruments come within a pre-specified distance from the vessel.[14,15]

Using audio data to ask and answer questions

Similar to the airline industry, ORs are being integrated with black boxes that continuously capture audio, and optionally, video and vital signs data.[16] However, to date, this technology has not been integrated with AI to provide real-time operative surveillance and assistance. In AI, speech-to-text and text-to-speech technologies are rather advanced. These methodologies enable the transcription of human conversation to text for computer analysis, as well as the conversion of computer-generated text to audio to enable computers to "speak." Using text generated by large language models (LLMs) such as generative pre-trained transformers (GPTs), a conversation back and forth between the surgeon and the AI system could improve surgical processes. Intraoperative surveillance data could be integrated into the system. While a surgeon could notify the AI about the situation and ask specific questions, AI surveillance systems could provide instant information based on the comprehensive audio, video and vital signs data it captures in real time.[17]

Anomaly detection in neurosurgery

Fortunately, complications and errors in neurosurgery are only a small minority of events. However, due to the resulting patient morbidity, mortality and increased costs, detecting and intervening in these suboptimal applications is highly important. AI offers a variety of solutions, such as unsupervised learning and clustering, to detect unusual patterns that may indicate suboptimal instances of events.[18] Increasing the awareness of the surgeon about these events, as well as triggering automated correction mechanisms, may increase the efficiency of the surgery and safety.

Predictive analytics for training and education

Traditional educational methodology and tools fall short in quantifying trainee surgical technical skills and providing objective and tailored feedback. AI has been shown to identify the year of neurosurgery residency training only by looking at trainee bimanual skills demonstrated during a simulated tumor resection task and providing more efficient feedback than human instructors.[19] These developments indicate that in the future, AI systems may exceed human performance in assessing actual operative skills in real time and become increasingly critical to teaching and evaluation of both learners and practicing surgeons. These systems can be deployed in simulation and real-life settings to enhance trainee engagement and learning, identify high-teaching utility events, and provide trainees with comprehensive information about their learning interaction.[20]

CURRENT EXAMPLES IN PRACTICE

There are multiple examples of AI-based predictive analytics using OR images or audio. Using pictures of surgical sponges/towels, CV systems are able to quantify the amount of blood lost during a case, and accurately guide blood transfusions.[21] These predictive analytics enable surgical teams to both resuscitate patients more accurately and prevent unnecessary waste. Other companies are building the infrastructure to record audio and video data systematically from the OR and provide insight into team communication, movement of team members and predictive analytics surrounding critical safety events. Granularly, companies are working on quantifying operative movements using CV and operative videos. These analytics are being used to assist in trainee development and provide quantitative data on surgical performance postoperatively.

FUTURE DIRECTIONS

Large language models and multimodal models

Due to popular innovations like ChatGPT, our field is increasing efforts to build predictive models that utilize both speech and language understanding.[22] Models which incorporate video, audio and/or speech are referred to as "multimodal models." Their utility within neurosurgery has been somewhat muted, however, there is a high likelihood we will see significant improvements in their functionality in the coming months to years.

Human-in-the-loop approach

One key forward-looking AI framework in medicine is the human-in-the-loop model. A human-in-the-loop approach allows AI-powered systems to function under the supervision of clinicians to ensure their effective and safe operation.[23] This model may be highly important in high-stakes clinical environments such as the OR where reliability and accuracy is at a premium. Often, these systems are not designed to replace human experts but rather to complement their judgment and focus their attention on critical elements that may be overlooked. Clinicians' oversight can play an important role in guiding these systems to adhere to clinical care standards and interpretations. In certain modes, these systems may reliably replicate expert decisions in an automated fashion to alleviate the demands on clinicians and increase their ability to assess and intervene in imperfect applications. AI-powered systems based on expert input may offer a more successful integration in clinical practice as they will offer a more relevant service in meeting the needs of the clinicians. The ability of future clinicians to efficiently utilize AI technologies may become a crucial factor in their productivity and accuracy.

Automated feedback

In high-pressure, minimal error environments such as the neurosurgical OR, critical feedback is integral for improvement as a trainee. However, following training, surgeons lose a critical feedback mechanism which training afforded. ML tools built on top of surgical video could allow for the thoughts of surgical mentors or experts to be applied to surgical video, enabling automated feedback even outside of training.

Potential pitfalls

Many AI models, particularly complex architectures such as DL models, operate as "black boxes," where model outputs are reported without revealing the underlying computations or reasoning that led to the outputs. This lack of transparency can be problematic in high-stakes fields, such as neurosurgery, where accountability, safety and trust are paramount.[24] Intraoperative video and audio information are inherently high-bandwidth modalities and DL systems often "learn" to make decisions utilizing this data-rich environment through methods that differ from human experts, increasing the complexity of the AI–human teaming process. Further, AI models are prone to acquire biases that might be difficult to identify. These biases may be acquired during data collection or AI model development and may be missed during testing and pilot applications. Biases result in suboptimal decision-making, and differences in performance between subgroups of patient cases. Last but not least, AI models may have significant challenges in generalizing to unseen data. An AI system developed in one clinical setting may not be reliably used in another clinical setting without fine-tuning and testing to achieve optimal accuracy across different clinical environments. Continued monitoring of production system performance will be increasingly important as more complex systems are developed and brought into the OR.

CONCLUSION

The neurosurgical OR contains rich potential data sources that are currently unstudied, including audio and video data. These data sources can be used to develop predictive analytics to improve surgical performance and optimize outcomes. We described the types of systems that can be implemented using existing technology to collect audiovisual data, process audiovisual signals and generate predictive analytics. In the coming years, as the value of these data are increasingly recognized, we anticipate continued proliferation of a variety of novel data collection and analysis systems. Surgeons should familiarize themselves with the opportunities, and pitfalls, of these systems and analytics as they increasingly become a part of daily surgical practice.

REFERENCES

1. Chadebecq F, Vasconcelos F, Mazomenos E, Stoyanov D. Computer vision in the surgical operating room. *Visc Med* 2020; 36(6): 456–62.
2. Hashimoto DA, Rosman G, Rus D, Meireles OR. Surgical video in the age of big data. *Ann Surg* 2018; 268(6): e47–e8.
3. van de Graaf FW, Eryigit Ö, Lange JF. Current perspectives on video and audio recording inside the surgical operating room: Results of a cross-disciplinary survey. *Updates Surg* 2021; 73(5): 2001–7.
4. Pangal DJ, Donoho DA. "Are we recording this?" Surgeons deserve next-generation analytics. *J Neurosurg* 2023; 139(6): 1792–5.
5. Green NE, Chen S-YJ, Hansgen AR, et al. Angiographic views used for percutaneous coronary interventions: A three-dimensional analysis of physician-determined vs. computer-generated views. *Catheter Cardiovasc Interv* 2005; 64(4): 451–9.

6. Al Abbas AI, Meier J, Daniel W, et al. Impact of team performance on the surgical safety checklist on patient outcomes: An operating room black box analysis. *Surg Endosc* 2024; 38(10): 5613–22.
7. Koskinen J. Computational evaluation of microsurgical skills, 2022. Available from: https://erepo.uef.fi/items/f3e8ca33-b78f-427a-8993-7cc3b0906c74 (Accessed May 2026).
8. Fuchtmann J, Riedel T, Berlet M, et al. Audio-based event detection in the operating room. *Int J Comput Assist Radiol Surg* 2024; 19(12): 2381–7.
9. Pangal DJ, Kugener G, Shahrestani S, et al. A guide to annotation of neurosurgical intraoperative video for machine learning analysis and computer vision. *World Neurosurg* 2021; 150: 26–30.
10. Esteva A, Chou K, Yeung S, et al. Deep learning-enabled medical computer vision. *NPJ Digit Med* 2021; 4(1): 5.
11. Yang JH, Goodman ED, Dawes AJ, et al. Using AI and computer vision to analyze technical proficiency in robotic surgery. *Surg Endosc* 2023; 37(4): 3010–17.
12. Yilmaz R, Bakhaidar M, Alsayegh A, et al. Real-time multifaceted artificial intelligence vs in-person instruction in teaching surgical technical skills: A randomized controlled trial. *Sci Rep* 2024; 14(1): 15130.
13. Tokuyasu T, Iwashita Y, Matsunobu Y, et al. Development of an artificial intelligence system using deep learning to indicate anatomical landmarks during laparoscopic cholecystectomy. *Surg Endosc* 2021; 35(4): 1651–8.
14. Donoho DA, Pangal DJ, Kugener G, et al. Improved surgeon performance following cadaveric simulation of internal carotid artery injury during endoscopic endonasal surgery: Training outcomes of a nationwide prospective educational intervention. *J Neurosurg* 2021; 135(5): 1347–55.
15. Kugener G, Pangal DJ, Cardinal T, et al. Utility of the simulated outcomes following carotid artery laceration video data set for machine learning applications. *JAMA Netw Open* 2022; 5(3): e223177-e.
16. Guerlain S, Adams RB, Turrentine FB, et al. Assessing team performance in the operating room: Development and use of a "black-box" recorder and other tools for the intraoperative environment. *J Am Coll Surg* 2005; 200(1): 29–37.
17. Hall A, Kawai K, Graber K, et al. Acoustic analysis of surgeons' voices to assess change in the stress response during surgical in situ simulation. *BMJ Simul Technol Enhanc Learn* 2021; 7(6): 471–7.
18. Samuel DJ, Cuzzolin F. Unsupervised anomaly detection for a smart autonomous robotic assistant surgeon (SARAS) using a deep residual autoencoder. *IEEE Robot Autom Lett* 2021; 6(4): 7256–61.
19. Yilmaz R, Winkler-Schwartz A, Mirchi N, et al. Continuous monitoring of surgical bimanual expertise using deep neural networks in virtual reality simulation. *NPJ Digit Med* 2022; 5(1): 54.
20. Yilmaz R. Development, validation, and testing of artificial intelligence systems for assessment and training of simulated surgical technical skills. McGill University, 2024. Available from: https://neurosim.mcgill.ca/wp-content/uploads/2024/07/THESIS-April-2024-FINAL-3.pdf (Accessed May 2026).
21. Holmes AA, Konig G, Ting V, et al. Clinical evaluation of a novel system for monitoring surgical hemoglobin loss. *Anesth Analg* 2014; 119(3): 588–94.
22. Guerra GA, Hofmann H, Sobhani S, et al. GPT-4 Artificial intelligence model outperforms ChatGPT, medical students, and neurosurgery residents on neurosurgery written board-like questions. *World Neurosurg* 2023; 179: e160–e5.
23. Wu X, Xiao L, Sun Y, et al. A survey of human-in-the-loop for machine learning. *Future Gener Comput Syst* 2022; 135: 364–81.
24. Rudin C. Why black box machine learning should be avoided for high-stakes decisions, in brief. *Nat Rev Methods Primers* 2022; 2(1): 81.

21

Advancing Basic Laboratory Research by Artificial Intelligence

ARMAN KOUL, ETHAN SCHONFELD AND ANAND VEERAVAGU

INTRODUCTION

Laboratory research has long been the cornerstone of medical innovation. Notable breakthroughs, such as the isolation and discovery of the unknown protein insulin from a dog's pancreas at the University of Toronto in 1921[1] to the stabilization and crystallization of the G protein-coupled receptor (GPCR) at Stanford in 2007 have revolutionized treatments for diabetes, cardiovascular disease and cancer.[2] Within neurosurgery, basic science research is responsible for the foundational knowledge that allow the surgical ability to modulate the brain. Landmark basic science findings in neurosurgery include Brodmann's cytoarchitectural mapping of the motor cortex[3] and Dandy's animal model studies demonstrating cerebrospinal fluid (CSF) production by the choroid plexus which allowed for the distinguishing of obstructive versus communicating hydrocephalus.[4] The importance of basic science within medicine, including neurosurgery, is just as paramount to this day. Powered by multi-omic technologies, the scale of data generated by and powering basic science is on an unprecedented scale. With the rise of artificial intelligence (AI), the integration of AI into laboratory research is generating significant optimism within the scientific community. This is due to AI's potential to identify signals within this big data, power high-throughput analysis, and eliminate inefficiencies in current research methodologies, significantly accelerating the pace of discoveries.

In traditional academic labs, researchers conduct experiments under a principal investigator's guidance, relying on research grants for funding. These experiments involve various tasks, from pipetting to working with animal models of disease, using specialized equipment like next-generation sequencing (NGS), polymerase chain reaction (PCR) systems and ultra-low temperature freezers. The data generated are meticulously analyzed to produce findings that may lead to clinical trials and eventual therapies that impact patients. This research process demands substantial time and financial resources. However, AI and automation have the potential to streamline and improve many aspects of the described scientific workflow, making it more cost-effective and efficient and ultimately allowing laboratories to operate more effectively. We have summarized the potential applications of AI in basic science research into three key areas:

1. Optimizing candidate selection and therapeutic development.
2. Automating experiments and related tasks.
3. Improving experimental data analysis.

Optimization of experiment selection and therapeutic development

When conducting research in a specific domain, scientists face endless possibilities and ideas to explore. They often narrow this vast sample space based on their mental models and previous

DOI: 10.1201/9781003471165-21

research, forming specific hypotheses. Moreover, these hypothesis are formed by analysis of preliminary data. However, given the vast amounts of multi-omic data and scientific discovery, AI offers a valuable tool for refining these hypotheses earlier in the process, allowing scientists to optimize their research approach and perform more informed experiments.

HIGH-THROUGHPUT SCREENING

Drug discovery is an incredibly lengthy and laborious process. A new medicine takes an average of 10–15 years and more than $2b before becoming available for patients.[5] High-throughput screening (HTS) was an early innovation that added more data to the decision-making process for selecting therapeutic candidates to pursue. Initially, drug discovery involved testing individually synthesized compounds on whole cells, tissue preparations or animal models.[6] HTS was created as a scalable process where compounds from a library could be efficiently tested on a common assay, generating large amounts of standardized data to refine drug development.[7] This process has become substantially more automated and optimized over time and today, automation allows for testing of over 100,000 samples per day against a singular target.[8] However, because of the extensive nature of the compound libraries, the hit rate for most assays is typically below 1%.[9] AI has emerged as a valuable tool to reduce costs and enhance the efficiency of HTS. For instance, iterative screening processes have been proposed that integrate AI-algorithmic filtering to decide what compounds should continue to be screened at each stage.[10] AI platforms like AtomNet developed by Atomwise use convolutional neural networks to analyze vast chemical libraries to help discover new small molecule medicines based on predicted structure.[11] Platforms like these lead some to suggest that AI could eventually replace HTS entirely given sufficient understanding of chemical structure spurred by the development of advanced reasoning models.

STRUCTURE-BASED DRUG DESIGN

Formulating research and developing chemical compound hypotheses based on our understanding of target structures is essential. While HTS excels at generating numerous candidates, simply increasing the number of samples tested is inefficient and costly. AI enables scientists to make more informed and effective attempts. Rather than simply taking more "shots on goal," AI can enable scientists to also take better "shots on goal." Structure-based drug design (SBDD) offers "intelligent" opportunities for drug discovery by using computational techniques such as virtual screening, molecular docking and dynamic simulations.[12] Virtual screening seems to virtually replicate HTS to evaluate drug candidates such as the previously described platform AtomNet. Here, AI automates the analysis of binding affinity through predictive algorithms. SBDD can also suggest the design of synthetically generated *de novo* drugs. These are novel compounds that have not yet been studied *in vitro* for binding to a specific target but are predicted to do so based on computational models. This is challenging due to the incredibly large search space of molecular structures and countless combinations they can form. Here, AI is invaluable in refining this complex process of synthetic drug synthesis. For instance, researchers at the Leiden Academic Centre for Drug Research developed a deep reinforcement learning framework to find a target for the adenosine A2A receptor.[13] The team began by creating a neural network to generate viable molecules, which they fine-tuned with bioactive molecules known to target the A2A receptor. They identified key binding features and used them as quality metrics. Reinforcement learning was used to evaluate the model's effectiveness in generating candidates with strong binding potential, with feedback loops incorporated to improve the generation of effective targets. To increase variability and prevent overfitting to known structures, two recurrent neural networks were integrated into the process. Finally, results showed a model proficient at generating novel viable molecules that have the desired binding characteristics. Projects like these, which harness existing scientific knowledge, well-defined problems, labeled datasets and AI techniques to significantly elevate the quality of future experiments, demonstrate how AI can drive a new era of scientific innovation.

Beyond the selection of initial candidates, SBDD also involves optimizing a hit's chances of success by analyzing their molecular interactions with the target, leading to the design of more potent and selective compounds.[14] Molecular docking is a virtual simulation technique used in SBDD to predict ligand conformation and binding within a target's active site. It involves multiple iterations to explore conformational space and uses scoring functions to rank ligands based on predicted binding energies and complex stability.[15] Various AI-based docking platforms, such as DiffDock,[16] RoseTTAFold All-Atom,[17] Alphafold3[18] and ArtiDock[19] have been developed, each with unique strengths and weaknesses. Since its first success in identifying protease inhibitors for HIV treatment in 1990,[20] SBDD has been instrumental in developing therapies for a wide range of diseases, from urinary tract infections (UTIs) to cancer. Similar applications of AI can be employed to develop similar compounds to known drugs that limit off target effects to reduce therapeutic side effects.[21,22] As AI work continues to advance, its integration with SBDD is expected to drive even more groundbreaking discoveries, ushering in a new era of precision medicine. The future of drug discovery lies not just in taking more shots, but in taking the right shots—SBDD, powered by AI, is poised to make this vision a reality.

Foundation models for biology

Foundation models are large-scale AI models trained on extensive, diverse datasets, enabling them to be fine-tuned for a wide array of applications. Whereas many applications of AI seek to solve one particular task like identifying clusters of samples or predicting the outcome of an intervention, foundation models are distinguished by their versatility and broad applicability, handling various tasks.[23] This is enabled by transfer learning (TL)—the ability of a model to apply knowledge from one task to another, related task. While the concept has existed for some time, recent computational advances have made foundation models more applicable to complex, data-rich fields like biology. Biology is inherently complex and multifaceted, yet it operates under fundamental natural laws. By embedding these principles within foundation models and applying them to various challenges, we can unlock the potential for groundbreaking scientific discoveries.

An example of a foundational model developed for biology is the interdisciplinary team of researchers at Stanford and the Chan Zuckerberg Initiative that developed the Universal Cellular Embedding (UCE) foundation model.[24] UCE provides a universal way to represent any cell, regardless of tissue or species, mapping new cells from previously unobserved organisms into the model's embedding space. Similarly, Evolutionary Scale's ESM3 model is designed to simulate the evolutionary process,[25] generating a novel green fluorescent protein with only 58% identity to a known protein, akin to 500 million years of evolution. These achievements highlight the capability of foundation models to explore vast, previously inaccessible areas of biological space, paving the way for novel and more efficient scientific discoveries. Other foundation models such as AlphaFold for protein structure prediction[26] and DeepNovo for peptide sequencing from mass spectrometry[27] further demonstrate the potential of AI in studying biology. These models act as a base layer that can be fine-tuned for specific applications. As more foundational models are developed in biology, they will pave the way for significant and impactful innovations in research and treatments for patients.

AUTOMATION IN EXPERIMENTS AND SUB-TASKS

Conducting experiments is extremely expensive, driven by the cost of equipment, materials and the training of researchers. Beyond financial costs, the considerable time scientists spend on manual, repetitive tasks detracts from their ability to explore innovative methods and engage deeply with the research questions they aim to answer. These costs, combined with the variability introduced by differing levels of human involvement in sample-handling procedures,[28] result in significant inefficiencies in the experimentation process across many laboratories.

AI-powered automation offers a potential solution to these challenges in both industry and academia. It allows for the routinization of complex but repetitive tasks essential to scientific experimentation. The HTS methods mentioned earlier serve as an excellent example of how automation can drive incredible efficiency upstream in the research process. Ongoing research into other automation techniques shows similarly promising potential.

AI-powered robotics

AI-powered robotic platforms have been developed to enhance timely and cost-efficient experimentation. The "Adam" and "Eve" robots, created at Aberystwyth and Manchester University, exemplify an early iteration of this innovation. "Adam" was constructed to conduct microbial and yeast-growth experiments, while "Eve" was meant to specialize in drug screening and design.[29] These robots are designed to interact with each other in an automated fashion and form a closed system of experimental performance and analysis. This serves to significantly increase the throughput of experiments performed and substantially accelerate the data generation process. Since their development, numerous teams have pursued robotic automation for experimental tasks. Pipetting workstations offer a straightforward solution for automating one of the most manual aspects of lab work—pipetting. These systems, which vary in price and size, help systematize the pipetting process and streamline library preparation for experiments.[30] Additionally, robotic arms like ThermoFisher's F5 Robot and Denso Robotic's VS series have been employed as automation tools for HTS, further enhancing laboratory efficiency. Beyond these more straightforward tasks, robotic automation has the capability to take on more difficult tasks normally reserved for seasoned researchers. A team at MIT successfully trained a robotic arm to carry out AI-planned synthetic routes for small-molecule targets and exhibited proficiency in complex stereochemical awareness.[31] As robots such as these become increasingly complex, they ultimately allow scientists to spend less time on manual experiments and more on ideation and method refinement.

Because of the multifactorial nature of experiments, scientists often have to move samples between different machines within a laboratory. These experiments may also require specialized environments like isolation from UV, noise and vibration.[32] Mobile robots allow for the performance of complex, coordinated tasks, adding another layer of automation to the laboratory setting. These robots have been integrated into various laboratories and have attracted investment from industrial manufacturers like KUKA and conventional biotechnology manufacturers like Thermo-Fisher.

The integration of mobile robots has been shown to greatly improve scientific experimentation, as evidenced by a team at the University of Liverpool that built a modular and automated "robotic chemist." This robot optimized photocatalyst mixtures for hydrogen production from water, achieving a sixfold increase in activity over initial formulations.[33] Advanced robotic systems like this have the potential to address increasingly complex problems across various scientific fields, freeing scientists from manual tasks and allowing them to focus more on ideation and method refinement.

AI-integrated labs

As robots and machines for conducting experiments become more complex, developing sophisticated and optimized infrastructure to run them becomes essential. Many academic and industry researchers are working on solutions to enhance current laboratory technologies while also creating systems that are well-suited for the future of laboratory automation. Open-source systems such as Aquarium have been developed to help labs integrate experimental design, inventory management, protocol execution and data capture into a unified source.[34] Systems like this leverage AI to help standardize workflows for labs without the hefty upfront cost that novel robotics will incur. There are a number of different companies that also offer similar offerings. Opentron's OT-2 robot was built with the intention of creating a personalized pipetting robot. It works through integrating a lab's existing labware, instruments, and protocols through open-source software. Because the software is open-source, the Opentrons OT-2 hardware is not explicitly necessary to use the platform and labs can integrate the automation suite with existing lab tools.[35] Strateos Lab Automation Software offers a modular platform that allows labs to manage and automate their own on-premise research operations through the cloud.[36] Modular automation of lab functions allows for more precise measurement and provides more levers to apply AI for optimization in the experimental process.

Distributed labs

Even with optimized and automated platforms, the cost of establishing and operating a lab remains high. The initial investment in equipment and training can be prohibitive, particularly for neurosurgeons involved in basic science research. "Cloud Labs" present an innovative solution by allowing scientists to design and deploy experiments remotely through the use of software. These experiments are then executed at a physical lab equipped with high levels of automation and AI-driven optimization, streamlining the research process. This innovation democratizes research, allowing a diverse range of clinicians to explore scientific questions crucial to patient care. Numerous instances exist of novel pharmaceutical agents being remotely created using AI integrated with these "Cloud Labs."[37–39]

In industry, innovation has traditionally favored larger companies, which have the resources to make significant capital investments in testing hypotheses and running experiments. These investments in equipment, labor and materials are justified as fixed costs that can be recouped through the resulting innovations. However, small companies often lack these resources, making it challenging to compete. Cloud labs provide an excellent alternative, enabling smaller companies to leverage their scientific creativity and ingenuity without the need for large upfront investments. There are a number of different offerings for the cloud lab service with varying interfaces for researchers to interact with including Strateos. These services include automated experimentation with machines that include liquid handlers, bioreactors and high content imagers.

In 2023, Emerald Cloud Lab (ECL) partnered with Carnegie Mellon University (CMU) to establish a $40 million cloud lab in Pittsburgh, the first of its kind in academia.[40] This facility enables CMU researchers to remotely access ECL's automated research environment, utilizing robotics and computer codes for conducting wet-laboratory experiments.[41] Similar collaborations with academic medical centers could provide clinicians the opportunity to engage in complex wet-lab research within their universities without significantly affecting their clinical responsibilities. Cloud labs democratize access to advanced research tools, enhancing reproducibility and enabling efficient, large-scale data generation.

IMPROVED ANALYSIS OF EXPERIMENTAL DATA

Enabling more experiments will significantly increase the volume of generated data, creating a greater need for extracting novel and computationally efficient insights. AI is transforming how researchers interact with these data, enabling meaningful scientific discoveries through advancements in data storage, interoperability, the quality of insights developed and the methods used to develop these insights.

Data storage

With the advent of new technologies, generating unprecedented volumes of biological data has become significantly easier and more cost-effective. NGS, particularly Illumina sequencing, has accelerated DNA and RNA sequencing while reducing costs. Advanced mass spectrometry and cryogenic electron microscopy (Cryo-EM) now enable detailed proteomic analyses and macromolecule visualization, respectively, deepening our understanding of biological systems.[42] These technologies have unlocked new insights from biological samples, allowing for data extraction in ways previously impossible. With the vast increase in data describing biological samples, there is a growing need for robust platforms to store and manage this information effectively.

Cloud computing platforms such as Microsoft Azure and Amazon Web Services (AWS) provide scalable and flexible resources to efficiently manage and analyze large-scale omics data generated through experimentation.[43] Utilizing these available resources has allowed for immense sharing across the scientific community. The Cancer Genome Atlas (TCGA) Program has used these tools to make multi-omic data spanning 33 cancer types available to researchers via application programming interface (API) access.[44]

Despite improvements in cloud-based data storage, some scientists lament that these advancements still fall short of capturing the intricacy and importance of multi-omic data. They have called for improved hosting options that can handle the complexity of multi-omics data, as well as the development of tools and guidelines for storing and sharing these datasets. Enhanced storage solutions could significantly improve the utilization of the new data being collected.[45]

Data interoperability

Beyond the omics data generated from experiments, vast amounts of information are now being produced across various healthcare modalities. These include physiological data from wearables, billing information from claims, EHRs from hospitals and lab results from consumer testing. Previously, these data sources existed in isolation due to protected health information (PHI) constraints, limiting integrated analysis. However, software engines like Datavant now enable the secure assignment of patient tokens to these data silos, allowing for their combination in a separate environment and facilitating comprehensive analysis and insights from diverse multimodal patient data and samples.[46,47]

This enhancement in interoperability facilitates the creation of comprehensive datasets that integrate both real-world and lab-generated data. The utilization of these multimodal datasets has significantly improved model performance in various health-related tasks, demonstrating their potential to advance research and applications within the health domain.[48] The Medical Information Mart for Intensive Care (MIMIC),[49] MedPix 2.0,[50] The Cancer Imaging Archive (TCIA),[51] and National COVID-19 Chest Imaging Database (NCCID) [52] all represent complex, multimodal, open-source datasets that have been made available due to advancements in data storage and interoperability. The availability of these data has allowed for significant strides to be made in the application of AI to medicine and biology.

Data insight quality

Significant advancements in data storage and interoperability have paved the way for unprecedented access to experimental and patient data. AI has rapidly transformed the speed and quality of insights scientists can extract from samples while also reducing the amount of data required for meaningful analysis. For example, flow cytometry is commonly used to analyze cellular characteristics, including tumor markers, through a staining process that can potentially alter cell signaling and viability. However, a UCLA team evidence the use of DL in combination with a novel label-free technique to extract the same information without the need for staining, preserving the natural state of the cells.[53] Similarly, spatial omics represent methods used to profile cells within their natural tissue context by measuring gene expression and regulation relative to a cell's spatial location within the tissue.[54] Other technologies like CODEX multiplexed tissue imaging allow for immunohistochemical staining of up to 60 markers.[55] These highly dimensional data can enable massive cataclysm of scientists' downstream ability to understand the development and function of entire organ systems and is largely being powered by the pairing of new imaging technology with AI for improved analysis and interpretability.[56]

The power of AI in analysis and interpretability is reflected in recent laboratory equipment integration of AI directly into their hardware to enable new and improved data collection. Leia Microsystems microscopes directly integrate with their AI software platform to perform tasks like cell detection and phenotyping.[57] AI enables the analysis of new modalities and views of samples through innovative data capture techniques, enhancing our understanding of biological complexity. Once these modalities of data are created, it further exacerbates the already challenging complexity and dimensionality of the biological and medical data. The diverse data collected from samples or patients offer multiple perspectives on biological phenomena, each with its own unique characteristics. Multimodal AI models integrate these different data "views"—such as genomics, epigenomics, metabolomics, metagenomics, transcriptomics and proteomics in biological samples providing a more comprehensive analysis. Multiple algorithms have been proposed to account for these unique modalities of data. Multiscale PHATE has been shown to be able to predict outcomes in patients with COVID–19.[58] Similarly, multimodal implementations of existing AI algorithms like support vector machines (SVMs),[59] multidimensional scaling,[60] spectral-embedding[61] and others have been created to allow scientists to preserve the uniqueness of different types of data in their joint analysis. Implementations of these algorithms have been open-sourced in publicly available python packages.[62]

Recent advancements in multimodal AI have largely been driven by the tech industry. The transformer architecture, introduced by a team of Google scientists in 2017[63] revolutionized AI performance by improving the accuracy and efficiency of processing sequential data.[64] While popularized by OpenAI's ChatGPT as an LLM, they have been instrumental in the creation of foundational multimodal models like VideoBert for video and text,[65] Contrast Language-Image Pre-Training (CLIP) for image and text.[66] More recently, Meta has proposed algorithms building on transformers specifically designed for multimodal inputs.[67]

These innovations have a profound impact on medicine and biology. While many models have been developed to address specific medical issues, the complexity of medicine demands the creation of broader foundational models. These models are necessary to tackle the diverse and interconnected challenges that arise in medical research and practice. Med-Palm 2 represents a multimodal foundational model explicitly meant to serve the purpose of answering expert-level medical questions.[68] There have also been proposed frameworks that call for foundation models that represent general medical artificial intelligence.[69] AI is allowing for more of the data generated from samples to be studied as the collective biological entities that they represent. This promises to enable massive improvements and discoveries in the near future.

Data analysis

Experimental data are typically analyzed using a range of tools tailored to the specific requirements of the analysis. These tools can include spreadsheet software like Microsoft Excel, statistical programs like R and Stata and programming languages like Python and SQL. Each tool requires a certain level of expertise and a learning curve to use effectively. Consequently, the ability to accurately analyze data can sometimes hinder scientific progress. However, AI has the potential to simplify the data analysis process, making it more accessible and accelerating scientific advancement. ChatGPT has introduced features that enable users to work with dynamic tables and charts by integrating with existing systems like Google Sheets and Microsoft Excel when provided with data uploads.[70] Likewise, tools like Julius.ai are meant to serve the role of a data analyst transforming conversational text and data-related queries into visualizations and concise data answers.[71] LLMs have become invaluable tools for enhancing researchers' coding efficiency and quality.[72] Trained on extensive datasets sourced from code repositories and user programming questions, AI assistants can significantly aid users in writing and optimizing code. Tools such as GitHub Copilot, Supermaven and Cursor are designed to improve coding speed and accuracy, allowing researchers to perform data analysis more effectively and efficiently.

As language models advance and computing costs decline, we can anticipate an increase in solutions that enable researchers to upload data to platforms and query them with conversational language for results. This will lead to quicker feedback cycles in understanding experimental outcomes, ultimately streamlining the scientific process and enhancing overall efficiency.

CONCLUSION

The integration of AI and automation into basic laboratory research is reshaping the future of scientific discovery, driving efficiency and innovation across multiple domains. As highlighted, automation allows scientists trying to discover new therapies to take "more shots on goal" and AI helps scientists refine hypotheses and take "better shots on goal." The confluence of these two allows for the substantial improvement of the drug discovery process.

The automation of complex tasks, such as HTS and AI-powered robotic platforms, not only reduces costs but also frees researchers from time-consuming manual labor, enabling them to focus on more creative and impactful aspects of their work. Additionally, AI-enhanced data storage and analysis tools are unlocking new dimensions of insight, allowing researchers to interact with their data in unprecedented ways.

As AI continues to advance, its applications in biology and medicine are set to expand, leading to more efficient and precise experimentation. The development of new foundation models in biology will likely deepen our understanding of how biological processes relate to patient outcomes. Research shows that TL can enhance drug response predictions with fewer *in vivo* samples by leveraging extensive *in vitro* data.[73] More recent studies have also used TL to improve patient drug response predictions from preclinical data, like organoid models.[74,75] Additionally, AI models have successfully been shown to predict appropriate dosing[76] and effective toxicity[77] of proposed therapeutics.

In neurosurgery, translational research is increasingly intersecting with "big data." For example, glioblastoma immunology lacks simple biomarkers for response to therapy, and is beginning to query complex signals in multiomics data for disease subtyping and therapy response. Perhaps no subfield of neurosurgery is more engrained with "big data" than functional neurosurgery. In both animal research models in basic science labs, as well as using data generated from sEEG in real patients, functional neurosurgeons must identify signals in complex dimensional data. In both these neurosurgical fields as well as all others, AI and automation, as described in this chapter, have the potential to enable neurosurgeons to address critical scientific questions with unprecedented ability and efficiency. These advancements not only streamline the scientific process but also democratize access to sophisticated research tools, enabling a wider range of researchers to contribute to critical innovations in neurosurgery. Ultimately, AI is not only accelerating the pace of discovery but also transforming the way science is conducted. This shift is paving the way for a new era of medical research and innovation, with the potential to significantly improve patient lives.

REFERENCES

1. Diem P, Ducluzeau PH, Scheen A. The discovery of insulin. *Diabetes Epidemiol Manag* 2022; 5: 100049.
2. Cherezov V, Rosenbaum DM, Hanson MA, et al. High-resolution crystal structure of an engineered human β2-adrenergic G protein–coupled receptor. *Science* 2007; 318(5854): 1258–65.
3. Amunts K, Zilles K. Architectonic mapping of the human brain beyond Brodmann. *Neuron* 2015; 88(6): 1086–107.
4. Dandy WE, Blackfan KD. An experimental and clinical study of internal hydrocephalus. *J Am Med Assoc* 1913; 61(25): 2216–17.
5. Berdigaliyev N, Aljofan M. An overview of drug discovery and development. *Future Med Chem* 2020; 12(10): 939–47.
6. Wildey MJ, Haunso A, Tudor M, et al. High-Throughput Screening. In: Goodnow RA (ed). *Annual Reports in Medicinal Chemistry*. San Diego: Academic Press; 2017, pp. 149–95.
7. Entzeroth M, Flotow H, Condron P. Overview of high-throughput screening. *Curr Protoc Pharmacol* 2009; 9: 9.4.
8. Liu B, Li S, Hu J. Technological advances in high-throughput screening. *Am J Pharmacogenomics* 2004; 4(4): 263–76.
9. Shun TY, Lazo JS, Sharlow ER, Johnston PA. Identifying actives from HTS data sets: Practical approaches for the selection of an appropriate HTS data-processing method and quality control review. *J Biomol Screen* 2011; 16(1): 1–14.
10. Dreiman GHS, Bictash M, Fish PV, et al. Changing the HTS paradigm: AI-driven iterative screening for hit finding. *SLAS Discov Adv Sci Drug Discov* 2021; 26(2): 257–62.
11. Wallach I, Bernard D, Nguyen K, et al. AI is a viable alternative to high throughput screening: A 318-target study. *Sci Rep* 2024; 14(1): 7526.
12. Batool M, Ahmad B, Choi S. A structure-based drug discovery paradigm. *Int J Mol Sci* 2019; 20(11): 2783.
13. Liu X, Ye K, van Vlijmen HWT, et al. An exploration strategy improves the diversity of de novo ligands using deep reinforcement learning: A case for the adenosine A2A receptor. *J Cheminformatics* 2019; 11(1): 35.
14. Wilson GL, Lill MA. Integrating structure-based and ligand-based approaches for computational drug design. *Future Med Chem* 2011; 3(6): 735–50.
15. Huang SY, Zou X. Advances and challenges in protein-ligand docking. *Int J Mol Sci* 2010; 11(8): 3016–34.
16. Corso G, Stärk H, Jing B, et al. DiffDock: Diffusion steps, twists, and turns for molecular docking. *arXiv:2210.01776v2*, 2023.
17. Krishna R, Wang J, Ahern W, et al. Generalized biomolecular modeling and design with RoseTTAFold All-Atom. *Science* 2024; 384(6693): eadl2528.
18. Abramson J, Adler J, Dunger J, et al. Accurate structure prediction of biomolecular interactions with AlphaFold 3. *Nature* 2024; 630: 493–500.
19. RECEPTOR.AI. Receptor.AI Introduces ArtiDock. Available from: https://www.receptor.ai/news-and-blogs/receptor-ai-introduces-artidock (Accessed May 2026).
20. Roberts NA, Martin JA, Kinchington D, et al. Rational design of peptide-based HIV proteinase inhibitors. *Science* 1990; 248(4953): 358–61.
21. Powers AS, Pham V, Burger WAC, et al. Structural basis of efficacy-driven ligand selectivity at GPCRs. *Nat Chem Biol* 2023; 19(7): 805–14.
22. Suomivuori CM, Latorraca NR, Wingler LM, et al. Molecular mechanism of biased signaling in a prototypical G protein–coupled receptor. *Science* 2020; 367(6480): 881–7.

23. Bommasani R, Hudson DA, Adeli E, et al. On the opportunities and risks of foundation models. *arXiv:2108.07258v3*, 2022.
24. Rosen Y, Roohani Y, Agarwal A, et al. Universal cell embeddings: A foundation model for cell biology, 2023. Available from: https://www.biorxiv.org/content/10.1101/2023.11.28.568918v1 (Accessed May 2026).
25. Hayes T, Rao R, Akin H, et al. Simulating 500 million years of evolution with a language model, 2024. Available from: https://www.biorxiv.org/content/10.1101/2024.07.01.600583v1 (Accessed May 2026).
26. Jumper J, Evans R, Pritzel A, et al. Highly accurate protein structure prediction with AlphaFold. *Nature* 2021; 596(7873): 583–9.
27. Tran NH, Zhang X, Xin L, et al. De novo peptide sequencing by deep learning. *Proc Natl Acad Sci* 2017; 114(31): 8247–52.
28. Polo SHL, Saravia-Butler AM, Boyko V, et al. RNAseq analysis of rodent spaceflight experiments is confounded by sample collection techniques. *iScience* 2020; 23(12): 101733.
29. Sparkes A, Aubrey W, Byrne E, et al. Towards robot scientists for autonomous scientific discovery. *Autom Exp* 2010; 2: 1.
30. Hess JF, Kohl TA, Kotrová M, et al. Library preparation for next generation sequencing: A review of automation strategies. *Biotechnol Adv* 2020; 41: 107537.
31. Coley CW, Thomas DA, Lummiss JAM, et al. A robotic platform for flow synthesis of organic compounds informed by AI planning. *Science* 2019; 365(6453): eaax1566.
32. Xie Y, Sattari K, Zhang C, Lin J. Toward autonomous laboratories: Convergence of artificial intelligence and experimental automation. *Prog Mater Sci* 2023; 132: 101043.
33. Burger B, Maffettone PM, Gusev VV, et al. A mobile robotic chemist. *Nature* 2020; 583(7815): 237–41.
34. Vrana J, de Lange O, Yang Y, et al. Aquarium: Open-source laboratory software for design, execution and data management. *Synth Biol* 2021; 6(1): ysab006.
35. Opentrons. GitHub Available from: https://github.com/Opentrons (Accessed May 2026).
36. Strateos Lab Control Software—Automated Workflow Execution. Available from: https://strateos.com/integrated-run-sample-and-reagent-management/ (Accessed May 2026).
37. Fitzpatrick DE, Battilocchio C, Ley SV. A novel internet-based reaction monitoring, control and autonomous self-optimization platform for chemical synthesis. *Org Process Res Dev* 2016; 20(2): 386–94.
38. Liang J, Xu S, Hu L, et al. Machine-learning-assisted low dielectric constant polymer discovery. *Mater Chem Front* 2021; 5(10): 3823–9.
39. Fitzpatrick DE, Maujean T, Evans AC, Ley SV. Across-the-world automated optimization and continuous-flow synthesis of pharmaceutical agents operating through a cloud-based server. *Angew Chem Int Ed* 2018; 57(46): 15128–32.
40. Arnold C. Cloud labs: Where robots do the research. *Nature* 2022; 606(7914): 612–13.
41. The Tartan. CMU Cloud Lab to bring remote science into mainstream, 2024. Available from: https://the-tartan.org/2024/02/19/cmu-cloud-lab-to-bring-remote-science-into-mainstream/ (Accessed May 2026).
42. Cook CE, Bergman MT, Finn RD, et al. The European Bioinformatics Institute in 2016: Data growth and integration. *Nucleic Acids Res* 2016; 44(D1): D20–6.
43. Koppad S, Annappa B, Gkoutos GV, Acharjee A. Cloud computing enabled big multi-omics data analytics. *Bioinforma Biol Insights* 2021; 15: 11779322211035921.
44. Tomczak K, Czerwińska P, Wiznerowicz M. The Cancer Genome Atlas (TCGA): An immeasurable source of knowledge. *Contemp Oncol* 2015; 19(1A): A68–77.
45. Conesa A, Beck S. Making multi-omics data accessible to researchers. *Sci Data* 2019; 6(1): 251.
46. Bernstam EV, Applegate RJ, Yu A, et al. Real-world matching performance of deidentified record-linking tokens. *Appl Clin Inform* 2022; 13: 865–73.
47. Kiernan D, Carton T, Toh S, et al. Establishing a framework for privacy-preserving record linkage among electronic health record and administrative claims databases within PCORnet®, the National Patient-Centered

Clinical Research Network. *BMC Res Notes* 2022; 15(1): 337.
48. Kline A, Wang H, Li Y, et al. Multimodal machine learning in precision health: A scoping review. *NPJ Digit Med* 2022; 5(1): 1–14.
49. Johnson AEW, Bulgarelli L, Shen L, et al. MIMIC-IV, a freely accessible electronic health record dataset. *Sci Data* 2023; 10(1): 1.
50. Siragusa I, Contino S, La Ciura M, et al. MedPix 2.0: A comprehensive multimodal biomedical dataset for advanced AI applications. *arXiv:2407.02994v5*, 2024.
51. Clark K, Vendt B, Smith K, et al. The Cancer Imaging Archive (TCIA): Maintaining and operating a public information repository. *J Digit Imaging* 2013; 26(6): 1045–57.
52. GigaScience. An overview of the National COVID-19 Chest Imaging database: Data quality and cohort analysis, 2021. Available from: https://academic.oup.com/gigascience/article/10/11/giab076/6437679 (Accessed May 2026).
53. Chen CL, Mahjoubfar A, Tai LC, et al. Deep learning in label-free cell classification. *Sci Rep* 2016; 6(1): 21471.
54. Bressan D, Battistoni G, Hannon GJ. The dawn of spatial omics. *Science* 2023; 381(6657): eabq4964.
55. Black S, Phillips D, Hickey JW, et al. CODEX multiplexed tissue imaging with DNA-conjugated antibodies. *Nat Protoc* 2021; 16(8): 3802–35.
56. Ertürk A. Deep 3D histology powered by tissue clearing, omics and AI. *Nat Methods* 2024; 21(7): 1153–65.
57. Leica Microsystems. Aivia AI image analysis software. Available from: https://www.leica-microsystems.com/products/microscope-software/p/aivia/ (Accessed May 2026).
58.Kuchroo M, Huang J, Wong P, et al. Multiscale PHATE identifies multimodal signatures of COVID−19. *Nat Biotechnol* 2022; 40: 681–91.
59. Xu J, Han J, Nie F, Li X. Multi-view scaling support vector machines for classification and feature selection. *IEEE Trans Knowl Data Eng* 2020; 32(7): 1419–30.
60. Bai S, Bai X, Latecki LJ, Tian Q. Multidimensional scaling on multiple input distance matrices. *Proc AAAI Conf Artif Intell* 2017; 31(1): 1.
61. Xia T, Tao D, Mei T, Zhang Y. Multiview spectral embedding. *IEEE Trans Syst Man Cybern Part B Cybern* 2010; 40(6): 1438–46.
62. Perry R, Mischler G, Guo R, et al. mvlearn: Multiview machine learning in python. *arXiv:2005.11890v4*, 2021.
63. Vaswani A, Shazeer N, Parmar N, et al. Attention is all you need. Advances in neural information processing systems, 2017. Available from: https://papers.nips.cc/paper_files/paper/2017/hash/3f5ee243547dee91fbd053c1c4a845aa-Abstract.html (Accessed May 2026).
64. Acosta JN, Falcone GJ, Rajpurkar P, Topol EJ. Multimodal biomedical AI. *Nat Med* 2022; 28(9): 9.
65. Sun C, Myers A, Vondrick C, et al. VideoBERT: A joint model for video and language representation learning. *arXiv:1904.01766v2*, 2019.
66. Radford A, Kim JW, Hallacy C, et al. Learning transferable visual models from natural language supervision. *arXiv:2103.00020v1*, 2021.
67. Baevski A, Hsu WN, Xu Q, et al. data2vec: A general framework for self-supervised learning in speech, vision and language. *arXiv:2202.03555v3*, 2022.
68. Singhal K, Tu T, Gottweis J, et al. Towards expert-level medical question answering with large language models. *arXiv:2305.09617v1*, 2023.
69. Moor M, Banerjee O, Abad ZSH, et al. Foundation models for generalist medical artificial intelligence. *Nature* 2023; 616(7956): 259–65.
70. Dursun O. ChatGPT now supports Google Drive and OneDrive, integrating interactive charts and tables. Neowin, 2024. Available from: https://www.neowin.net/news/chatgpt-now-supports-google-drive-and-onedrive-integrating-interactive-charts-and-tables/ (Accessed May 2026).
71. Julius AI. Your AI Data Analyst. Available from: https://julius.ai (Accessed May 2026).
72. Cooper N, Clark AT, Lecomte N, et al. Harnessing large language models for coding, teaching and inclusion to empower

research in ecology and evolution. *Methods Ecol Evol* 2024; 15(10): 1757–63.
73. Ma J, Fong SH, Luo Y, et al. Few-shot learning creates predictive models of drug response that translate from high-throughput screens to individual patients. *Nat Cancer* 2021; 2(2): 233–44.
74. Kong J, Lee H, Kim D, et al. Network-based machine learning in colorectal and bladder organoid models predicts anti-cancer drug efficacy in patients. *Nat Commun* 2020; 11(1): 5485.
75. Logun M, Wang X, Sun Y, et al. Patient-derived glioblastoma organoids as real-time avatars for assessing responses to clinical CAR-T cell therapy. *Cell Stem Cell* 2025; 32(2): 181–190.e4.
76. Blasiak A, Khong J, Kee T. CURATE.AI: Optimizing personalized medicine with artificial intelligence. *SLAS Technol* 2020; 25(2): 95–105.
77. Basile AO, Yahi A, Tatonetti NP. Artificial intelligence for drug toxicity and safety. *Trends Pharmacol Sci* 2019; 40(9): 624–35.

Index

Note: Page numbers in *italic* refer to tables; those in **bold** refer to figures

C

T

For Product Safety Concerns and Information please contact our
EU representative GPSR@taylorandfrancis.com Taylor & Francis
Verlag GmbH, Kaufingerstraße 24, 80331 München, Germany